SCHIZOPHRENIA AND AFFECTIVE DISORDERS

BIOLOGY AND DRUG TREATMENT

EDITED BY

ARTHUR RIFKIN

John Wright • PSG Inc
Boston Bristol London
1983

Library of Congress Cataloging in Publication Data
Main entry under title:

Schizophrenia and affective disorders.

Bibliography: p.
Includes index.
1. Schizophrenia—Chemotherapy. 2. Schizophrenia—Physiological aspects. 3. Affective disorders—Chemotherapy. 4. Affective disorders—Physiological aspects. I. Rifkin, Arthur. [DNLM: 1. Affective disorders—Drug therapy. 2. Schizophrenia—Drug therapy. 3. Affective disorders—Physiopathology. 4. Schizophrenia—Physiopathology. 5. Psychopharmacology. WM 207 S337]
RC514.S3345 1983 616.89'8206 83-5941
ISBN 0-7236-7054-4

Published simultaneously by:
John Wright • PSG Inc, 545 Great Road, Littleton, Massachusetts 01460, U.S.A.
John Wright & Sons Ltd, 823–825 Bath Road, Bristol BS4 5NU, England

Printed in the United States of America.

International Standard Book Number: 0-7236-7054-4

Library of Congress Catalog Card Number: 83-5941

To my Family, Eva, William and
Deborah, for their tolerance
and encouragement.

CONTRIBUTORS

GREGORY M. ASNIS, MD
Director, Psychopharmacology Clinic
Montefiore Medical Center
Associate Professor of Psychiatry
Director of Behavioral Endocrinology
Albert Einstein School of Medicine
Bronx, New York

JOHN M. DAVIS, MD
Director of Research
Illinois State Psychiatric Institute
Professor of Psychiatry
University of Chicago
Chicago, Illinois

KENNETH L. DAVIS, MD
Chief, Psychiatry Service
Veterans Administration Medical Center
Bronx, New York
Associate Professor of Psychiatry
Mt. Sinai School of Medicine
New York, N.Y. 10029

JOHN M. KANE, MD
Director, Psychiatric Research
Long Island Jewish–Hillside Medical Center
Glen Oaks, New York
Associate Professor of Psychiatry
School of Medicine
Health Science Center
State University of New York at Stony Brook
Stony Brook, New York

BRUCE J. KINON, MD
Director, Laboratory for Neuropsychopharmacology Research
Long Island Jewish–Hillside Medical Center
Glen Oaks, New York
Assistant Professor of Psychiatry
School of Medicine
Health Science Center
State University of New York at Stony Brook
Stony Brook, New York

DONALD F. KLEIN, MD
Director of Research
New York State Psychiatric Institute
Professor of Psychiatry
College of Physicians and Surgeons
Columbia University
New York, New York

MICHAEL I. LEVY, MD
Director, Special Treatment Unit
Veterans Administration Medical Center
Bronx, New York
Assistant Professor of Psychiatry
Mount Sinai School of Medicine
New York, New York

KATHERINE M. NOLL, PhD
Research Consultant
Illinois State Psychiatric Institute
Assistant Professor of Psychology
Department of Psychology
Elmhurst College
Elmhurst, Illinois

ROBERT F. PRIEN, MD
Chief, Affective Disorders Section
Pharmacologic and Somatic Treatments Research Branch
National Institute of Mental Health
Rockville, Maryland

FREDERIC M. QUITKIN, MD
Director, Depression Evaluation Service
New York State Psychiatric Institute
Associate Professor of Psychiatry
College of Physicians and Surgeons
Columbia University
New York, New York

JUDITH G. RABKIN, PhD
Research Scientist
New York State Psychiatric Institute
Adjunct Assistant Professor of Public Health (Epidemiology) in Psychiatry
Columbia University
New York, New York

ARTHUR RIFKIN, MD
Director, Division of Clinical Psychopharmacology Research
Mount Sinai Hospital
Associate Professor of Psychiatry
Mount Sinai School of Medicine
New York, New York

NEIL D. RYAN, MD
Instructor of Psychiatry
College of Physicians and Surgeons
Columbia University
New York, New York

SAMUEL G. SIRIS, MD
Associate Director
Division of Clinical Psychopharmacology Research
Mount Sinai Hospital
Assistant Professor of Psychiatry
Mount Sinai School of Medicine
New York, New York

THEODORE VAN PUTTEN, MD
Staff Psychiatrist
Veterans Administration Medical Center
Brentwood Division
Professor of Psychiatry
Neuropsychiatric Institute
UCLA School of Medicine
Los Angeles, California

CONTENTS

ACKNOWLEDGMENTS

I gratefully acknowledge the editorial assistance of Gerard Reardon, MSW, and the secretarial help of Lois Silver, Kimberly Green and Maria Gonzalez.

PREFACE

The three essentials for any clinical discipline are patient care, training, and research, with each component having an impact on the other. Research is required for the better understanding of etiological factors involved in illness, more efficient treatment procedures, and more effective preventive measures. A variety of research strategies, as well as serendipity, has led to achieving these goals in a range of medical disorders.

In the mid-1950s major changes in psychiatry occurred in the approach to the treatment of mental illness. The availability of neuroleptic and antidepressant medications provided a means of treating and managing many psychotic patients who in the past had been doomed to a lifetime in a custodial hospital or, at best, a life with much unhappiness and suffering. In recent years the results of clinical trials and outcome studies investigating various treatment modalities have been incorporated into the treatment of mental illness. This book provides a current appraisal and review of the current state of knowledge in the treatment of schizophrenia and affective disorders which are the major psychiatric illnesses of public health concern.

Simultaneously, with the availability of psychopharmacologic treatment for psychiatric disorders, major advances have been made in the past several decades in the area of neurobiology which has expanded the understanding of brain and behavior. The effectiveness of chemical agents in the treatment of mental disorders naturally led to the investigation of the role of possible underlying neurobiological deficits in schizophrenia and affective disorders. With the explosion of both knowledge and techniques in the neurosciences, research concerned with putative neurobiological processes involved in the etiology, course, and outcome of schizophrenia and affective disorders has provided the basis for a new era in the biological understanding of mental illness. The chapters in this volume provide a succinct review of the current state of the art in biological psychiatry for readers immersed in the field, and for those with only a limited amount of background.

As so eloquently pointed out by Dr. Rifkin, the treatment of psychiatric disorders is not as yet based upon the understanding of underlying neurobiological processes in schizophrenia and affective disorders. It may be too soon for such clinical and scientific criteria to be met. It has been pointed out that the successful treatment of an infectious disorder with penicillin would not lead to the conclusion that the signs and symptoms of the infection were due to a deficiency in penicillin. On the other hand, if considerable knowledge about bacteria as an etiological factor in infection were not known, successful treatment with penicillin would provide a probe to begin to understand some of the etiologic processes involved with the ultimate isolation of the bacteria and the effect of penicillin on the chemistry and metabolism of the organism. Psychopharmacologic treatment has served not only as a means of alleviating the symptoms of psychiatric disorders, but also as a stimulus to further investigation of neurobiological phenomenon which may be related to etiology. It is important and critical to separate these two major advances in psychiatry, but also to recognize the promise the future holds as a result of basic and clinical research for the understanding of the pathogenesis of schizophrenia and affective disorders and the treatment and prevention of these illnesses. It matters not if the initial impetus is chance which leads to knowledge, and, as stated by Marcus Aurelius, "The world is either the effect of contrivance or chance; if the latter, it is a world for all that—that is to say, it is a regular and beautiful structure."

MARVIN STEIN, MD
Esther and Joseph Klingenstein Professor
Chairman, Department of Psychiatry
Mount Sinai School of Medicine

INTRODUCTION

This book is intended for a reader who is knowledgeable about the fundamentals of psychiatry, and, in particular, about the psychopathology of schizophrenia and affective disorders. Also, it assumes a reader who has some understanding of the physiology and biochemistry of the brain. Further, I imagine the best reader of the volume to be a nonspecialist in the areas covered. The person seeking further details about the current frontiers of our subject, or a wider range within each area, must seek it in more comprehensive books or journals. The reader who will profit most from this book is the psychiatrist, psychiatric resident, and perhaps other mental health professionals, who want a less-than massive view of where the field of biological psychiatry now stands in its attempt to understand and treat schizophrenia and affective disorders.

If nothing else is accomplished by this book, I can assert confidently that it has broadened the editor's understanding of the task of educating busy professionals in areas that cry out for fuller treatment. In editing the manuscripts of others, and in co-authoring several chapters myself, I realize the immensity of the gap between what is known and what may reasonably be expected to be of sufficient interest to the clinician who does not have the luxury of sufficient time to pore over original papers. To present a catalogue of facts would be merely soporific; to summarize a field with entertaining, even epigrammatic assertions, not documented by reference to original data, is to force the writer's biases on a readership that is not trusted with any responsibility of evaluating facts and arriving at its own conclusions. My aim is to steer between these unwanted extremes, which invites the danger of the compromise—too factual for readability and too opinionated to allow scope for the intellectual integrity of the reader. I am certain that this book contains interesting and useful facts. I hope the presentation and integration of them is suitable to the audience we intend.

In a certain sense this book is a failure. Its existence and its title suggest the close association of knowledge about drug treatment and biology of these disorders. We would like to think that the field of biological psychiatry progresses in a tidy fashion, in which the results of drug studies lead to revealing research in the basic mechanisms of psychopathology, which leads to the development of new drugs and better clinical results. Of course, the start of this benign spiral may be at any point.

Unfortunately, the reality is messier and frustrating. These two major aspects of biological psychiatry—clinical psychopharmacology and basic mechanisms of brain function—have, largely, proceeded separately. Each aspect can claim marvellous advances. For anyone who needs reminding about the advances in treatment of schizophrenia and affective disorders I recommend the experience I had of reading the case records of the "Iowa-500" in a basement office at the University of Iowa (courtesy of Dr. Tsuang). These records were of patients admitted to the, then, Iowa Psychopathic Hospital, during the 1930s and 1940s. The uniqueness of these records is in their completeness. Each patient was extensively evaluated by a psychiatrist and social worker who left voluminous typewritten reports (and even a photograph). The stories of the impact of chronic disorders on these patients and their families is heartrending, especially in comparison to what we could do at present for them.

Similarly, reading scientific journals of that era makes us realize how recent is much of our knowledge of brain function. The increase of knowledge has been called, rightly, an explosion.

Yet, quite unexpectedly, psychopharmacological and brain function research have gone on different tracks. The development of all important drugs in psychiatry has been based on enlightened serendipity and not on predictions from biochemical knowledge. Chlorpromazine was found largely because of the mistaken notion that the sedation caused by antihistamines was different from that caused by barbiturates, and it would "tranquilize" untranquil people. As it turned out, the sedation of antipsychotics is not qualitatively different, and their antipsychotic action is not related to their soporific action since the two actions can be dissociated.

Lithium was tried because Cade thought it calmed rodents, when in fact it had made them stuporous—an achievement well within the capability of almost any chemical given in sufficient dose. Monoamine oxidase inhibitors was found to be an antidepressant as a spinoff of its use as an antitubercular drug. The prototypical tricyclic antidepressant—imipramine—was made to be a congener of chlorpromazine, and was predicted to be antipsychotic. Fortunately, Kuhn also tested it in patients with depression.

Once a successful drug is found, most additional drugs have been developed on the principle of making a compound similar to the prototype in chemical structure, and/or pharmacological effect in animals. The discovery of the original drug and of later similar ones did not depend on the explosion of knowledge about brain function. Such knowledge has been used to explain how the drugs work, but such theories have not been established firmly, and have not predicted new drugs or new uses for existing drugs.

Each field—clinical psychopharmacology and mechanisms of brain function—had advanced; but there are few bridges between. Eventually, the two must meet and even overlap. On that day, there will not be a need, perhaps, for separate chapters in a book like this, for the biochemistry of a disorder and its drug treatment. But, at present, the reader must turn from one to the other with few linkages and wait for the future.

Some are impatient and try to force the future by asserting that it is here. They act as if drug treatment can be chosen according to biochemical understanding of psychopathology, or that the known pharmacological properties of effective drugs are adequate explanations for the biochemical abnormality which we assume is present in schizophrenia and affective disorders. We must be wary of such people. Too many false "eurekas" discredit the entire enterprise and cause clinical rigidities. A healthy skepticism which should engender humility is required. This book presents a great deal of information and offers provocative theories, but the astute reader will notice how much we do not know. In the face of the continuing terrible morbidity from schizophrenia and depression we cannot tolerate acceptance of our present knowledge of their treatment and biology. Reading these chapters should arouse the urge to do further research, to follow the leads that have opened. Let us hope the people and the resources will be available.

ARTHUR RIFKIN, MD

CHAPTER 1

THE NEUROENDOCRINOLOGY OF DEPRESSION

MICHAEL I. LEVY
KENNETH L. DAVIS

CURRENT METHODOLOGIES

The Dexamethasone Suppression Test

The hypothalamopituitary-adrenal (HPA) axis has been studied more than any other neuroendocrine system in patients with psychiatric disorders. This may result from the clinically evident association of adrenal steroids with psychiatric symptoms. Psychosis is reported in 20% of cases of Cushing's disease, depression being the most common manifestation.[1,2] Manic-like symptoms are less common in Cushing's disease, but may occur during treatment with exogenous steroids.[1] Both types of reaction are prominent and seem to be specific to these conditions rather than general reactions to illness or treatment.

Investigations of the HPA system's role in major depressive illness (Research Diagnostic Criteria) have utilized two types of strategies.[3] The first has been to sample various biological fluids and determine baseline levels of corticosteroids and related compounds. A large literature reporting plasma and urinary measurements of 17-hydroxycorticosteroids (17-OCHS) has appeared in the past 25 years. Plasma 17-OCHS levels taken from 9:00 AM blood samples were elevated in depressives compared with levels in both normal persons and with levels from the same patients after successful treatment.[4,5] Elevations were correlated with the severity of illness. Measurements of urinary 17-OCHS did not correlate well with diagnosis or severity of illness.[6–8] However, many of these earlier studies did not control for use of medication. Both phenothiazines and tricyclic antidepressants interact in the once-prevalent Porter-Silber reaction to produce artificially low 17-OCHS values.[9] Additionally, the marked diurnal variation of plasma corticosteroid levels suggests that single sampling protocols may be inadequate to demonstrate differences among groups.[10] Controlling for drug intake and sampling plasma frequently over a 24-hour period has produced the most consistent data. Patients with severe depression have markedly elevated cortisol levels that revert to normal after treatment and resolution of the episode.[10–13] Extremely anxious or psychotic depressives account for most corticosteroid hypersecretion, whereas the seemingly affectively nonaroused depressives tend to have normal cortisol levels.[10]

Cortisol levels have also been examined in the cerebrospinal fluid of depressives. Group comparisons with controls have generally revealed no differences, although one report showed elevated cerebrospinal fluid cortisol in depressives.[14–16]

The second major research strategy has been to perturb the HPA system and compare its response in patients and control subjects. This latter strategy has produced some of the most consistent data about the neurobiology of depression. The dexamethasone suppression test (DST) was reported as a marker for affective disorder by Carroll and co-workers.[17] Subjects are given an oral dose of dexamethasone (usually 1–2 mg) at approximately midnight and then have serial blood samples drawn during the following day. A rise in plasma cortisol above a level of 5 or 6 μg/dL in any sample is said to represent escape from cortisol suppression that is normally seen after administration of dexamethasone. Suppression for approximately 24 hours after the oral dexamethasone is considered a normal response.[18] A modified procedure in which only one blood specimen is drawn 16 hours after dexamethasone administration still detects 80% of abnormal responses.[18]

The DST was initially applied to a variety of psychiatric disorders. Patients meeting research criteria for major depression were compared with groups with schizophrenia, organic brain syndromes, anxiety neurosis, depressive neurosis, and personality disorders.[19] An abnormal DST was seen in approximately 50% of the major depression group and only a few percent from the other groups. Significantly, no patient with depressive neurosis had an abnormal DST, suggesting a basic distinction between these and patients with "endogenomorphic" features.[20] Approximately half of major depressives in other similar studies have shown this "escape" from dexamethasone suppression.[21,22] One recent report, however, demonstrated abnormal dexamethasone suppression in 9 of 17 patients with primary dementia, suggesting that the test may not be useful in separating primary dementias from "pseudodementias" associated with depression.[23]

The DST has been used to biologically distinguish between the primary and secondary subtypes of major depressive disorder. Secondary refers to depressive disorders preceded by schizophrenia, obsessive compulsive disorder, phobic disorder, antisocial personality, drug use disorder, schizoaffective disorder, panic disorder, Briquet's disorder, alcoholism, anorexia nervosa, organic brain syndrome, or preferential homosexuality.[3] It could be expected that depressive illness as a disease entity might be biologically distinct from changes in mood that follow other psychiatric or medical illnesses. Specific signs and symptoms have not been reliable in distinguishing these subtypes of depression.[24] The sensitivity of the DST has been demonstrated in studies with large numbers of patients where few or none of the secondary depressive group escaped suppression, whereas 40% to 60% of primary depressives were nonsuppressors.[22,25,26] Thus, the observation of nonsuppression in a patient may perhaps be taken as evidence in ruling out the above-mentioned conditions which by definition precede secondary depressive illness. Use of the DST to identify depressives who met DSM-3 criteria for melancholia yielded a sensitivity of 67% (nonsuppressors) and a specificity of 96%.[27]

Identifying affective illness in patients whose clinical presentation suggests a schizophreniform illness is a potential use of the DST. A salutory response to thymoleptics was correctly predicted with the DST in 10 of 10 patients from a larger group with marked psychotic features such as catatonia and paranoia.[28] By clinical judgment, only 8 of the same 10 were correctly predicted to respond to thymoleptics.

Anorexia nervosa, which can be an antecedent of secondary depression, has been shown to be associated with nonsuppression of the DST.[29] This may be an example of biology ultimately invalidating nosology, since anorexia is usually associated with depressed mood and vegetative symptoms, and there is genetic and electrophysiological evidence suggesting a link between anorexia nervosa and primary depression.[30,31] Abnormal dexamethasone suppression was not evident in schizophrenics who had starved themselves to a comparable degree.[32]

The heterogeneity of depressive illness is supported by the DST. Differing rates of escape have been reported in three putative subtypes of primary unipolar depressive illness.[22,33,34] Familial pure depressive disease, in which the proband has a first-degree relative with depression, but no first-degree relative with either alcoholism, antisocial personality disorder, or mania, is associated with a 76% rate of escape. Sporadic depressive disease, in which a proband has no first-degree relative with a psychiatric illness, yields a 44% rate of escape. Only 7% escape occurs in depression spectrum disease, which is defined as depression in a proband who has a first-degree relative with alcoholism, antisocial personality disorder, or both. Stronger family loading for depressive illness would seem, then, to predict nonsuppression and may isolate a biologically distinct and perhaps "purer" form of the illness. Perhaps depression spectrum disease is less a genetic illness than a common psychological response to the familial conditions (alcoholism and sociopathy) which define it. However, the finding of varied DST abnormality in genetic subtypes has been inconsistently replicated in subsequent studies.[27,35,36]

Predicting response to treatment as well as prognosis is of theoretical and practical interest. The DST has yielded conflicting data when correlated with treatment response. Nonsuppression was initially reported to be associated with poor response to antidepressant treatment, but the opposite has been found in more recent reports.[26,37] Treatment was more standardized, however, in the earlier report. Clearly, further research is needed to clarify this important question. Less controversial is the relationship of DST to the course of the illness. Resolution of a depressive episode is usually associated with normalization of the DST.[26,38,39] Where normalization does not occur, there is a greater likelihood of early relapse, and there may be indication for further acute treatment despite apparent clinical improvement.[38,40]

Predicting response to a particular antidepressant by using the DST was attempted in one very preliminary report.[41] Patients who were nonsuppressors tended to improve more with imipramine or desipramine treatment than with clomipramine or amitriptyline, and suppressors had the opposite response. The more noradrenergic effect of the former two drugs, compared with the more serotenergic effect of the latter two, suggests that DST nonsuppression may be reflecting decreased noradrenergic inhibition of the HPA axis.[42,43] However, the results were based on global impressions, whereas changes in the Hamilton and Beck depression scales were not statistically significant.

The DST seems to be an extremely safe test. Adverse side effects of the DST have not been reported.[19] Major psychotropic drugs, including tricyclic antidepressants, neuroleptics, monoamine oxidase inhibitors, lithium carbonate, and benzodiazepines, do not interfere with the test.[17,44] An increased rate of nonsuppression is not a consequence of normal aging.[45]

The TRH/TSH Stimulation Test

Hypothalamic thyrotropin-releasing hormone (TRH), pyroglutamyl-histidyl-prolinamide, has been administered as a putative treatment as well as a diagnostic test for depressive illness. An extrapituitary role for TRH is suggested by its relatively widespread (ie, beyond the hypothalamus) distribution in the brain and its interactions with noradrenergic neurotransmitters.[46–48]

Initial interest in TRH as a treatment for depression resulted from work demonstrating a synergistic effect of thyroid-stimulating hormone (TSH) with the antidepressant activity of tricyclic antidepressants.[49–51] The phenomenon was more evident in women than in men and is presumed to be an effect of the hormones on noradrenergic and possibly serotonergic neurotransmission.

TRH was initially used as a treatment for depression by Prange and co-workers.[52] Injection of 600 μg intravenously decreased Hamilton depression scores significantly for several days in a group of 10 depressive women with initial Hamilton scores of at least 18. This finding was replicated in several trials with comparable doses of TRH with small groups of patients.[53-56] However, studies with larger populations employing similar methodology failed to demonstrate any therapeutic effect of TRH alone or with a tricyclic antidepressant.[57-61] TRH infusion produced in some patients physical sensations, such as a metallic taste on the tongue, which may have stimulated a placebo response in the positive studies.

A serendipitous finding in the TRH treatment trials was decreased release of TSH after TRH infusion in depressed patients compared with controls.[52-54,56,58,62-76] Approximately 33% of euthyroid major depressives have a blunted TSH response to TRH as ascertained by measuring TSH at intervals over one hour after infusion of 400–600 μg of TRH in bolus form. A change in TSH level less than 5.0 mIU/mL above baseline is the most commonly employed criterion for blunting. Using 7.0 mIU/mL as the cutoff in one report, however, resulted in a diagnostic sensitivity of 56% and a specificity of 93%.[77] The low sensitivity of this test has led to efforts to identify subgroups of depressives based on response. Although 31 of 32 unipolar depressives had blunted TSH response in one report, compared with 1 of 12 bipolar depressives, bipolar patients in both manic and depressed conditions had blunted TSH response to TRH in other reports.[78-80] Further work is needed to evaluate the nosological utility of TRH responsiveness.

GROWTH HORMONE STIMULATION TESTS

Interest in growth hormone (GH) responsiveness in depressives developed from evidence implicating biogenic amines in GH release and regulation.[81-83] Progress in research had been tentative because of the many factors which can affect GH secretion. These include sex, menopausal status, medications, diet, stress, and sleep.[81,82,84] Meaningful data can be obtained when these factors are controlled for in research studies.

GH responsiveness has been measured by provocative challenge with levodopa and by response to the hypoglycemia induced by insulin. Decreased release of GH in response to insulin-induced hypoglycemia in depressives compared with controls has been reported by several groups.[85-87] However, the finding was not seen in all patients studied. Nevertheless, a subgroup demonstrated this abnormality in what were generally very carefully controlled studies.

Growth hormone release occurs in normal persons after the oral administration of levodopa, probably as a result of increased central dopamine activity.[88] No differences in GH release between controls and depressives after a 500 mg oral dose of levodopa were found in several studies, although increased GH release in bipolar compared with unipolar depressives and controls has been reported.[89–91] The distinction between unipolar and bipolar depressives was reported in a study in which patients were fed controlled-monoamine-level diets, which may produce more stable baseline hormone levels. In any event, no firm conclusion has emerged from studies of levodopa and GH in depressives.

NEUROTRANSMITTER BASIS OF HORMONE REGULATION

The neuroendocrine abnormalities in the foregoing section are of interest not only because they aid in identifying depression but also because they presumably reflect underlying regulatory defect in the central nervous system. They are easily measurable parameters that may correspond to changes in the activity of whatever chemical or chemicals mediate the signs of depressive illness. Current hypotheses of the etiology of depression are primarily concerned with neurotransmitters.[92–94] Any relationship between the neurotransmitters most likely implicated in depressive illness and the neuroendocrine abnormalities under discussion would support a possible etiology of depression. However, an essential prerequisite to such analysis is a careful elucidation of the relationships between specific endocrine parameters and neurotransmitters. Unfortunately, as will become clear, a simple relationship between an endocrine measure and a neurotransmitter rarely exists.

Norepinephrine

Norepinephrine has not definitely been shown to regulate cortisol secretion, though there is evidence of a tonic inhibitory effect mediated through corticotropin-releasing factor.[95] There is indirect evidence in that a plot of the diurnal variation of brain norepinephrine is the mirror image of the normal cortisol diurnal variation, suggesting inhibition of cortisol release by norepinephrine.[96,97] Norepinephrine stimulation of GH release has been demonstrated in animal studies.[98] Indirect pharmacological evidence suggests α-adrenergic stimulation and β-adrenergic inhibition of GH release in humans.[99] Norepinephrine most likely stimulates TSH release, although the regulation of this hormone is quite complex.[99] Release of TRH after dopamine infusion is blocked by pretreatment with disulfiram, which prevents conversion of dopamine to norepinephrine.[100] TRH release is blocked by reserpine, which depletes catecholamine stores.[100]

Serotonin

Cortisol levels are increased by augmented serotonergic activity, probably through stimulation of adrenocorticotropic hormone (ACTH) release. Intrahypothalamic injection of serotonin in animals leads to elevated plasma corticosteroid levels.[101] In humans, administration of the serotonin precursor 5-hydroxytryptophan raises ACTH levels.[102] 5-Hydroxytryptophan administration in humans also stimulates GH release, suggesting a serotonergic mechanism.[103] This effect is blocked by cyproheptadine, a serotonin antagonist.[104] Serotonin probably inhibits TSH release, as evidenced by the lowering of TSH after 5-hydroxytryptophan administration.[78]

Dopamine

Dopaminergic regulation of cortisol release has not been clearly demonstrated. Single oral daily doses of levodopa had no effect on ACTH levels in humans, and dopamine had no effect on stress responsiveness in dogs at less than pharmacological doses.[101,105] However, stimulation of GH release by levodopa is an established phenomenon.[88] Mediation of this effect by dopamine rather than norepinephrine is evidenced by failure of fusaric acid, a dopamine β-hydroxylase inhibitor, to block it.[88] Apomorphine, a direct dopamine receptor agonist, also increases GH levels.[106] Dopamine and levodopa affect TSH variably depending on the thyroid status of the subject. Suppression of TSH by levodopa occurs in chronically hypothyroid subjects, but no effect on TSH has been shown in euthyroid subjects.[107] As mentioned previously, dopamine-induced release of TRH is blocked by disulfiram, suggesting little, if any, role for this neurotransmitter in TSH regulation.

Acetylcholine

Increased release of cortisol by cholinergic agents such as carbachol, pilocarpine, and nicotine has been reported.[108–110] Physostigmine, a cholinesterase inhibitor, elevated plasma cortisol levels as well as GH and prolactin only in patients who became nauseated during infusion, suggesting that cholinergic drugs may increase cortisol as part of a nonspecific stress response.[111,112] Atropine, an anticholinergic agent, blocks ACTH and cortisol release in animals.[101,103] Except during the stress described above, specific cholinergic regulation of GH secretion has not been clearly shown, although the increase of GH release during sleep is diminished by methscopolamine, a cholinergic antagonist.[114] Cholinergic regulation of TSH has not been established.

Cortisol—Possible Effects on Other Neuroendocrine Tests

The neuroendocrine tests considered here have been discussed as if they were independent of each other. However, similarly to neurotransmitters which can only be understood in relationship to each other, hormonal systems may interact so that permutations in one are reflected in others. The possibility that elevated plasma corticosteroid levels lead to the other neuroendocrine abnormalities discussed has been suggested.[115]

Deficient GH response to hypoglycemia correlated with high endogenous cortisol production in a group of 13 hospitalized depressives.[116] In these patients one abnormality was seldom seen without the other. A causal relationship is suggested in several reports of exogenous steroid administration leading to decreased GH responsivity.[117-121] These reports involve a wide range of corticosteroid doses and marked decreases in GH release. Patients with Cushing's disease whose mean plasma cortisol levels are comparable with those seen in depressive illness also demonstrate decreased GH response to hypoglycemia, although there is not a correlation in all cases.[122]

Corticosteroids influence TSH response to TRH depending on daily and total dose. Lower doses and shorter periods of duration seem to produce variable effects, whereas longer-term administration leads to suppression of TSH response to TRH.[123-125] A suppressed response is also seen in patients with Cushing's disease. However, two reports with a total of 70 major depressive subjects did not indicate a correlation between the DST and TRH test results.[126,127]

In summary, several provocative neuroendocrine tests have been generally considered as largely independent phenomena, perhaps reflecting a particular neurotransmitter abnormality. There is some evidence suggesting that the TSH and GH abnormalities may be epiphenomena, secondary to increased corticosteroid levels. However, nearly all of this evidence has been gathered from nondepressed subjects and should be considered tentative. Clinical studies of depressives thus far indicate that the phenomena are not completely linked to elevated corticosteroid production.

IMPLICATIONS FOR HYPOTHESES OF DEPRESSIVE ILLNESS

Biogenic Amine Hypothesis

The hypothesis that depression results from insufficient release of neurotransmitter at synapses of central cathecholaminergic and/or serotonergic neurons is supported by a large body of mainly pharmacologic evidence.[92,128-131] Much of this evidence is based on the presumed mechanisms of action of known antidepressant drugs such as the tricyclics and monoamine oxidase inhibitors.[128] However, these drugs are not without effect on other neurotransmitter systems, and recent human studies of novel antidepressants as well as animal studies measuring receptor changes cast doubt on the hypothesis as originally stated.[132-135] While hormonal regulation involves a complex, incompletely understood interaction of at least several neurotransmitters, it is a somewhat more naturalistic "window" through which information about the nature of depression can be gleaned.

An abnormal DST is consistent with the cathecholamine hypothesis of depression. The tonic-inhibitory effect that norepinephrine apparently exerts on ACTH secretion may be abated in patients with depression if there is a pervasive central deficit of this neurotransmitter. How dexamethasone acts to suppress corticosteroid release is not fully understood, but norepinephrine may play a role in this phenomenon.[136] Another feature of corticosteroid regulation is periodicity. Serotonin, along with norepinephrine, is thought to contribute to maintenance of the diurnal variation of corticosteroid release, which is disturbed in many depressed patients, suggesting altered serotonergic function in depressive illness.[96,137]

The blunted response of TSH in response to TRH may be consistent with the biogenic amine hypothesis in that norepinephrine and serotonin modulate thyroid function. Norepinephrine stimulates TRH release and also may act further along the hormone's axis in potentiating the effect of TSH or release of thyroid hormone.[138] However, decreased norepinephrine activity along this axis might be expected to decrease TRH release and perhaps enhance the sensitivity of TSH release to exogenous TRH. The TRH test data are at variance with this relatively simple model and may not support the hypothesis.

The decreased responsiveness of growth hormone to hypoglycemia is ostensibly compatible with this hypothesis. Both norepinephrine and serotonin stimulate GH release, and a blunted response may indicate diminished stores of one or both of these neurotransmitters.

Cholinergic Hypothesis

Much of the pharmacologic evidence supporting the catecholamine hypothesis of depression also supports the hypothesis that depression results from increased central cholinergic activity.[132,139] Reserpine, which was central to the conception of the catecholamine hypothesis, produces numerous physiological effects, suggesting cholinergic activity.[108] The anticholinergic "side effects" shared by the tricyclic antidepressants are perhaps less an annoyance than peripheral reflections of how these drugs may in part work in the brain to alleviate depression. Pharmacologic studies of drugs affecting cholinergic activity in both depressed and manic patients add further support to the cholinergic hypothesis, as do electrophysiological studies of rapid eye movement sleep latency in depressives and in normal persons treated with cholinergic drugs.[132,139–142]

The correlation of increased and decreased cortisol release with corresponding changes in cholinergic activity is compatible with a cholinergic hypothesis of depression. Autonomously aberrant acetylcholine release might increase HPA activity in such a way as to render it less subject to feedback regulation by endogenous steroids or exogenously administered dexamethasone. A correlation between escape from dexamethasone administration and response to particularly anticholinergic antidepressants might then be expected, but has not been demonstrated.

GH regulation has not been convincingly shown to be regulated by acetylcholine, though there is some evidence.[143] Tests of GH response to hypoglycemia induced by insulin probably reflect abnormalities in central adrenergic and noradrenergic more than cholinergic function. Perhaps the majority of depressives who do *not* show abnormal GH response to hypoglycemia represent a subgroup with disturbed cholinergic activity. This may be a productive area for future work.

SUMMARY

The methodologies used to investigate the nature of depressive illness and to diagnosis it cover an extremely broad spectrum. They include invasive and complicated neurobiological tests such as lumbar punctures, sleep electroencephalography, and protracted urine collections, as well as time-consuming structured interviews based on diagnostic inventories and rating scales.

In the context of current clinical practice, these procedures are cumbersome at best, if not completely impractical to administer. The lack of an easily administered "assay" which would add objectivity to acumen has separated psychiatry from other medical specialties.

The neuroendocrine parameters discussed here indicate that psychiatry is well on its way toward developing a clinically meaningful blood test for depressive illness. The DST is a safe, simple procedure which identifies about 50% of major depressives with high specificity. Its administration can be simplified so that only one afternoon blood test need be drawn after taking a pill at bedtime the previous night.[27] The TRH test and GH stimulation test identify smaller percentages of this population. The data are encouraging, but not enthralling, since it is not yet clear how nonresponders differ from responders. Outcome studies are needed to sort out the issue of predicting treatment response. More vigorous studies addressing the selection of specific drugs or other treatment modalities will be extremely valuable.

The theoretical implications of these tests await a better understanding of the neural regulation of hormonal release. Catecholamines, indoleamines, and acetylcholine are not independent of each other, but rather function as counterbalances of each other, so that "too much acetylcholine" or "too little norepinephrine" become relative terms which may have little absolute meaning. Current theoretical models have obvious heuristic value, but may be wishful thinking in an extremely complex field. Perturbing only one part of a regulatory system may result in a nearly complete compensatory response, so that the result is barely perceptible or difficult to interpret. Combination drug studies which maximally adjust an endocrine system in one direction or another may generate more conclusive data.

REFERENCES

1. Reichlin S: Neuroendocrinology, in Williams RH (ed): *Textbook of Endocrinology*. Philadelphia, WB Saunders Co, 1968, pp 1007–1008.
2. Michael R, Gibbons JL: Interrelationships between the endocrine system and neuropsychiatry. *Int Rev Neurobiol* 1963;5:243–302.
3. Spitzer R, Endicott J, Robins E: *Research Diagnostic Criteria for a Selected Group of Functional Disorders*. ed 2. New York, Biometrics Research, New York State Psychiatric Institute, 1978.
4. Board F, Wadeson R, Persky F: Depressive affect and endocrine functions. *Arch Neurol Psychiatry* 1957;76:612.
5. Gibbons JL, McHugh PR: Plasma cortisol in depressive illness. *J Psychiatr Res* 1962;1:162–171.
6. Gibbons JL, Gibson JG, Maxwell AE, et al: An endocrine study of depressive illness. *J Psychosomat Res* 1960;5:32–41.
7. Pryce IG: The relationship between 17-hydroxycorticosteroid excretion and glucose utilization in depression. *Br J Psychiatry* 1964;110:90–94.
8. Stenback A, Jackobson T, Rimon R: Depressive and anxiety ratings in relation to the excretion of total urinary 17-OCHS in depressive subjects. *J Psychosomat Res* 1966;9:355–362.
9. Sachar EJ: Corticosteroids in depressive illness. A reevaluation of control issues and the literature. *Arch Gen Psychiatry* 1967;17:544–553.
10. Sachar EJ, Hellman L, Fukushima DK, et al: Cortisol production in depressive illness. *Arch Gen Psychiatry* 1970;23:289–298.
11. McClure DJ: The effects of antidepressant medication on the diurnal plasma cortisol levels in depressed patients. *J Psychosomat Res* 1966;10:197–202.
12. Sachar EJ: Corticosteroids in depressive illness. II. A longitudinal psychoendocrine study. *Arch Gen Psychiatry* 1967;17:554–567.
13. Sachar EJ, Hellman L, Roffwarg HP, et al: Disrupted 24 hour patterns of cortisol secretion in psychotic depression. *Arch Gen Psychiatry* 1973;28:19–24.
14. Coppen A, Brooksbank BWL, Noguera R, et al: Cortisol in the cerebrospinal fluid of patients suffering from affective disorders. *J Neurol Neurosurg Psychiatry* 1971;34:432–435.
15. Jimerson DC, Post RM, Van Kammer DP, et al: Cerebrospinal fluid cortisol levels in depression and schizophrenia. *Am J Psychiatry* 1980;137:979–980.
16. Träshman L, Tybring G, Asberg M, et al: Cortisol in the CSF of depressed and suicidal patients. *Arch Gen Psychiatry* 1980;37:761–767.
17. Carroll BJ, Curtis GC, Mendels J: Neuroendocrine regulation in depression. I. Limbic system—adrenocortical dysfunction. *Arch Gen Psychiatry* 1976;33:1039–1044.
18. Carroll BJ, Feinberg M, Greden JF: Neuroendocrine diagnostic criteria for depression. *Psychopharmacol Bull* 1980;16:42–44.
19. Carroll BJ, Curtis GC, Mendels J: Neuroendocrine regulation in depression. II. Discrimination of depressed from nondepressed patients. *Arch Gen Psychiatry* 1976;33:1051–1058.

20. Klein DF: Endogenomorphic depression: A conceptual and terminological revision. *Arch Gen Psychiatry* 1974;31:447–454.
21. Brown WA, Johnston R, Mayfield, D: The 24 hour dexamethasone suppression test in a clinical setting: Relationship to diagnosis, symptoms, and response to treatment. *Am J Psychiatry* 1979;136:543–547.
22. Schlesser MA, Winokur G, Sherman BM: Hypothalamic-pituitary-adrenal axis activity in depressive illness. Its relationship to classification. *Arch Gen Psychiatry* 1980;37:737–743.
23. Spar JE, Gerner R: Does the dexamethasone suppression test distinguish dementia from depression? *Am J Psychiatry* 1982;139:238–239.
24. Nelson JC, Charney DS: The symptoms of major depressive illness. *Am J Psychiatry* 1981;138:1–13.
25. Brown WA, Shuey I: Response to dexamethasone and subtype of depression. *Arch Gen Psychiatry* 1980;37:747–751.
26. Brown WA: Studies of response to dexamethasone in psychiatric patients. *Psychopharmacol Bull* 1980;16:44–45.
27. Carroll BJ, Feinberg M, Greden JF, et al: A specific laboratory test for the diagnosis of melancholia. *Arch Gen Psychiatry* 1981;38:15–22.
28. Carman JS, Hall K, Wyatt ES, et al: Dexamethasone nonsuppression: Predictor of thymoleptic response in catatonic and schizoaffective patients. *Society of Biological Psychiatry Scientific Proceedings,* 1980, p 36.
29. Walsh BT, Katy JL, Levin J, et al: Adrenal activity in anorexia nervosa. *Psychosomat Med* 1978;40:499–506.
30. Winokur A, March V, Mendels J: Primary affective disorder in relatives of patients with anorexia nervosa. *Am J Psychiatry* 1980;137:695–698.
31. Cantwell DP, Struzenberger S, Burroughs J, et al: Anorexia nervosa: An affective disorder. *Arch Gen Psychiatry* 1977;34:1087–1093.
32. Gerner RH, Gwirtsman HE: Abnormality of dexamethasone suppression tests and urinary MHPG in anorexia nervosa. *Am J Psychiatry* 1981;138: 650–653.
33. Winokur G, Behan D, Van Valkenburg C, et al: Is a familial definition of depression both feasible and valid? *J Nerv Ment Dis* 1978;166:764–768.
34. Winokur G: Unipolar depression: Is it divisible into autonomous subtypes? *Arch Gen Psychiatry* 1979;36:47–52.
35. Coryell W, Gaffney G, Burkhardt PE: The dexamethasone suppression test and familial subtypes of depression—a naturalistic replication. *Biol Psychiatry* 1982;17:33–40.
36. Rudorfer MV, Hwu HG, Clayton PJ: Dexamethasone suppression test in primary depression: Significance of family history and psychosis. *Biol Psychiatry* 1982;17:41–48.
37. McLeod WR: Poor response to antidepressants and dexamethasone nonsuppression, in Davies B, Carroll BJ, Mowbray RW (eds): *Depressive Illness: Some Research Studies.* Springfield, Charles C Thomas, 1972, pp 202–206.
38. Greden JF, Albala AA, Haskett RF, et al: Normalization of dexamethasone suppression test: A laboratory index of recovery from endogenous depression. *Biol Psychiatry* 1980;15:449–458.
39. Gold MS, Pottash ACC, Extrin I, et al: Dexamethasone suppression tests in depression and response to treatment. *Lancet* 1980;1:1190.
40. Albala AA, Greden JF, Tarika J, et al: Changes in serial dexamethasone suppression tests among unipolar depressives receiving electroconclusive treatment. *Biol Psychiatry* 1981;16:551–560.
41. Brown WA, Haier RJ, Qualls CB: Dexamethasone suppression test identifies subtypes of depression which respond to different antidepressants. *Lancet* 1980;1:928–929.

42. Sachar EJ: Neuroendocrine abnormalities in depressive illness, in Sachar EF (ed): *Topics in Psychoendocrinology.* New York, Grune & Stratton, 1975, pp 145–146.
43. Van Loon GR: Brain catecholamines and ACTH secretion, in Gawong FW, Martini L (eds): *Frontiers in Neuroendocrinology.* New York, Oxford, 1973, pp 209–247.
44. Amsterdam JD, Winokur A, Caroff S: Effect of tricyclic antidepressant on the dexamethasone suppression test. *Am J Psychiatry* 1981;138:1245–1246.
45. Tourigny-Rivard MF, Raskind M, Rivard D: The dexamethasone suppression test in an elderly population. *Biol Psychiatry* 1981;16:1177–1184.
46. Winokur A, Utiger RD: Thyrotropin releasing hormone: regional distribution in rat brain. *Science* 1974;185:265–267.
47. Reichlin S, Jackson IMD, Seyler LE: Regulation of the secretion of TRH and LHRH, in Seeman P, Brown GM (eds): *Frontiers in Neurology and Neuroscience Research.* Toronto, University of Toronto Press, 1974, pp 48–59.
48. Brown BM, Krigstein I, Dankova J, et al: Relationship between hypothalamic and median eminence catecholamines and thyroid function. *Neuroendocrinology* 1972;10:207–217.
49. Prange AJ, Wilson IC, Rabon AM, et al: Enhancement of imipramine antidepressant activity by thyroid hormone. *Am J Psychiatry* 1969;126:457–469.
50. Wheatley D: Potentiation of amitriptyline by thyroid hormone. *Arch Gen Psychiatry* 1972;26:229–233.
51. Coppen A, Whybrow PC, Noguera R, et al: The comparative antidepressant value of L-tryptophan and imipramine with and without attempted potentiation by Liothyromine. *Arch Gen Psychiatry* 1972;26:234–241.
52. Prange AJ, Wilson IC, Lara PP, et al: Effects of thyrotropin releasing hormone in depression. *Lancet* 1972;2:999–1002.
53. Kastin AJ, Ehrensing RH, Schalch DS, et al: Improvement in mental depression with thyrotropin-releasing hormone. *Lancet* 1972;2:740–742.
54. Itil TM, Patterson CD, Polvan V, et al: Clinical and CNS effects of oral and i.v. thyrotropin releasing hormone (TRH). *Psychopharmacol Bull* 1975;11: 29–30.
55. Tiway CM, Frais JL, Rosenbloom AL: Response to thyrotropin in depressed patients. *Lancet* 1972:2:1086.
56. Van der Vis-Melsen MJE, Weiner JD: Improvement in mental depression with decreased thyrotropin response after administration of TRH. *Lancet* 1972;2:1415.
57. Coppen A, Montgomery S, Peet M: Thyrotropin releasing hormone in the treatment of depression. *Lancet* 1966;2:433–434.
58. Hollister LE, Berger P, Ogle FL, et al: Protirelin (TRH) in depression. *Arch Gen Psychiatry* 1974;31:468–470.
59. Hall R, Hunter PR, Price JS, et al: Thyrotropin releasing hormone in depression. *Lancet* 1975;1:162.
60. Takahashi S, Kondo H, Yoshimura M, et al: Antidepressant effect of thyrotropin releasing hormone (TRH) and the plasma thyrotropin levels in depression. *Folia Psych Neurol Jpn* 1973;27:305–314.
61. Amsterdam J, Winokur A, Caroff S, et al: Thyrotropin releasing hormone's mood-elevating effects in depressed patients, anorectic patients, and normal volunteers. *Am J Psychiatry* 1981;138:115–116.
62. Kirkegaard C, Norlem N, Lauridsen VB, et al: Protirelin stimulation test and thyroid function during treatment of depression. *Arch Gen Psychiatry* 1975; 32:1115–1118.
63. Maeda K, Yuyuru K, Ohgo S, et al: Growth hormone and prolactin release after injection of thyrotropin releasing hormone in patients with depression.

J Clin Endocrinol Metab 1975;40:501–505.
64. Chazot G, Chalumean A, Aimard G, et al: Thyrotropin releasing hormone and depressive states: From agroanoninines to TRH. *Lyon Med* 1974;231: 831–836.
65. Ehrensing RH, Kastin AJ, Schalch DS, et al: Affective state and thyrotropin and prolactin responses after repeated injections of thyrotropin-releasing hormone in depressed patients. *Am J Psychiatry* 1974;131:714–718.
66. Takahashi S, Kondo H, Yoshimura M: Thyrotropin responses to TRH in depressive illness. *Folia Psychiatr Neurol Jpn* 1974;28:355–565.
67. Widerloo E, Sjostrom E: Effects of thyrotropin releasing hormone on endogenous depression. *Nord Psychiatr Tidskift* 1975;29:5103–5120.
68. Pecknold LL, Ban TA: TRH in depressive illness. *Pharmacopsychiatry* 1977;12:166–173.
69. Loosen PT, Prange AJR, Wilson IC, et al: Thyroid stimulating hormone response after thyrotropin releasing hormone in depressed, schizophrenic and normal women. *Psychoneuroendocrinology* 1977;2:137–148.
70. Gregoire F, Brauman H, de Buch R, et al: Hormone release in depressed papients before and after recovery. *Psychoneuroendocrinology* 1977;2:303–312.
71. Vogel HP, Benkert O, Allig R, et al: Psychoendocrinological and therapeutic effects of TRH in depression. *Acta Psychiatr Scand* 1977;46:223–232.
72. Hatotani N, Nomura J, Yagamuchi T, et al: Clinical and experimental studies on the pathogenesis of depression. *Psychoneuroendocrinology* 1977;2: 115–130.
73. Brambilla F, Emeraldi E, Sacchetti E, et al: Deranged anterior pituitary responsiveness to hypothalamic hormones in depressed patients. *Arch Gen Psychiatry* 1978;35:1231–1238.
74. Tsuitsui S, Yamayahu Y, Namba T: Combined therapy of T3 and antidepressants in depression. *Arch Int Med Res* 1979;7:138–146.
75. Loosen PT, Prange AJ: TRH: A useful tool for psychoendocrine investigation. *Psychoneuroendocrinology* 1980;5:63–80.
76. Asnis GN, Nathan IS, Halbreich U, et al: TRH tests in depression. *Lancet* 1980;1:424–425.
77. Extein I, Pottash ALC, Gold MS: The thyrotropin-releasing hormone test in the diagnosis of unipolar depression. *Psychiatry Res* 1981;5:311–316.
78. Gold MS, Pottash ALC, Davies RK, et al: Distinguishing unipolar and bipolar depression by thyrotropin release test. *Lancet* 1979;2:411–412.
79. Kirkegaard C, Bjrum N, Cohn D, et al: Thyrotropin releasing hormone (TRH) stimulation test in manic-depressive illness. *Arch Gen Psychiatry* 1978;35:1017–1026.
80. Extein I, Pottash ALC, Gold MS, et al: Differentiating mania from schizophrenia by the TRH test. *Am J Psychiatry* 1980;137:981–982.
81. Martin JB: Neural regulation of growth hormone secretion. *N Engl J Med* 1973;288:1384–1393.
82. Brown G, Reichlin S: Psychologic and neural regulation of growth hormone secretion. *Psychosomat Med* 1972;34:45–61.
83. Chambers JW, Brown GM: Neurotransmitter regulation of growth hormone and ACTH in the rhesus monkey: Effects of biogenic amines. *Endocrinology* 1976;98:420–428.
84. Ettigi PG, Lal S, Martin JB, et al: Effect of sex, oral contraceptives and glucose loading on apomorphine induced growth hormone secretion. *J Clin Endocrinol Metab* 1975;40:1094–1098.
85. Gruen PH, Sachan EJ, Altman N, et al: Growth hormone response to hypoglycemia in postmenopausal depressed women. *Arch Gen Psychiatry* 1975;32:31–33.

86. Garver DL, Pandey GN, Dekirmenjian H, et al: Growth hormone and catecholamines in affective disorders. *Am J Psychiatry* 1975;132:1149–1154.
87. Sachar EJ, Finkelstein J, Hellman C: Growth hormone responses in depressive illness. *Arch Gen Psychiatry* 1971;25:263–269.
88. Boyd AE III, Lebovitz HE, Pfeiffer JB: Stimulation of human growth hormone secretion by L-Dopa. *N Engl J Med* 1970;283:1425–1429.
89. Sachar EJ, Altman NK, Gruen PH, et al: Human growth hormone response to levodopa. *Arch Gen Psychiatry* 1975;32:502–503.
90. Maany I, Mendels J, Frazer A: Apomorphine: Effect on growth hormone. *J Endocrinol Metab* 1975;40:162–163.
91. Gold PW, Goodwin FK, Wehr T, et al: Growth-hormone and prolactin response to levodopa in affective illness. *Lancet* 1976;2:1308–1309.
92. Schildkraut JJ: The catecholamine hypothesis of affective disorders: A review of supporting evidence. *Am J Psychiatry* 1965;122:509–522.
93. Coppen A, Prange AJ Jr, Whybrow PC: Abnormalities of indoleamines in affective disorders. *Arch Gen Psychiatry* 1972;26:474–478.
94. Janowsky DS, El-Yousef MK, Davis JM, et al: A cholinergic-andrenergic hypothesis of mania and depression. *Lancet* 1972;2:632–635.
95. Jones MT, Hillhouse E, Burden J: Secretion of corticotropin releasing hormone in vitro, in Martimi L, Ganong WF (eds): *Frontiers in Neuroendocrinology,* vol 4. New York, Raven Press, 1976, pp 194–226.
96. Reis DJ, Wurtman RJ: Diurnal changes in brain noradrenaline. *Life Sci* 1968;7:91–98.
97. Sachar EJM, Asnis G, Halbreich U, et al: Recent studies in the neuroendocrinology of major depressive disorders. *Psychiatr Clin North Am* 1980;3: 313–326.
98. Toivola PTK, Gale CC: Stimulation of GH release by microinfusion of norepinephrine into hypothalamus of baboons. *Endocrinology* 1972;90: 895–902.
99. Frohman LA, Stachura ME: Neuropharmacologic control of neuroendocrine function in man. *Metabolism* 1975;24:211–234.
100. Ettigi PG, Brown GM: Psychoneuroendocrinology of affective disorder. *Am J Psychiatry* 1977;134:493–501.
101. Kreiger DT: Neurotransmitter regulation of ACTH release. *Mt Sinai J Med (NY)* 1973;40:302–314.
102. Imura H, Nakai Y, Kato Y, et al: Effect of andrenergic agents on growth hormone and ACTH secretion, in Scow RO (ed): *Endocrinology.* Amsterdam, Excerpta Medica, 1973, pp 156–162.
103. Imura H, Nakai Y, Yoshima T: Effect of 5-hydroxyptophan on growth hormone and ACTH release in man. *J Clin Endocrinol Metab* 1973;36:204–206.
104. Nakai Y, Imura H, Sakurai H, et al: Effect of cyproheptadine on human growth hormone secretion. *J Clin Endocrinol Metab* 1974;38:446–449.
105. Eddy RL, Jones AC, Chakmakjian ZH, et al: Effect of levodopa (L-DOPA) on human hypophyseal trophic hormone release. *J Clin Endocrinol Metab* 1973;33:709–712.
106. Lal S, de la Vega EE, Sourkes TL, et al: Effect of apomorphine on growth hormone, prolactin, leutinizing hormone, and follicle stimulating hormone in human serum. *J Clin Endocrinol Metab* 1973;37:719–724.
107. Rapoport B, Refetoff S, Fang VS, et al: Suppression of serum thyrotropin (TSH) by L-DOPA in chronic hypothyroidism: Interrelationships in the regulation of TSH and prolactin secretion. *J Clin Endocrinol Metab* 1973;36: 256–262.
108. Krieger HP, Krieger DT: Chemical stimulation of the brain: Effect on adrenal corticoid release. *Am J Physiol* 1970;216:1632–1641.

109. Suzuki T, Abe K, Hirose T: Adrenal cortical secretion in response to pilocarpine in dogs with hypothalamic lesions. *Neuroendocrinology* 1975; 17:75–82.
110. Balfour DJK, Khyllar AK, Longden A: Effects of nicotine on plasma corticosterone and brain amines in stressed and unstressed rats. *Pharmacol Biochem Behav* 1975;3:179–182.
111. Davis BM, Davis KL: Cholinergic mechanism and anterior pituitary hormone secretion. *Biol Psychiatry* 1980;15:303–310.
112. Janowsky DS, Risch C, Parker D, et al: Increased vulnerability to cholinergic stimulation in affective disorder patients. *Psychopharmacol Bull* 1980;16:29–31.
113. Kahara GB, Stark E: The effects of cholinomimetic drugs and atropine on ACTH release. *Neuroendocrinology* 1976;21:31–41.
114. Daughaday WH, Cryer PE: Growth hormone hypersecretion and acromegaly, in Krieger DT, Hughes JC (eds): *Neuroendocrinology.* Sunderland, Mass, Sinauer, 1980, pp 293–298.
115. Kendler KS, Davis KL: Elevated corticosteroids as a possible cause of abnormal neuroendocrine function in depressive illness. *Commun Psychopharmacol* 1977;1:183–194.
116. Sachar EJ, Finkelstein J, Hellman L: Growth hormone responses in depressive illness. *Arch Gen Psychiatry* 1971;25:263–269.
117. Hartog M, Guafar MA, Fraser R: Effect of corticosteroids on serum growth hormone. *Lancet* 1964;2:376–378.
118. Frantz AG, Rabkin MT: Human growth hormone. Clinical measurement, response to hypoglycemia and suppression by corticosteroids. *N Engl J Med* 1964;271:1375–1381.
119. Daly JR, Fletcher MR, Glass D, et al: Comparison of effects of long-term corticotrophin and corticosteroid treatment on responses of plasma growth hormone, ACTH, and corticosteroid to hypoglycemia. *Br Med J* 1974;2: 521–524.
120. Copinschi G, L'Hermite M, Ledercq R, et al: Effects of glucocorticoids on pituitary hormonal responses to hypoglycemia. Inhibition of prolactin release. *J Clin Endocrinol Metab* 1975;40:442–449.
121. Donald RA, Espiner EA: The plasma cortisol and corticotropin response to hypoglycemia following adrenal steroid and ACTH administration. *J Clin Endocrinol Metab* 1975;41:1–6.
122. Krieger DT, Glick SM: Growth hormone and cortisol responsiveness in Cushing's syndrome. *Am J Med* 1972;52:25–40.
123. Otsuki M, Dahoda M, Baba S: Influence of glucocorticoids on TRF-induced TSH response in man. *J Clin Endocrinol Metab* 1973;36:95–102.
124. Vanhaelst L, Golstein J, L'Hermite M, et al: Effects of dexamethasone and secobarbital on the pituitary response to thyrotropin releasing hormone (TRH) in man: Synergistic inhibition of thyrotropin (TSH) release. *Neuroendocrinology* 1974;16:282–292.
125. Re RN, Kouride IA, Ridgway EC, et al: The effect of glucocorticoid administration on human pituitary secretion of thyrotropin and prolactin. *J CLin Endocrinol Metab* 1976;43:338–346.
126. Davis KL, Hollister LE, Math AA, et al: Neuroendocrine and neurochemical measurements in depression. *Am J Psychiatry* 1981;138:1555–1562.
127. Extein I, Pottash ALC, Gold MS: Relationship of TRH test and dexamethasone suppression test abnormalities in unipolar depression. *Psychiatry Res* 1981;4:49–53.

128. Baldesarini RJ: An overview of the basis for amine the hypothesis in affective illness, in Mendels J (ed): *The Psychobiology of Depression.* New York, Spectrum Publications, 1975, pp 69–83.
129. Bunney WE Jr, Davis JM: Norepinephrine in depressive reactions. *Arch Gen Psychiatry* 1965;13:483–494.
130. Prange AJ Jr: The pharmacology and biochemistry of depression. *Dis Nerv Syst* 1964;25:217–221.
131. Davis JM: Theories of biological etiology of affective disorders. *Int Rev Neurobiol* 1970;12:145–175.
132. Janowsky DS, El-Yousef MK, Davis JM: A cholinergic-adrenergic hypothesis of mania and depression. *Lancet* 1972;2:632–635.
133. Zis AP, Goodwin FK: Novel antidepressants and the biogenic amine hypothesis of depression. *Arch Gen Psychiatry* 1979;36:1097–1107.
134. Wang RY, Aghajanian GK: Enhanced sensitivity of amygdaloid neurons to serotonin and norepinephrine after chronic antidepressant treatment. *Commun Psychopharmacol* 1980;4:83–90.
135. Vetulani J, Stawarz RJ, Dingell JV, et al: A possible common mechanism of action of antidepressant treatments. *Naunyn Schmiedebergs Arch Pharmacol* 1976;293:109–114.
136. McEwen BS: The brain as a target organ of endocrine hormones, in Krieger DT, Hughes JC (eds): *Neuroendocrinology.* Sunderland, Mass, Sinauer, 1980, pp 33–42.
137. Hollister LE, Davis KL, Davis BM: Hormones in the treatment of psychiatric disorders. *Hosp Pract* 1975;10:103–110.
138. Mowbray JF, Peart WS: Effect of noreadrenaline and adrenaline on the thyroid. *J Physiol* 1960;151:261–271.
139. Davis KL, Berger P: Pharmacological investigations of the cholinergic imbalance hypotheses of movement disorders and psychosis. *Biol Psychiatry* 1978;13:23–49.
140. Rountree DW, Nevin S, Wilson A: The effects of diisopropylfluorophosphonate in schizophrenia and manic depressive psychosis. *J Neurol Neurosurg Psychiatry* 1950;13:47–62.
141. Janowsky DS, El-Yousef MK, Davis JM, et al: Cholinergic reversal of manic symptoms. *Lancet* 1972;1:1236–1237.
142. Kupfer DJ: REM latency. A psychobiologic marker for primary depressive disease. *Biol Psychiatry* 1976;11:159–174.
143. Leviston SA, Cryer PE: Endogenous cholinergic modulation of growth-hormone secretion in normal and acromegalic humans. *Metabolism* 1980;29:703–706.

CHAPTER 2

HYPOTHESES REGARDING THE MECHANISM OF ACTION OF ANTIDEPRESSANT DRUGS: NEUROTRANSMITTERS IN AFFECTIVE DISORDERS

JOHN M. KANE

Since the introduction of effective pharmacologic agents for the treatment of depression, considerable research has been directed toward understanding the mechanism of action of antidepressants and utilizing these drug effects as a guide to the elucidation of the etiology and pathophysiology of affective illness.

A basic assumption in behavioral neurochemistry is that specific substances, neurotransmitters, play a key role in impulse transmission through intricate networks of neurons in the central nervous system. The interconnections between neurons consist primarily of anatomical and chemical synapses at which point a variety of factors come into play which can modify a neuronal current.

There are numerous compounds which act as neurotransmitters, substances which have specific receptors and fulfill the criteria outlined by Barchas et al in Table 2-1.[1] In addition, a more recent concept has evolved regarding neuromodulators, substances that do not fulfill the criteria for neurotransmitters in that they do not directly convey nerve signals from the presynaptic to the postsynaptic receptor, but are capable of altering neuronal activity in other ways (Table 2-1).

Historically, the characteristics of neurotransmitters have been best studied and most widely understood in catecholamine, indoleamine, and

Table 2-1
Criteria for Establishing the Identity of a Neuroregulator in the Nervous System

Neurotransmitter

The substance must be present in presynaptic elements of neuronal tissue, possibly in an uneven distribution throughout the brain.

Precursors and synthetic enzymes must be present in the neuron, usually in close proximity to the site of presumed action.

Stimulation of afferents should cause release of the substance in physiologically significant amounts.

Direct application of the substance to the synapse should produce responses which are identical to those of stimulating afferents.

There should be specific receptors present which interact with the substance; these should be in close proximity to presynaptic structures.

Interaction of the substance with its receptor should induce changes in postsynaptic membrane permeability leading to excitatory or inhibitory postsynaptic potentials.

Specific inactivating mechanisms should exist which stop interactions of the substance with its receptor in a physiological reasonable time frame.

Interventions at postsynaptic sites or through inactivating mechanisms; the effects of stimulation of afferents or of direct application of the substance should be equally responsive.

Neuromodulator

The substance is not acting as a neurotransmitter, in that it does not act transsynaptically.

The substance must be present in physiological fluids and have access to the site of potential modulation in physiologically significant concentrations.

Alterations in endogenous concentrations of the substance should affect neuronal activity consistently and predictably.

Direct application of the substance should mimic the effect of increasing its endogenous concentration.

The substance should have one or more specific sites of action through which it can alter neuronal activity.

Inactivating mechanisms should exist which account for the time course of effects of endogenously or exogenously induced changes in concentrations of the substance.

Interventions that alter the effects on neuronal activity of increasing endogenous concentrations of the substance should act identically when concentrations are increased by exogenous administration.

Reprinted with permission from Barchas JD, et al: Behavioral neurochemistry: Neuroregulators and behavioral states. *Science* 1978;200:964–973.

cholinergic systems; however, many questions remain to be answered despite the literally thousands of investigations that have been carried out to better understand these systems. The function and regulation of neuromodulators are less well understood, the whole concept being a relatively recent one. However, this adds an enormous dimension both to the complexity of behavioral neurochemistry and to the potential for therapeutic intervention.

Unfortunately, much of what we know about these systems must be learned from animal studies or studies of peripheral tissue in humans, thus making inferences regarding links between behavior and neurochemistry quite difficult. The human brain is extraordinarily complex, and the techniques which generally have evolved to study neurotransmission are too invasive or too destructive to be applied to the human central nervous system. Despite this, intriguing lines of evidence have accumulated to implicate neurochemical systems in specific behavioral conditions, mood states, and psychiatric illnesses.

Historically, the catecholamine hypothesis of affective disorders was the first to be widely explored. Everett and Tolman[2] may have made the first statement of the catecholamine hypothesis, but it was subsequently tied more directly to affective illness by Schildkraut[3] and independently by Bunney and Davis.[4] The early support for this hypothesis (and the indoleamine hypothesis, which is combined with the catecholamine hypothesis under the broader rubric of the "biogenic amine hypothesis") rests on the observation that reserpine (derived from the plant *Rauwolfia serpentina* and used in India for many years) was capable of producing in animals a syndrome that included sedation and motor retardation.[5] In addition, when reserpine was used to treat hypertension, a subgroup of patients developed clinical depression.[6] It was not clear until a prospective study was conducted to what extent underlying predisposition or vulnerability to depression might play a role in reserpine induced depression, but it appears that reserpine is certainly not associated with depression in all patients receiving it. Those with a previous history or a family history of depression appear more vulnerable, and it has been suggested that reserpine is capable of precipitating a depression rather than producing it de novo.[6] The subsequent discovery that reserpine is capable of depleting central neuronal stores of serotonin, norepinephrine, and dopamine suggested a possible link between these neurotransmission systems and depression.

In addition, when the drug iproniazid was used in the treatment of tuberculosis, some patients developed elevation of mood and increased activity. Pharmacologically, this agent was shown to be a potent inhibitor of the enzyme monoamine oxidase (MAO) and to increase central nervous system concentrations of norepinephrine and serotonin.[7] Subsequently, this drug and other MAO inhibitors were shown to have therapeutic activity in the treatment of depression.[8]

Tricyclic antidepressants were introduced as a modification of the phenothiazine nucleus, but were found to have antidepressant rather than antipsychotic properties.[9] These compounds were thought to act by preventing the reuptake of biogenic amines into presynaptic nerve terminals, thereby increasing functional activity at the synapse.[3,4]

These observations served as the background for further elaboration of the catecholamine and indoleamine hypotheses. Numerous problems remain in attempting to validate these hypotheses, but they have served a very useful function in stimulating clinical and preclinical research.

A variety of strategies have been employed to study the catecholamine hypothesis. Drugs which effect catecholamine anabolism or catabolism or receptor activity have frequently been studied clinically to determine their effect in precipitating or alleviating mania or depression. In addition, dopamine and norepinephrine, their metabolites, and enzymes involved in their synthesis or breakdown have been studied in depressed and manic patients both during an episode and when well. Generally, plasma, urine, or cerebrospinal fluid (CSF) has been the source of measurement; however, some brain tissue has been studied from autopsy material.

An example of such attempts to test the catecholamine hypothesis includes the assessment of noradrenergic activity by measuring metabolites of norepinephrine, particularly 3-methoxy-4-hydroxyphenylglycol (MHPG), a norepinephrine metabolite in urine, plasma, or CSF. Some reports[10,11] suggested that MHPG is reduced in patients with depression; however, these findings are not consistent, and the extent to which urine MHPG (the most frequently utilized measure) reflects central rather than peripheral noradrenergic activity remains controversial.[12]

It should be kept in mind throughout this review, however, that affective illnesses are heterogenous, and different neurochemical abnormalities may be present in subgroups of depressed patients, making the clear identification of neurochemical abnormalities in patient samples which are likely to be etiologically heterogenous difficult at best.

Norepinephrine is a catecholamine which is derived from tyrosine, an amino acid. Tyrosine is converted by the enzyme tyrosine hydroxylase to 3,4-dehydroxyphenylalanine (levodopa). Levodopa is in turn decarboxylated by dopa decarboxylase to form dopamine. Dopamine (a neurotransmitter in many brain systems) is, in noradrenergic systems, converted to norepinephrine by the enzyme dopamine beta-hydroxylase. Receptors which are stimulated by norepinephrine are pharmacologically classified into subtypes, alpha or beta, depending upon their response to specific sympathomimetic amines. For example, alpha receptors respond preferentially to agonists such as phenylephrine or methoxamine and are blocked by phentolamine. Beta receptors respond preferentially to isoproterenol and are blocked by propranolol. These subtypes may be further divided on the basis of location (presynaptic or postsynaptic) or preferential response to specific agonists or antagonists. The regulation of neurotransmission is extraordinarily complex and will only be highlighted. Factors that affect the activity in a specific system include the following: (1) the rate of synthesis of the neurotransmitter, which can be affected by a rate limiting step, the availability of the precursor, the presence or absence of enzyme cofactors, etc; (2) the firing rate of the neuron, which depends upon incoming stimuli; (3) the rate of release of the neurotransmitter, which may be effected by neuronal autoreceptors (presynaptic receptors); (4) the rate of reuptake of the neurotransmitter from the synapse back into the nerve terminal; (5) the rate of degradation or inactivation in the synaptic cleft or intraneuronally with different enzymes playing different roles in each case (for example, in noradrenergic systems catechol-*o*-methyl transferase plays the predominant role extraneuronally, and monoamine oxidase plays the predominant role intraneuronally); and (6) the responsitivity of the receptors (both presynaptic and postsynaptic). This responsitivity can be effected by chronic administration of agonists or antagonists and, in addition, by so-called neuromodulators, which do not act as agonists or antagonists themselves but may alter the state of the receptor.

It is clear from this brief summary that there are numerous possibilities for defects or shifts in this system, and when one considers the possibility of multiple alterations that may offset or potentiate each other, as well as interaction with other neurochemical systems, the identification of single or simple "abnormalities" can conceivably be quite difficult.

A long series of drugs which are considered to increase functional catecholaminergic transmission have been studied in the treatment of depression. Levodopa, a precursor of both dopamine and norepinephrine, has been given in high doses (eg, 7 g per day for four weeks), but has generally not been associated with good therapeutic response.[13]

Amphetamine increases release of norepinephrine and dopamine and has some effect in blocking their reuptake. In addition, amphetamine inhibits MAO to some extent and has some direct stimulatory effect on catecholamine receptors. Amphetamine is generally not associated with good antidepressant effect, although it can produce transient improvement in some patients.[14,15] Piribedil and bromocriptine, both of which are dopamine agonists, have been reported to have antidepressant properties in some studies; however, further work is necessary to clarify these effects.[16,17]

Cocaine, which blocks the reuptake of norepinephrine and dopamine, has been tried in the treatment of depression with negative results; however, the number of patients studied was small, and the drug was administered for a briefer period than tricyclic drugs would be in the treatment of depression.[18]

The administration of agents which block or reduce the synthesis of catecholamines would be expected to produce or exacerbate depression or even to reverse the effects of a successful course of antidepressant treatment. Alpha-methyl-para-tyrosine (AMPT), which blocks the rate-limiting step in the synthesis of dopamine and norepinephrine has been associated with worsening of depression in some patients, but not in others.[19] AMPT has also been given to manic patients with the assumption that if mania is due to an excess of catecholamines, AMPT should be an effective treatment. Some decrease in manic symptoms has been reported in patients receiving AMPT, but the effects have not been consistent and this strategy has not been widely studied.[20]

The pharmacologic treatments which are most effective in mania, lithium and neuroleptics, may affect catecholamines in ways that are consistent with the catecholamine hypothesis. Neuroleptics are potent blockers of dopamine receptors and have some effect in blocking adrenergic (norepinephrine) neurotransmission as well. These effects would be expected to reduce manic symptomatology; however, one might also expect a worsening of depressive symptoms among depressed patients receiving the drugs, and this is not a frequent occurrence. Lithium is thought to decrease the release of norepinephrine in some brain preparations and to increase the uptake of norepinephrine into synaptosomes.[21,22] This would be consistent with an antimanic effect, but is difficult to explain as the mechanism of lithium's antidepressant effect in bipolar patients or its reasonably well-established efficacy in the prophylaxis of unipolar depression. Lithium's mechanism of action is far from clear, however, and a variety of other neurochemical effects have been suggested.[23]

Precursor loading is another strategy that has been used to test the catecholamine hypothesis. The use of levodopa was alluded to previously, but tyrosine has been utilized as well in an attempt to increase catecholamine synthesis. Originally, it was felt that this would not have an effect on catecholamine synthesis, but recent studies indicate that it can. In addition, some preliminary results suggest a clinical therapeutic effect.[24]

Serotonin is synthesized from L-tryptophan. The first and possible rate-limiting step is the conversion of L-tryptophan to 5-hydroxytryptophan (5HTP) by the enzyme tryptophan hydroxylase. The enzyme 5HTP decarboxylase then converts 5HTP to serotonin (5-hydroxytryptamine). Within the neuron, serotonin is degraded by monoamine oxidase to 5-hydroxyindoleacetic acid (5HIAA). It has now been suggested that different isoenzymes of MAO have relative specificity for specific biogenic amines (MAO type A appears to show specificity for the oxidative deamination of serotonin). As is the case with dopamine and norepinephrine, serotonin appears to also have multiple receptors, presynaptic and postsynaptic. As described above, numerous factors affecting synthesis, storage, release, reuptake, breakdown, and receptor sensitivity could alter the functioning of serotonergic systems.

The indoleamine hypothesis suggests that a reduction in functional serotonin occurs during depression. Most antidepressants have similar effects on serotonin reuptake or degradation (in the case of MAO inhibitors) as they do on norepinephrine or dopamine. Some antidepressants have more effect on one system than another, and this has led some to postulate a preferential role for specific antidepressants in subgroups of depressions (those with low dopamine or norepinephrine as compared with those with low serotonin); however, the evidence supporting this is not consistent or impressive at the present time.[25,26] The major metabolite of serotonin (5HIAA) has been shown to be reduced in some, but not all, human postmortem studies of depressed patients who committed suicide.[27–30] However, the number of factors that may effect these postmortem measures is enormous.

Some investigators have reported decreased levels of 5HIAA in CSF among depressed patients as compared with that in normal controls.[31] However, others have failed to confirm this.[32] Asberg et al[33] have suggested a bimodal distribution of CSF 5HIAA among depressed patients, and they have also suggested that those patients with the lower values of this serotonin metabolite are more likely to make serious or violent suicide attempts.

Tryptophan is the amino acid from which serotonin is formed. Tryptophan competes with other neutral amino acids for transport into the brain. Several investigators have suggested that the administration of 1-tryptophan (or 5HTP) has antidepressant effects.[34,35] In addition, other studies which have combined 1-tryptophan or 5HTP with antidepressants (particularly those antidepressants with relatively high potency for blocking serotonin reuptake, such as clomipramine) have suggested that antidepressant activity is potentiated by the concurrent administration of these serotonin precursors.[36,37] (One study that explored the maintenance and prophylactic efficacy of 5HTP in depressed patients who had responded to clomipramine demonstrated a superiority of 5HTP over placebo in reducing depressive relapse rate in a double-blind crossover design.[38])

In a strategy analogous to the use of AMPT in testing the catecholamine hypothesis, parachlorophenylalanine has been used to test the indoleamine hypothesis.[39] Parachlorophenylalanine is an inhibitor of tryptophan hydroxylase, the rate-limiting enzyme in serotonin synthesis. One report suggested that parachlorophenylalanine could reverse the antidepressant effect of imipramine and tranylcypromine (an MAO inhibitor).[40]

We are not aware of any attempts to replicate these findings, however, and parachlorophenylalanine is not an easy drug to work with since it produces a variety of unpleasant side effects.

Some other findings which are supportive of an indoleamine hypothesis include decreased free plasma tryptophan concentrations in some depressed patients[41,42] (however, others failed to replicate this[43,44]) and a reduced rate of serotonin uptake into platelets from patients with affective disorder.[45]

Although much research is the psychobiology of affective disorders has focused on catecholamine or indoleamine systems a cholinergic-adrenergic balance hypothesis was proposed by Janowsky et al.[46] This hypothesis suggests that mood or affective state may be controlled by a balance between central cholinergic and adrenergic neurotransmitter activity, with depression resulting from cholinergic predominance and mania from adrenergic predominance. (An example of a similar balance is seen in the extrapyramidal system where either anticholinergic or dopaminergic agents can be used to treat Parkinson's disease, although the basic defect appears to be in dopaminergic systems.)

When centrally active sympathomimetic drugs are administered to animals (increasing central adrenergic function), an activated or excited state with increased self-stimulation and motor activity can be produced (a state that may be a model to some extent for behavioral aspects of mania). This type of hyperactivity, however, can be antagonized by centrally acting cholinomimetics.[47] In addition, the administration of cholinolytic agents can also produce behavioral activation.[48] Animal studies such as these have lent support to this type of balance hypothesis.

The observation that in human subjects the administration of irreversible cholinesterase inhibitors could produce a depressed-like clinical picture lent further support to this hypothesis.[49] It was subsequently shown that physostigmine (but not neostigmine, which does not cross the blood brain barrier) could produce a state of lethargy, social withdrawal fatigue, and constricted effect.[50] In addition, physostigmine, when administered to manic patients, brought about some reduction in manic symptoms such as overtalkativeness, euphoria, grandiosity, and flight of ideas and at times produced a depressed state with sadness and crying.[51]

Other studies have found physostigmine capable of increasing depressive symptoms in patients already suffering from depression or producing a depressed mood in euthymic individuals with a previous history of depression.[52]

Cholinergic mechanisms appear to be implicated in a well-established phenomenon regarding sleep architecture. Depressed individuals have been found to have a shorter duration of sleep before the onset of rapid eye movements (referred to as REM latency), as compared with controls. It has been suggested that this change in sleep pattern may reflect a cholinergic receptor hypersensitivity.[53] The ability of cholinomimetic agents to reduce REM latency appears to be increased in patients with affective illness (regardless of present mood state) as compared with normal controls.[53]

The hypothesis discussed so far generally revolve around the notion of a monoamine deficiency at the synapse playing a role in the pathophysiology of depression and the therapeutic activity of antidepressant drugs depending upon their ability to increase the availability of biogenic amines at the synapse either through high-affinity reuptake inhibition (tricyclic antidepressants) or inhibition of catabolism (MAO inhibitors).

A series of studies have shown that a high-affinity binding site for [^{3}H]imipramine exists in rat brain and in human platelets.[54–56] Raisman et al[55] have reported that depressed patients have significantly lower levels of [^{3}H]imipramine binding to platelet membranes than do controls. Although binding was reported to be lower, there was no apparent change in affinity. It has been suggested that the binding site for [^{3}H]imipramine is related to the presynaptic uptake site for serotonin, since Paul et al[57] have reported that tricyclic antidepressants share similar relative potencies in the blocking of serotonin reuptake presynaptically and the inhibition of [^{3}H]imipramine binding. These findings could be used to support the indoleamine hypothesis of depression as well.

The change found in this binding characteristic among patients with a history of depression may not be related to current mood state, since attempts at correlating this measure with measures of depressed mood have so far been unsuccessful.[55] In addition, the binding properties are not altered as a function of treatment outcome. A recent report[58] of imipramine binding in postmortem frontal cortex of suicides and matched controls found significantly lower binding (ie, reduction in binding sites) in the suicides.

One of the difficulties with the biogenic amine hypothesis as its evolved over the past 20 years is that several days and frequently two to four weeks (or even more) of antidepressant drug treatment are necessary to produce remission,[9] whereas the drug-induced neurochemical effects that were felt to be the mechanism of action occur much more rapidly and may be seen after a single administration of the drug.[59] In addition, several newer antidepressants (eg, iprindole, mianserin, and bupropion) do not exhibit the "classic" neuropharmacologic profile of the tricyclic antidepressants (however, since these drugs are not presently marketed in the United States, we may not have had a sufficient experience to assess their relative efficacy). Other drugs which are effective inhibitors of presynaptic biogenic amine uptake, such as amphetamine or cocaine, do not appear to be useful antidepressants.

Research has shifted to some extent in recent years from studying the relatively "acute" presynaptic effects of antidepressants to studying the adaptive changes which may occur in receptors (either presynaptic or postsynaptic). Advances in the application of neurotransmitter receptor binding techniques, single unit electrophysiologic studies, and the measurement of adenylate cyclase activity have contributed to the ability to study changes in receptor function which may play a role in depression and which are brought about by administration of antidepressant medications (or electroconvulsive therapy).

The adaptive changes in serotonin and norepinephrine systems after long-term administration of antidepressant drugs have been the subject of numerous reports.[60] It appears that the long-term administration of different classes of antidepressants has variable effects on norepinephrine and serotonin (5HT) turnover. Studies that have involved metabolite changes and clinical responses (eg, MHPG and 5HIAA levels) have also been inconsistent.

These findings would suggest considerable heterogeneity in specific biogenic amine involvement or a need for more attention to be focused on receptor function and adaptation.

The evidence that cyclic adenosine 3′,5′-monophosphate (cAMP) participates in some contexts as a "second messenger," mediating the effect of postsynaptic receptor stimulation, has provided a new tool in studying receptor function. It has been suggested that changes in the sensitivity of a receptor might be evidenced by changes in the capability of a specific neurotransmitter to stimulate the production of cAMP when applied to that receptor.[61]

Several studies have examined the effect of antidepressant treatment (including tricyclic antidepressants, MAO inhibitors, and electroconvulsive therapy) to alter the sensitivity of receptors to norepinephrine. It has been suggested that all effective somatic treatments for depression reduce norepinephrine-stimulated cAMP accumulation. In addition, the time course of this effect correlates well with the time course of clinical antidepressant treatment response.[61]

One possible explanation for this reduction in receptor sensitivity is that an increase in the norepinephrine available at the synapse brought about by reuptake blockade leads to a "down regulation" of the postsynaptic receptor. However, atypical antidepressants such as iprindole or bupropion do not have significant uptake blocking ability, but do have similar effects as other more "typical" antidepressants in desensitizing the norepinephrine-stimulated cAMP system.[62]

A major problem remains in this model of drug action in that it is not clear which adrenergic receptors are involved in this process.[60] It appears that the beta-adrenergic component (which can be assessed with the beta-agonist isoproterenol) does not account for the full decrease in norepinephrine receptor response. Therefore, as Charney et al [60] suggest, a non-beta component must be involved.

Two other "atypical" antidepressants, mianserin and zimelidine, appear to selectively reduce the sensitivity of the non-beta component after long-term treatment. Despite the variety of antidepressant treatments that appear to have this effect, a problem remains in that some drugs that do not have clear-cut antidepressant activity (eg, chlorpromazine and amphetamine) are able to produce a similar effect. Further caution is needed in extrapolating from these models, given the nature of the tissue

preparations used in these studies and other factors that may play a role in cAMP metabolism.

Another strategy that has been applied to study antidepressant action involves the effect of antidepressant treatment on receptor binding. Numerous studies (see Charney et al[60] for review) in recent years have reported reduction in the density of beta-adrenergic receptors in rat brain after long-term treatment with tricyclic antidepressants as well as MAO inhibitors and electroconvulsive therapy. Again, the fact that this change requires relatively long-term rather than acute treatment supports its relevance to antidepressant efficacy. In addition, deprivation of REM sleep, which has been suggested to have an antidepressant effect, also results in down regulation of beta-adrenergic receptors.[63] It is not clear whether there are meaningful exceptions to this proposed model. Results with bupropion have been inconsistent.[62] Some reports [64,65] suggest that mianserin does not produce this effect, and other reports suggest that amphetamine does.[66] The results from studies of alpha-adrenergic receptor binding after antidepressant treatment are far less consistent.[60] The alpha receptors have been divided into $alpha_1$ and $alpha_2$ binding sites.

Receptor systems for serotonin are also of considerable interest given the evidence alluded to above implicating this system in the pathophysiology of affective illness. Serotonin receptors have been described which are labeled by serotonin and referred to as 5HT receptors. Those which are labeled by tritiated spiperone (a neuroleptic) are referred to as $5HT_2$ receptors, though the specificity of this receptor remains to be established. A variety of tricyclic antidepressants and MAO inhibitors have been reported to decrease the density of $5HT_2$ receptors;[67,68] however, it appears that electroconvulsive therapy may not have this effect.[69]

The mechanism involved in this effect remains far from well established. The possibility that increased availability of 5HT or norepinephrine at the synapse results in a desensitization would be appealing if all antidepressant treatments resulted in this functional increase in 5HT or norepinephrine, but this appears not to be the case, since several effective drugs do not appear to block reuptake or degradation.

A very sophisticated technique has been developed which allows for single-unit electrophysiological measurement of response to neurotransmitters after chronic treatment with antidepressants. As Charney et al[60] suggest in their review, these single-unit studies generally find enhanced serotonergic and $alpha_1$-adrenergic response in several postsynaptic brain regions. These findings, therefore, are different from the neurochemical studies described above, and those differences remain to be reconciled.

In conclusion, this area of research has become increasingly sophisticated and complex. The hope remains that a final common pathway for effective antidepressant treatment will be found; however, this expectation may be inconsistent with assumptions that depression is a clinically and biologically heterogenous disorder.

At present, the attempts to relate pretreatment levels of biogenic amine metabolites to treatment response are inconsistent. It is extremely difficult to measure relevant receptor functions in depressed patients before and after treatment, and this remains an enormous challenge. Neuroendocrine tests which have been employed in this context are very nonspecific, since production and release of a given hormone may be controlled by several neurotransmitters.

Clearly, further research is needed to determine the relevance of the phenomena we have described. Hopefully, new clinical strategies will be developed to further explore the role of changes in receptor function in depression and its treatment.

REFERENCES

1. Barchas JD, Akil H, Elliot GR, et al: Behavioral neurochemistry: Neuroregulators in behavioral states. *Science* 1978;200:964–973.
2. Everett GM, Tolman JP: Mode of action of Rauwolfia alkaloids and motor activity, in Masderman J (ed): *Biological Psychiatry.* New York, Grune and Stratton, 1959, pp 75–81.
3. Schildkraut JJ: Catecholamine hypothesis of affective disorders: A review of supporting evidence. *Am J Psychiatry* 1965;122:509–522.
4. Bunney WE Jr, Davis JM: Norepinephrine in depressive reactions: A review. *Arch Gen Psychiatry* 1965;13:483–494.
5. Weiskrantz L, Wilson WA: The effects of reserpine on emotional behavior on normal and brain operated monkies. *Ann NY Acad Sci* 1955;61:36.
6. Goodwin FK, Ebert MH, Bunney WE Jr: Mental effects of reserpine in man: A review, in Shader RI (ed): *Psychiatric Complications of Medical Drugs.* New York, Raven Press, 1972, pp 73–101.
7. Davidson AN: Physiological role of monoamine oxidase. *Physiol Rev* 1958; 38:729–747.
8. Pare CMB, Sandler MJ: A clinical and biochemical study of a trial of iproniazid in the treatment of depression. *J Neurol Neurosurg Psychiatry* 1959;22:247–251.
9. Klein DF, Gittelman R, Quitkin F, et al: *Diagnosis and Drug Treatment of Psychiatric Disorders: Adults and Children.* ed 2. Baltimore, The Williams & Wilkins Co, 1980.
10. Goodwin FK, Cowdry RW, Webster MH: Predictors of drug response in the affective disorders: Toward an integrated approach, in Lipton MA, DiMascio A, Killam KF (eds): *Psychopharmacology: A Generation of Progress.* New York, Raven Press, 1978, pp 1277–1288.
11. Maas JW: Biogenic amines in depression: Biochemical and pharmacological separation of two types of depression. *Arch Gen Psychiatry* 1975;32:1357–1361.
12. Blombery PA, Kopin I, Gordon EK, et al: Conversion of MHPG to vanillylmandelic acid. *Arch Gen Psychiatry* 1980;37:1095–1098.

13. Goodwin FK, Murphy DL, Brody HKH, et al: L-dopa, catecholamines, and behavior: A clinical and biochemical study in depressed patients. *Biol Psychiatry* 1970;2:341–366.
14. Silberman EK, Reus VI, Jimerson DC, et al: Heterogeneity of amphetamine response in depressed patients. *Am J Psychiatry* 1981;138:1302–1307.
15. Bann TA: The use of amphetamines in adult psychiatry. *Semin Psychiatry* 1969;1:129–143.
16. Post RM, Gerner RH, Carman JS, et al: Effects of a dopamine agonist piribedil in depressed patients. *Arch Gen Psychiatry* 1978;35:609–615.
17. Waehrens J, Gerlach J: Bromocriptine and imipramine in endogenous depression: A double-blind controlled trial in outpatients. *J Affective Disord* 1981;3:193–202.
18. Post RM, Kotin J, Goodwin FK: Effects of cocaine in depressed patients. *Am J Psychiatry* 1974;131:511–517.
19. Brody HKH, Murphy DL, Goodwin FK, et al: Alpha-methyl-para-tyrosine in affective illness, in Vinar O, Vatava A, Bradley PB (eds): *Advances in Neuropharmacology.* Amsterdam, North Holland Publishers, 1971, pp 114–141.
20. Brody HKH, Murphy DL, Goodwin FK, et al: Catecholamines and mania: The effect of alpha-methyl-para-tyrosine on manic behavior and catecholamine metabolism. *Clin Pharmacol Ther* 1971;12:218–224.
21. Katz RI, Chase T, Kopin I: Evoked release of norepinephrine in serotonin from brain slices: inhibition by lithium. *Science* 1968;162:466–467.
22. Colburn R, Goodwin FK, Bunney WE Jr, et al: The effect of lithium on the uptake of norepinephrine by synaptosomes. *Nature* 1967;215:1395–1398.
23. Pert A, Rosenblatt JE, Sivit C, et al: Long-term treatment with lithium prevents the development of dopamine receptor supersensitivity. *Science* 1978;201:171–173.
24. Gellenberg AJ, Wojcik JD, Growdon JH, et al: Tyrosine for the treatment of depression. *Am J Psychiatry* 1980;137:622–623.
25. Asberg M, Bertilsson L, Tuck D, et al: Indoleamine metabolites in the cerebrospinal fluid of depressed patients before and during treatment with nortriptyline. *Clin Pharmacol Ther* 1972;14:277–286.
26. Bertilsson L, Asberg M, Thoren P: Differential effect of chorimipramine and nortriptyline on cerebrospinal fluid metabolites of serotonin and noradrenalin in depression. *Eur J Clin Pharmacol* 1976;21:194–200.
27. Shaw DM, Camps FEA, Eccleston EG: 5-Hydroxytryptamine in the hind brain of depressive suicides. *Br J Psychiatry* 1967;113:1407–1411.
28. Cochran E, Robbins E, Grote S: Regional serotonin levels in brain: A comparison of depressive suicides and alcoholic suicides with controls. *Biol Psychiatry* 1976;11:283–294.
29. Beskow J, Gottfries GG, Roos BE, et al: Determination of monoamine and monoamine metabolites in the human brain: Post mortem studies in a group of suicides and in a control group. *Acta Psychiatr Scand* 1976;53:7–20.
30. Pare CMB, Yeung DPH, Price K, et al: 5-Hydroxytryptamine noradrenalin and dopamine in brain stem, hypothalamus and caudate nucleus of controls and of patients committing suicide by coal gas poisoning. *Lancet* 1969;2: 133–135.
31. VanPraag HM, Korf J: Endogenous depressions with and without disturbances in the 5-hydroxytryptamine metabolism: A biochemical classification? *Psychopharmacologia* 1971;19:148.
32. Vestergaard P, Sorenson T, Hoppe E, et al: Biogenic amine metabolites in cerebral spinal fluid of patients with affective disorders. *Acta Psychiatr Scand* 1978;58:88–96.

33. Asberg M, Bertilsson L, Ringberger V, et al: "Serotonin Depression"—A biochemical subgroup within the affective disorder? *Science* 1976;191:478–480.
34. Coppen A: Indoleamine and affective disorders. *J Psychiatr Res* 1972;9: 163–171.
35. Brody HKH, Sack R, Siever L: Clinical studies of L-5-hydroxytryptophan in depression, in Barchas J, Usdin E (eds): *Serotonin and Behavior.* New York, Academic Press, Inc, 1973, pp 549–559.
36. Walinder J, Skott A, Carlsson A, et al: Potentiation of the antidepressant action of clomipramine by tryptophan. *Arch Gen Psychiatry* 1976;33:1384–1389.
37. VanPraag HM, VanDen Burg W, Bos ERH, et al: 5-Hydroxytryptophan in combination with clomipramine in therapy-resistant depression. *Psychopharmacologia* 1974;38:267–269.
38. VanPraag HM, Haan S: Central serotonin metabolism and frequency of depression. *Psychiatry Res* 1979;1:219–224.
39. Koe BK, Weissman A: PCPA: A specific depletor of brain serotonin. *J Pharmacol Exp Ther* 1966;154:499–516.
40. Shopsin B, Freedman E, Gershon S: Parachlorophenylamine reversal of tranylcypromine effects in depressed patients. *Arch Gen Psychiatry* 1976;33: 811–819.
41. Coppen A, Prange AJ Jr, Whybrow PC, et al: Abnormalities of indoleamines in affective disorders. *Arch Gen Psychiatry* 1972;26:474–478.
42. Coppen A, Wood JK: Tryptophan and depressive illness. *Psychol Med* 1978; 8:49–57.
43. Niskanen P, Huttunen M, Tamminen T, et al: The daily rhythm of daily plasma tryptophan and tyrosine in depression. *Br J Psychiatry* 1976;128:67–73.
44. Reily GJ, Shaw DM: Total and non-bound tryptophan in unipolar illness. *Lancet* 1976;2:1249.
45. Tuomisto J, Tukiainen E, Ahlfors VG: Decreased uptake of 5-hydroxytryptamine from blood platelets in patients with endogenous depression. *Psychopharmacology* 1979;65:141.
46. Janowsky DS, El-Yousef MK, Davis JM, et al: A cholinergic-adrenergic hypothesis of mania and depression. *Lancet* 1972;2:632–635.
47. Janowsky DS, El-Yousef MK, Davis JM, et al: Cholinergic antagonism of methylphenidate-induced stereotyped behavior. *Psychopharmacologia* 1972; 27:295–303.
48. Fibiger HC, Lytle LD, Campbell BM: Cholinergic modulation of adrenergic arousal in the developing rat. *J Comp Physiol Psychol* 1970;72:384–389.
49. Gershon S, Shaw FH: Psychiatric sequelae of chronic exposure to organophospherous insectides. *Lancet* 1961;1:1371–1374.
50. Davis KL, Hollister LE, Overall J, et al: Physostygmine effects on cognition and affect in normal subjects. *Psychopharmacologia* 1976;51:23–27.
51. Janowsky DS, El-Yousef MK, Davis JM, et al: Parasympathetic suppression of manic symptoms by physostygmine. *Arch Gen Psychiatry* 1973;28: 542–547.
52. Janowsky DS, Risch SC, Parker D, et al: Increased vulnerability to cholinergic stimulation in affective disorder patients. *Psychopharmacol Bull* 1980;16:29–31.
53. Sitaram N, Nurnberger J, Gershon E, et al: Faster cholinergic REM sleep induction in euthymic patients with primary affective illness. *Science* 1980;208: 200–202.

54. Langer SZ, Zarifian E, Briley M, et al: High-affinity binding of ^{3}H-imipramine in brain and platelets and its relevance to the biochemistry of affective disorders. *Life Sci* 1981;29:211–220.
55. Raisman R, Sechter D, Briley MD: High-affinity ^{3}H-imipramine binding in platelets from untreated and treated depressed patients compared to healthy volunteers. *Psychopharmacology* 1981;75:368–371.
56. Langer SZ, Briley M: High affinity ^{3}H-imipramine binding. A new biological tool for studies in depression. *Trends Neuro Sci* 1981;4:28–31.
57. Paul SM, Rehavi M, Skolnick P, et al: Demonstration of specific "high affinity" binding sites for ^{3}H-imipramine on human platelets. *Life Sci* 1980;26:953–959.
58. Stanley M, Virgilio J, Gershon S: Tritiated imipramine binding sites are decreased in the frontal cortex of suicides. *Science* 1982;216:1337–1339.
59. Iverson LL, McKay AVP: Pharmacodynamics of antidepressants and antimanic drugs, in Paykel ES, Coppen A (eds): *Psychopharmacology of Affective Disorders.* New York, Oxford University Press, 1979, pp 60–90.
60. Charney DS, Mankes DB, Henninger GR: Receptor sensitivity and the mechanism of action of antidepressant treatment. *Arch Gen Psychiatry* 1981;38:1160–1180.
61. Sulser F: New perspectives on the mode of action of antidepressant drugs. *Trends Pharmacol Sci* 1979;1:92–94.
62. Sulser F: Review of the mode of action of antidepressant drugs. Presentation at Meeting An Approach to Dilemmas in the Pharmacotherapy of Depression, Feb 4 and 5, 1982. Lake Buena Vista, Fla.
63. Mogilnicka E, Arbilla S, Depoortere H, et al: Rapid-eye-movement sleep deprivation decreases the density of ^{3}H-dihydroalprenolol and ^{3}H-imipramine binding sites in the rat cerebral cortex. *Eur J Pharmacol* 1980;65:289–292.
64. Sellinger-Barnette MM, Mendels J, Frazer A: The effect of psychoactive drugs on beta-adrenergic receptor binding sites in rat brain. *Neuropharmacology* 1980;19:447–454.
65. Clements-Jewery S: The development of cortical beta-adrenoceptor subsensitivity in the rat by chronic treatment with trazadone, doxepin and mianserin. *Neuropharmacology* 1978;17:779–781.
66. Selinger M, Sarai K, Frazer A, et al: Beta adrenergic receptor binding in rat cerebral cortex after repeated administration of psychotropic drugs. *Fed Proc* 1978;37:309.
67. Tang SW, Seeman P, Kwan S: Effect of chronic tricyclic antidepressant treatment on serotinergic and histaminergic receptors. *Neurosci Abstr* 1980;6:861.
68. Mann E, Enna SJ: Neurochemical and behavioral correlates of antidepressant drug action. *Neurosci Abstr* 1980;6:800.
69. Kellar KJ, Kascio CS, Butler JA, et al: Differential effects of electroconvulsive shock and antidepressant drugs on serotonin to receptors in rat brain. *Eur J Pharmacol* 1981;69:515–518.

CHAPTER 3

SOMATIC TREATMENT OF ACUTE DEPRESSION*

JUDITH G. RABKIN
DONALD F. KLEIN
FREDERIC M. QUITKIN

Depressive disorders are the most prevalent of psychiatric illnesses. They seem to have multiple causes, including biological, psychosocial, and behavioral components, are expressed through a variety of symptoms, and cover a wide range of severity, disability, and duration. Depressive symptoms may signify the presence of a full psychiatric syndrome of affective disorder or may accompany other psychiatric or medical conditions simply as signals of distress and demoralization. Although as many as one in five people in the general population is apt to express some symptoms of depression at any one point in time, only about 1 in 20 will have the full psychiatric syndrome of depressive disorder.

In the general psychiatric literature, depression characteristically is portrayed as a phasic disorder with illness episodes separated by months or years of normal functioning. It is estimated that 65% to 80% of patients have acute illnesses followed by recovery. In the remainder, there is a chronic course with significant residual symptomatic and social impairment. For those with phasic illness, episodes are usually believed to range from 6 to 12 months in untreated cases. Recent data such as those of Shapiro and Keller[1] suggest, however, that even treated patients who respond to therapeutic intervention remain symptomatic for longer periods of time than formerly believed. Such evidence reinforces the indications for active and prompt treatment programs for depressive disorders.

The first task of the clinician is to clarify the nature of the depressive symptoms of the patient and to make a differential diagnosis. Diagnostic

*Portions of this chapter have appeared in Rabkin JG, Klein DF: The biological therapies, in Lewis J, Usdin G (eds): *Treatment Planning in Psychiatry*. Washington, DC, American Psychiatric Association, 1982.

guidelines are available both in the general clinical literature (DSM-III)[2] and in the research literature (the Feighner Criteria[3] or Research Diagnostic Criteria [RDC][4] for selected disorders including schizophrenia and affective disorders). In general, research criteria are more stringent, thereby creating a larger group of patients with residual or unclassified disorders. This is acceptable for research, but less helpful for clinical purposes. Both clinical and research diagnostic guidelines provide definitions of type, number, and severity of symptoms characterizing various psychiatric disorders.

CLINICAL SYMPTOMS OF DEPRESSIVE DISORDER

In addition to pervasive dysphoric mood, which may be expressed as sadness, tearfulness, or irritability, behavioral and cognitive alterations are usually reported. These include loss of interest in usual activities, inability to respond even transiently to pleasant events or situations (referred to as mood autonomy), distinct changes in sleep, eating, energy level, and motor activity, and feelings of guilt, recurrent thoughts of death, and impaired concentration. The distinction between acute depressive illness, the subject of the present chapter, and chronic depression is a relative one based on duration, the patient's subjective sense of whether or not the illness is phasic with better and worse interludes, and whether the dysphoria is sustained over a period of years.

The RDC were developed by Spitzer et al[4] to provide a consistent set of criteria for investigators participating in a multicenter study focusing on affective disorders, sponsored by the Clinical Research Branch of the National Institute of Mental Health. The goal of the RDC is to identify relatively homogeneous groups of patients who meet specified diagnostic criteria. They are organized on the principle that, for research purposes, it is better to avoid false-positives (cases incorrectly included as having a particular condition) than false-negatives (cases incorrectly excluded). In this diagnostic system, all diagnoses are judged to be either absent ("no"), probable, or definite. "Probable" implies more than 50% certainty, and usually requires that fewer explicit criteria be met than those needed to make a "definite" diagnosis.

The RDC distinguish among major, intermittent, and minor depressive disorders. Within the category of major depressive disorder, 10 overlapping subtypes are delineated, including the primary-secondary distinction and recurrent unipolar, endogenous, psychotic, agitated, retarded incapacitating, situational, and simple depression.

According to the DSM-III nomenclature, depressive disorders are grouped into three categories: major affective disorders, where a full unipolar or bipolar syndrome is manifested; other affective disorders, in which there is only a partial syndrome; and a residual category of atypical affective disorders.

The DSM-III category of major depressive episode is derived from and largely equivalent to the RDC of major depressive disorders, "definite." The subtype of "melancholia" is similar to the RDC subtype of "endogenous." The DSM-III subtype is, however, more stringently defined since it requires mood autonomy as an *essential* characteristic which the RDC definition does not. In both RDC and DSM-III definitions, "major" episodes include both psychotic and nonpsychotic, reactive or precipitated as well as "nonreactive" or apparently spontaneous episodes, and primary as well as secondary disorders. "Neurotic" or "atypical" (in the sense originated by English psychiatrists) as well as the traditional endogenous symptom constellations may meet either RDC or DSM-III criteria for major depressive disorder. (There is a terminology problem here since the adjective "atypical" is regularly used throughout DSM-III to demarcate residual, poorly defined categories. Unfortunately, in the area of affective disorder, the term "atypical" has a specific historical meaning that will be discussed below.)

Other DSM-III depressive diagnoses are cyclothymic disorder, dysthymic disorder, and atypical depression. Cyclothymic disorder refers to a long-term illness of at least two years' duration with either sustained or intermittent periods of both depressive and manic symptoms which are not sufficiently severe to meet criteria for major depressive or manic episodes. Dysthymic disorder or "depressive neurosis" is a chronic mild disturbance involving either depressed mood or anhedonia (loss of interest or pleasure in usual activities) of at least two years' duration. Atypical depression, as the term is used in DSM-III, is a residual category for those whose depressive symptoms cannot otherwise be classified. The term atypical depression is used by others, including ourselves, not as a residual category but to describe patients with a specific symptom constellation including the essential feature of mood reactivity. We currently define the syndrome as present when, in addition to mood reactivity, patients also manifest two of four associated features of oversleeping, overeating and/or weight gain, extreme lethargy ("leaden paralysis"), and pathologic rejection sensitivity, especially in the context of a romantic relationship. We will discuss this syndrome further with respect to treatment indications for monoamine oxidase inhibitors (MAOIs).

Overall, although differing in the rigor of their criteria, the diagnostic distinctions in both the RDC and DSM-III are based on number, type, and severity of symptoms present within a specified time frame. Because it is the official diagnostic nomenclature, the DSM-III nosology is the one used routinely in clinical settings, but it is important for clinicians to be acquainted with the RDC system as well, since it has become the standard research nosology in studies of affective disorders published in American scientific journals.

In general, it is appropriate to consider somatic treatment for patients whose symptoms have persisted unabated for at least three weeks, whose social, familial, or occupational functioning is impaired by these symptoms, and who meet DSM-III diagnostic criteria for some form of depressive disorder. Antidepressant medication is generally considered the treatment of choice only for patients with major depression. Although their unequivocal efficacy has been established only for this group, other patients with moderate or even mild depression may be suitable candidates for pharmacotherapy either initially or after other therapeutic approaches have failed.

DIFFERENTIAL DIAGNOSIS

Depressed mood characterizes several other conditions which must be distinguished from primary depressive disorder because they respond to different treatment strategies. Grief reactions often entail the same symptoms, but are considered illness episodes only when the intensity and duration of reaction clearly exceed the characteristic grief behavior of the individual's social group. Grief reactions are usually self-limiting. Demoralization also differs from depression, although it may be a consequence of depression or other psychiatric and medical disorders. Demoralization is a failure of self-confidence, a loss of faith in one's competence. Both depressed and demoralized people feel sad, lonely, hopeless, blocked, worried, low in energy, and possibly tense. However, unlike the former, the demoralized person can enjoy himself in low-demand situations where there is no opportunity for failure. Behavioral rather than psychotropic treatments seem indicated in the management of demoralization.

Patients with depressed mood may have another disorder, psychiatric or medical, preceding the depression. As many as 3 in 10 medical patients with chronic disorders such as hypertensive disease and arthritis have been described as depressed,[5] although it is not clear whether they have depressive symptoms or a full syndrome. The distinction between such secondary depressions and primary depressive disorder is useful in some cases in which treatment of the primary disease may lead to amelioration of the depressive symptoms. In addition, the clinician must differentiate primary depression from organic or drug-induced depression. Some medications, such as reserpine, may induce depression. In such cases, the first step in management is to address the cause (if possible terminating the medication in question) rather than to treat the symptoms.

It is not unusual for patients to display symptoms of both depression and anxiety; some meet diagnostic criteria for both disorders. DSM-III rules for diagnostic classification exclude diagnosis of an anxiety disorder if these symptoms only appear together with affective disorder and not between affective episodes. Some interesting new evidence from genetic studies calls into question these taxonomic rules. Patients with simultaneous manifestations of anxiety and depression have higher rates of *both* disorders in their first-degree relatives than do "pure" depressed patients.[6] Perhaps both syndromes are indeed present in such patients even if they occur only simultaneously; further research is expected to clarify the issue.

TREATMENT PLANNING

Pretreatment Evaluation

All psychiatric patients, whether or not they are to receive somatic treatment, should have a detailed medical workup. The clinician should also obtain a comprehensive medical history, determination of current medical status and medications being taken, a family history of psychiatric illness, and a personal developmental and psychiatric history. If the patient has received previous treatment, details about type, duration, and outcome should be elicited.

Medical data are needed both to assess contributing factors to current illness and for selection of safe treatment methods. In patients who may receive somatic treatments, special consideration should be given to those conditions which may affect the safety of treatment; cardiovascular, renal, hematological, hepatic, and metabolic function warrant particular attention. In view of the range of toxic effects of neuroleptics, tricyclic antidepressants (TCAs), and MAOIs, the examining physician should consider the presence of cardiac decompensation, arrhythmia, conduction defects, hypertension or hypotension, renal disease, and any metabolic disorders which may affect speed of drug clearance.

Because of the possibility of negative interactions with other medications and medical conditions, a complete enumeration of current medications should be elicited from the patient and, if possible, any treating physician. Psychotropic drugs can interact with those prescribed for medical conditions with potentially grave consequences. Psychotropic medications may also aggravate existing medical conditions apart from the medications used to treat them. TCAs lower the threshold for major convulsions; therefore, epileptic patients so treated require particularly close supervision. They also may exacerbate preexisting glaucoma because of their anticholinergic effects so, again, close monitoring and appropriate consultation are indicated.

Overall, for both therapeutic and legal reasons, a meticulous medical workup, backed up where possible with medical records from other physicians and institutions, is a prerequisite to the initiation of somatic treatment for psychiatric disorder.

Clinical history This area of inquiry is a key determinant in treatment planning, providing guidelines in the setting of reasonable therapeutic goals as well as effective means of achieving them. Issues included here are developmental history, premorbid social adjustment, prior psychiatric illnesses, and previous treatment experiences.

In general, it is helpful to use a structured form or checklist to cover these areas. Without systematic procedures it is too easy to miss large areas of potential relevance. A specific checklist for note taking is an aid to the novice and a useful reminder to the experienced clinician. Such an outline need not be gone through in any mechanical order, but by the end of the assessment all areas should have been covered.

The patient's previous efforts to cope with illness, either in the current episode or an earlier one, are of interest in treatment planning. It is seldom the case that someone goes directly to a psychiatrist without first attempting other solutions. Even if these efforts were ultimately unsuccessful, as is evidently the case at least for the current episode, they may provide leads regarding potentially available ancillary resources.

Perhaps the most immediately useful material the patient can supply is a detailed description of previous treatment, including nature of response or lack of response. In addition to the patient's report, records of all previous care should be obtained, if possible. Reactions to somatic therapies are of particular interest. As a rule, medication that was previously successful for a comparable illness episode is the treatment of choice for the current episode. Patients usually respond to successive courses of electroconvulsive therapy (ECT) as they did earlier (barring changes in cerebral function), both in type of response, number of treatments, and stability.

Although a report of past positive drug response is generally valid and can be accepted at face value, reports of negative outcome do not necessarily mean that the medication previously used should be disqualified from consideration in the current episode. Although previous negative experiences may actually indicate that the medication is not useful for a particular patient, it is also possible that the drug was prescribed incorrectly or the patient's compliance was inadequate. Unfortunately, it is not uncommon to find that presumably appropriate medication fails because it was prescribed at levels high enough to elicit side effects but insufficient to attain a therapeutic level, or else the trial was too brief to assess the drug's efficacy. A third possibility is that the wrong medication was chosen as, for example, the prescription of benzodiazepines for patients who are equally anxious and depressed.

If the correct drug was prescribed at appropriate dose levels for a sufficient period of time and the patient failed to respond, it is possible that he or she did not take the medication as directed. In this context, both the patient and family members must be interviewed to assess the degree of the patient's cooperation with taking prescribed medication. Often patients do not accurately report what happened. Simply asking the patient whether he or she took the medication regularly will not suffice; patients may say they took their medication regularly and by this mean only once a week. One should ask specific questions such as how many pills were taken how many times a day. Further, patients often report that they had bad reactions to certain drugs or were allergic to them. This is often an inaccurate representation of the facts, and detailed reviews are necessary to avoid discarding potentially useful interventions. It is also possible that averse drug reactions did occur that could be modified with suitable ancillary treatment.

If the correct drug was prescribed at suitable doses, and the patient followed the regimen correctly, had a diagnosis compatible with a specific drug benefit, but reported a poor response to treatment, one other consideration may be relevant. The diagnosis must then be reviewed with particular emphasis on the possibility of histrionic personality disorder or malingering.

Finally, one should determine the nature of the patient's past experience with drugs having addictive potential as well as any history of drug dependence and alcoholism. MAOIs should be used cautiously in patients with such a recent history.

In summary, identification of previously effective treatment for a similar illness episode would indicate its use in the present. On the other hand, prescription of medication similar to medications that have already failed is only occasionally useful. Apart from probable lack of efficacy and delay in relieving the patient's symptoms, there is the problem of further demoralization and loss of hope by the patient who experiences multiple ineffective therapeutic trials.

Family history In view of increasingly persuasive evidence of familial or genetic patterns of illness, a family history of psychiatric disorder is often useful. Family histories are usually sought for first-degree relatives: parents, siblings, and offspring. Diagnostic and prognostically relevant information may be generated by a knowledge of illness in relatives and the nature of their clinical response to specific somatic therapies if they were treated.

Although the evidence is suggestive rather than definitive, bipolar disorder is widely believed to have a genetic component.[2] Even if a patient's only illness is depression, a bipolar diagnosis may be suspected if there is a family history of bipolar illness. The biological substratum of this syndrome is suggested not only by the nature of the symptoms themselves but also by the remarkable success of lithium in its treatment.

Suicide also runs in families and seems to be either genetically or socially transmitted. A family history of suicide has specific and immediate implications for patient care.

With the possible exception of bipolar disorder, family history is not customarily considered in arriving at a diagnosis. However, one group of investigators has developed a classification of depressive subtypes based entirely on such data. Winokur and colleagues[7] have delineated three subtypes of unipolar depressive disorder based on the presence and type of psychiatric disorder found among first-degree relatives. Based on small samples, these investigators have tentatively identified differential responses to medical treatment and variations in neuroendocrine characteristics. If these findings are substantiated, then family history will prove to have major significance in treatment planning beyond that already recognized.

Family histories can provide an additional dimension with respect to the patient's and relatives' assets as well as their individual and collective pathology. Patients interviewed when ill may be unable to realistically appraise their abilities and strengths when well, whereas relatives can provide this perspective. They can also present their own positive strengths and their attempts to cope with the patient and help him deal with the illness.

Use of biological tests in pretreatment evaluation Exciting leads have been generated by the identification of specific deviant neuroendocrine responses in patients during illness episodes. Two of the most widely studied procedures are the dexamethasone suppression test (DST), developed by Carroll, and the thyrotropin-releasing hormone–thyroid-stimulating hormone (TRH–TSH) test. In addition, sleep parameters have been shown to differentiate between depressed and other psychiatric patients. All of these tests are still experimental, essentially of heuristic rather than clinical importance at the present time, and do not yet have a role in the practical management of depressed patients.

DST After administration of an oral dose of the synthetic steroid dexamethasone, investigators have found that a sizeable number of patients with melancholia have higher plasma cortisol levels than normal persons, whose cortisol levels are "suppressed" by the ingestion of dexamethasone. This abnormality is related to abnormal hypothalamic-pituitary-adrenal regulation in depressed patients.[8] The DST identifies very few "false-positives" in the sense that almost all nonsuppressors are indeed depressives; its specificity rate is about 96%. However, a fair number of depressed patients are "false-negatives" in that they do suppress cortisol output after dexamethasone administration.[9] The test's sensitivity or ability to identify true negatives is about 45% for outpatient endogenous depressives and 67% for inpatient endogenous depressives. It is considerably less useful in identifying depression in less severly ill patients and those without endogenous symptoms. In our own work with "atypical" or "neurotic" depressive patients, only a small fraction have been nonsuppressors. In general, we do not recommend application of the DST in clinical practice as a routine test. If, however, special indications suggest its use, we suggest that only clinical laboratories familiar with DST analyses for psychiatric diagnosis be used since there are probably many false-positive DST results produced by other laboratories. We wish to emphasize that negative findings do not rule out depression, but that positive findings are typically valid.

TRH test TRH stimulates release of the hormone TSH by the pituitary gland. A number of investigators have found that, as a group, patients with major depressive disorder have a reduced or "blunted" TSH response to the administration of TRH. This observation fits with other observations of abnormal functioning of the hypothalamic-pituitary-adrenal axis in depressive disorder. Some investigators (eg, Gold et al[10]) believe this response to be characteristic of unipolar depressed patients in contrast to other depressed patients, but this claim has been challenged by others (eg, Loosen and Prange[11]). Additional research is required to clarify the utility of the TRH test in the diagnosis of depression and depressive subtypes.

Sleep measures Sleep disorders are widespread among psychiatric patients in virtually all diagnostic categories; 70% to 80% exhibit some kind of sleep disturbance. In addition, distinctive and consistent deviations specifically identify depressed patients. The most striking is shortened rapid eye movement (REM) latency (shorter period between onset of sleep and start of the first REM period), which in normal adults is about 70 to 90 minutes and in depressed patients is less than 60 minutes. Other distinctive and deviant sleep characteristics of depressed patients include more frequent sleep interruptions, less deep sleep, and more densely concentrated eye movements during REM sleep. At this time, as Kupfer and colleagues[12] have noted, "the existence of a sleep disorder in depression is no longer in question." Issues remaining to be clarified include the relationship of sleep abnormalities to depressive subtype, to clinical status, and to treatment outcome. Most research to date has been conducted with acutely ill endogenous depressed patients so that its application to outpatients and those with chronic disorders remains to be demonstrated.

Sleep measures and the other biological tests may some day provide laboratory measures of specific forms of psychopathology in the same way that urine tests can signify the presence of diabetes. At the present time, these tests are not clinically useful in routine practice, and their application in treatment planning is not indicated. Nevertheless, this is a rapidly developing area, and the potential for such objective diagnostic tests is great.

Assessing Severity of Illness

Evaluation of suicide risk Most severely depressed patients have some thoughts about suicide, and it is estimated that about 15% of those with primary affective disorder eventually kill themselves.[13] Consequently, the risk always warrants careful consideration and discussion with patient and family. Expression of vague thoughts of death in the absence of specific plans are of comparatively less concern than are specific plans or feelings of marked hopelessness. When appraising risk, one should consider the availability of adequate family supervision and whether the patient lives alone, drinks, or has a history of previous suicide attempts. Patients with severe agitation are at greater risk than others.

Hospitalization Except for acute mania, there are no diagnostic classifications which almost always mandate hospitalization. The three major clinical justifications for inpatient care are to protect the patient (eg, the suicidal patient), to protect others (eg, the belligerently assaultive psychotic patient), or to provide necessary medical supervision and care (eg, the elderly, depressed patient with cardiovascular disease). These indications cut across diagnostic categories and may include patients with schizophrenia, schizoaffective and affective disorders, as well as acute organic and other conditions.

In addition to these clinical indications, the decision to hospitalize is often influenced by social contingencies (eg, geographical proximity to a hospital or nature of insurance coverage) and treatment considerations (eg, use of investigational drugs or drug combinations). These issues are considered elsewhere in the chapter.

Hospitalization has the advantages of providing maximal protection and medical supervision. Its drawbacks include the possibility of stigma for the discharged patient who seeks to resume his normal life in the community and discontinuities of psychiatric care and clinical supervision after discharge.

Assessment of Psychosocial Supports

Family composition, marital status, occupation, organizational affiliations, and social and financial resources affect treatment planning in the sense that they reflect the patient's current living arrangements, life style, and social network. Especially with more seriously ill patients, the entire design of treatment may be contingent on the availability of sympathetic relatives or friends to support the patient before medication becomes effective, to supervise medication compliance and doctor visits, to report adverse drug reactions or illness exacerbations, and to provide supervision and guidance during acute episodes. Except for frankly suicidal or acutely manic patients for whom hospitalization is nearly always indicated, the presence or absence of close relatives, friends, religious advisors, or other competent, caring people may be the determining factor in making custodial arrangements. Close, continuous observation and companionship are necessary for the patient's morale and protection during the customary two- to three-week drug lag and become critical when either drug reactions or illness symptoms may impair the patient's judgment. For example, one sign of lithium toxicity is clouding of consciousness so that the patient may not be able to recognize the need to seek immediate medical care. On the other hand, patients entering a manic episode see no need for psychiatric treatment, and such a determination becomes the responsibility of concerned others.

Knowledge of a patient's job and the significance of income for the family's functioning may influence not only decisions about hospitalization, but sometimes also other treatment strategies. For example, ECT often requires time off from work, whereas antidepressant medication usually does not. The decision to discontinue lithium after a period of well being would also be influenced by the degree of disruption, both financial and social, that might ensue if an illness episode were thus precipitated.

In general, life circumstances, social supports, and family composition influence the clinician's willingness to treat patients on an outpatient basis, to use medications that entail risk of major adverse reactions, or, in the case of treatment refractory patients, to use unusual medication or treatment combinations that have higher probabilities of benefit as well as risks.

Indications and Treatment Goals for Drug Therapy

Patients with acute depression are candidates for antidepressant medication. Although there are far fewer complications with medically healthy patients, physical status alone seldom rules out the use of psychotropic drugs. With the exceptions noted in the following discussion, TCAs are usually the treatment of choice for a first drug trial.

Numerous clinical trials have shown that somewhere between 20% and 40% of depressed patients respond to placebo or remit spontaneously during a four- to six-week drug trial. About 70% of patients (including placebo responders) respond to TCAs, all of which are generally equivalent in efficacy. Another 10% to 15% of depressed patients respond to subsequent strategies after TCAs were not effective; these strategies include MAOIs, ECT, and nonstandard drugs and drug combinations. Overall, approximately 85% of patients with acute depressive illness do respond to somatic treatments, a proportion unsurpassed for any other patient group or treatment modality according to available empirical evidence.

Treatment goals When patients are described as drug responders, rated as improved, and considered less symptomatic after a course of medication, the base line for such assessment is their former level of functioning, not some hypothetical concept of positive mental health. That is, the goal and usual achievement of drug therapy is restoration to the patient's preillness status, not "cure." If the patient's premorbid level of adjustment was impaired or if he has experienced an acute exacerbation in the context of a chronic dysphoric condition, restoration to former level of functioning will not be equivalent to cure. This perspective is essential for adequate treatment planning concerning aftercare and provision of ancillary therapeutic, vocational, or support services.

Role of psychotherapy We want to emphasize that use of psychotropic drugs does not preclude concomitant or subsequent psychotherapy, either with the same or another clinician. In this context, we use the term "psychotherapy" to refer to a specific treatment plan using nonsomatic techniques, not the more general development of a therapeutic relationship between doctor and patient which is an integral component of any psychiatric treatment. Indeed, in the absence of a therapeutic alliance, psychopharmacological treatment is unlikely to succeed. Contrary to popular sociology, most Americans do not regard pills as wonderful magical remedies. In fact, the majority of patients initially are resistant to the notion of medication and generally require persuasion to cooperate. Without a therapeutic relationship, many patients probably would not agree to try medication, would not comply with the medication schedule, and certainly would not continue to do so during the three- to four-week drug lag in the absence of clear-cut mood improvement.

Apart from the therapeutic alliance that is integral to pharmacological treatment, a course of nonsomatic treatment may be indicated. Especially in cases of recurrent unipolar depression or bipolar disorder, it is quite likely that the illness episodes create disruptions in family relationships, friendships, and occupational performance. In addition, demoralization secondary to a depressive episode is not uncommon. Removal of depressive symptoms and restoration of euthymic mood may not lead to resolution of these other problems.

In the last 10 years, several new short-term methods of psychotherapy have been developed which are reportedly effective in the treatment of depression. These include cognitive therapy developed by Beck,[14] interpersonal therapy developed by DeMascio et al,[15] and behavioral techniques including the pleasant events schedule associated with Lewinsohn and Arconad.[16] These methods usually consist of weekly sessions for three to six months, require specific training in techniques that are spelled out in treatment manuals, and have specified and measurable goals. If the treating physician is not trained in one of these or other appropriate therapeutic techniques, referral may be indicated during or after somatic treatment. However, it is not demonstrated that the specific components of these treatments are actually responsible for their beneficial effects.

The balance of this chapter is devoted to a review of specific somatic treatments for depressive disorder. The three standard therapies currently used in clinical practice, TCAs, MAOIs, and ECT, are reviewed first. For each procedure we offer an overview of its development, associated risks and risk management, and treatment applications including indicators, pretreatment steps, guidelines for prescribing, and choice within category where applicable. In addition, we describe the clinical status of patients for whom this is the treatment of choice. After these three sections on standard therapies, we review a number of procedures to be considered for those patients who respond minimally or not at all to them. The final section is devoted to a brief review of new antidepressant drugs, which either have been approved recently by the Food and Drug Administration (FDA) for routine clinical practice or whose approval is anticipated in the near future.

In this chapter routine procedures and standard practices will be noted. However, prescription of medication is an extraordinarily individualized undertaking, determined not only by the guidelines but by illness stage, severity, and spectacular biological variations in individual drug tolerance. For example, some patients can tolerate only 25 mg of chlorpromazine a day, whereas others can tolerate 10,000 mg a day. Consequently, drug dosage must be adjusted to individual needs, and each patient should receive as much medication as is needed for clinical improvement as long as the side effects are manageable. Since nearly all psychotropic drugs, and indeed most active drugs of any kind, are likely to elicit some kind of side effect, the issue is not their appearance but their severity, duration, and reversibility. Caution should be used concerning the underprescription of psychotropic drugs, both in dose and duration, that so often characterizes their use and which may stem in part from excessive reliance on general guidelines.

TRICYCLIC ANTIDEPRESSANTS

History and Description

Antidepressants fall into two major categories: TCAs and MAOIs, which will be discussed in the next section. Drugs in the TCA category are those most widely used for the treatment of depression.

The first TCA identified as having antidepressant properties was imipramine, whose efficacy has been equalled but never surpassed by any antidepressant subsequently developed. Imipramine was derived in the 1940s as a modification of chlorpromazine. In 1958 Kuhn tested it with psychotic patients. Unlike the phenothiazines, imipramine had no effect of psychotic symptoms, but Kuhn noticed that it made depressed schizophrenic patients less depressed. He proceeded to study the drug with depressed patients and established it as an effective antidepressant. Today it remains the standard to which all newer drugs may be compared.

Since 1958, more than a dozen other antidepressants have been developed, and to date about half have been approved by the FDA for the treatment of depression. These include amitriptyline, desipramine, nortriptyline, protriptyline, trimipramine, amoxapine, and doxepin. All seem interchangeable in terms of their efficacy for depression, although their side effects vary somewhat.

TCAs can be grouped in terms of chemical structure as having one methyl group or two. The former are referred to as secondary amines and include desipramine, nortriptyline, and protriptyline. Those with two methyl groups are referred to as tertiary amines and include imipramine, amitriptyline, doxepin, trimipramine, and clomipramine. The last of these is still classified as an investigational drug. These groups differ in their action on the metabolism of central nervous system neurotransmitters. Tertiary amines are metabolized into secondary amines.

All of the drugs in this category produce little effect other than sedation in people who are not depressed. The tertiary amines tend to have greater sedative properties than the secondary amines, and within this group, amitriptyline and doxepin more so than imipramine.

In addition to these approved drugs, a number of others are in various stages of development and testing. Investigators are trying to develop antidepressants with more rapid onset of action, greater biologic specificity, fewer side effects, and efficacy for patients refractory to available treatments. New and promising drugs include TCAs such as maprotiline and mianserin and serotonergic antidepressants such as fluoxetine and others which are described below.

Risks and Risk Management

Overdose of TCAs can be lethal, a major drawback for medication prescribed for depressed and possibly suicidal patients. Even when taken in prescribed doses, both minor and potentially serious medical complications may ensue. Common unpleasant side effects include dry mouth, fatigue, constipation, sweating, tremor, nausea, drowsiness, and insomnia among others. It is important to note, however, that all of these problems are also symptoms of depression and may have been present before treatment or appear subsequently without being drug related. Nevertheless, TCAs do cause such anticholinergic effects. Extrapyramidal reactions are very rare. The range of side effects is wide, varies only slightly among TCAs, and often inconveniences the patient at least mildly.

Although these common side effects are not medically serious, they can interfere with drug compliance or dose increments. For most patients, they can be managed effectively with a variety of techniques. For example: sugarless chewing gum usually ameliorates the nuisance side effect of dry mouth, surgical elastic stockings reduce dizziness associated with postural hypotension, and water-retaining laxatives are helpful with constipation. Sometimes ancillary drugs are useful. Medications which enhance cholinergic effects such as neostigmine may help patients with marked sensitivity to a range of anticholinergic side effects. Ancillary prescription of propranolol is often useful for patients with persistent and troublesome tachycardia resulting from TCAs. An alternative strategy for this side effect if a tertiary amine (eg, imipramine) has been prescribed, is to substitute a secondary amine (eg, desipramine). For a more detailed presentation of the management of side effects of TCAs, the reader is referred to the discussion of Klein and colleagues.[17]

More serious are potential cardiovascular effects associated with TCAs, particularly for older patients with preexisting heart disease. TCAs slow conduction rate and may exacerbate cardiomyopathies and congestive heart failure. Nevertheless, as Kantor et al[18] have demonstrated, TCAs can be used safely for some cardiac patients with careful medical supervision and regular monitoring with serial electrocardiograms and may actually benefit dysrhythmias. In therapeutic doses, TCAs are not associated with cardiac complications in healthy young and middle-aged patients.

TCAs interact with several widely used drugs, including alcohol and antihypertensives. Their simultaneous use potentiates the effects (and side effects) of each so that, for example, patients who use both TCAs and alcohol more quickly become intoxicated, and TCA side effects are likely to be enhanced. TCAs alone sometimes induce orthostatic hypotension, so that their use in conjunction with antihypertensive medication can lead to excessive drop in blood pressure. The anticholinergic activity of TCAs makes it important to monitor functioning if they are used together with antiparkinsonian agents, phenothiazines, or other compounds that also have antimuscarinic effects. As a rule, combining antipsychotic and antidepressant drugs requires specific indications.

Finally, it is generally believed that TCAs may induce a switch to mania in some bipolar patients. New data reported by Lewis and Winokur[19] suggest that "the rate of induction of mania by TCAs is not greater than what one would expect from the natural history of the illness." This issue remains a matter of controversy. In addition, TCAs may induce confusional states and delirium, especially in older patients. These drug-related symptoms are sometimes misinterpreted as being illness manifestations, and so it is important to recognize their association with medication.

Risk management Suicide risk is reduced if only small amounts of medication (up to 1.25 g) are dispensed to acutely depressed patients. It has been reported that in most series, about two-thirds of patients with TCA overdose ingested other drugs as well, most often benzodiazepines or alcohol.[20] In cases of overdose, cardiac toxicity is the greatest hazard.

Immediate admission to an intensive care unit with equipment for continuous cardiac monitoring, defibrillation, and resuscitation is indicated. Once vital functions are stabilized, the next essential step is removal of unabsorbed drug from the gut as soon as possible. With respect to confusional or delirious reactions, the best first step is to stop the antidepressant. Physostigmine salicylate sometimes can alleviate many of the antimuscarinic, cardiotoxic, and neurotoxic features associated with TCA overdose. This drug itself can be toxic, however, particularly when large doses are given rapidly, so that its administration by an experienced clinician is indicated. Negative drug interactions are minimized by getting a careful history of other medications and, if their use is necessary, maintaining medical surveillance. Administration of medication before bedtime reduces the discomfort of some of the minor but annoying side effects.

Treatment Applications

Based on cumulative evidence from more than 100 studies, the efficacy of TCAs for the treatment of depressive disorder has been decisively established. The research evidence shows that the response to placebo is between 20% and 40%, and response to TCAs is about 70% to 80%. In other words, about one-third of patients get better without medication, another third are effectively treated with antidepressants, and the rest respond partially, transiently, or not at all.

TCAs are considered the pharmacologic treatment of choice for patients with major depressive disorders and for patients with approximately equivalent manifestations of anxiety and depression. Their utility has also been demonstrated for patients with panic disorder and agoraphobia.

Pretreatment evaluation Patients should be given a complete physical examination. A careful history should cover a review of other medications currently prescribed, evidence of substance abuse, prior treatment for depression, and cardiac status.

Guidelines for prescribing TCAs As with other drugs, treatment failures are not uncommonly due to the use of insufficient doses for inadequate periods of time. Imipramine and amitriptyline are the two most commonly prescribed TCAs. Initial doses of 50 mg in a single evening dose may be increased every four days to a ceiling of 300 mg. Dosage increments should be halted at the point of major improvement even if this occurs at a lower dose level. Some patients can only tolerate incremental raises of 50 mg per week. We have found that for such patients, a slower rate of increase can attain higher eventual dose levels than would be the case if a more rapid dose increase were attempted.

The ceiling level we suggest is higher than the maximum of 200 mg of imipramine per day for outpatients listed in the *Physicians' Desk*

Reference[21] or *The Pharmacological Basis of Therapeutics,*[22] but there is no evidence to show that outpatients require lower doses. Higher levels are often effective for patients who do not respond to lower doses.

Acute and continuation treatment As a rule, treatment with TCAs consists of two phases: acute and continuation. In addition, prophylactic treatment sometimes is indicated. In the acute phase, when the patient is actively symptomatic, medication is prescribed in the doses cited for a minimum of five weeks before it is concluded that the drug is ineffective. Some evidence suggests that amitriptyline is a useful sedative and may be preferable for older patients. After substantial improvement is achieved, medication is usually continued for six months at about half the acute dose level. The rationale is that medication suppresses but does not cure the symptoms, and that the underlying pathophysiology lasts for about this length of time. Patients who are asymptomatic can be seen infrequently during this treatment phase. After six months, a continuation regimen is considered to become prophylactic. Although we believe that all patients should receive continuation treatment, prophylaxis is indicated only for those with a short cycle length, history of frequent relapse, or previous serious suicide attempts. Lithium rather than TCAs is usually used prophylactically.

Patients for Whom TCAs Are the Treatment of Choice

In standard psychopharmacology textbooks, TCAs are recommended as the treatment of choice for severely depressed patients with endogenous symptoms. Almost all of the controlled clinical trials demonstrating the superior efficacy of TCAs over placebo were conducted with such patients. These patients would have met RDC and DSM-III criteria for major depressive disorder, endogenous (or melancholic) subtype. The major features of the clinical picture are persistent dysphoric mood or pervasive loss of interest or pleasure, accompanied by impairment in daily functioning and symptoms of the depressive syndrome. These include diurnal variation with mood worse in the morning, middle insomnia or early morning awakening, poor appetite, weight loss, and psychomotor agitation or retardation. Other symptoms characteristic of major depression are impaired concentration, loss of energy, and recurrent thoughts of death. According to DSM-III criteria, but not the RDC, lack of reactivity to environmental change ("mood autonomy") must be present to warrant the diagnosis of endogenous or "melancholic" major depression.

Patients with major depressive disorder who are good candidates for TCAs may have either unipolar or bipolar affective disorder. The illness episode need not be precipitated by an identifiable stressor, nor is the presence of psychotic symptomatology necessary. This diagnostic category overlaps with the concept of vital depression, with the "endogenomorphic" depression of Klein et al,[17] and with the notion of vegetative symptoms. All of these labels refer to patients who have a clear-cut phasic illness, who are quite severely depressed, who show behavioral as well as mood alterations, and who are in general responsive to TCA treatment.

MONOAMINE OXIDASE INHIBITORS

History and Description

MAOIs include a heterogeneous group of drugs having in common the ability to block oxidation of monoamines in the brain and various organs. Iproniazid was the first MAOI marketed for the treatment of depression. It was originally developed for the treatment of tuberculosis, and a mood-elevating effect was observed fortuitously. In the 1950s it was found to inhibit the enzyme MAO. In 1957 it was applied in psychiatry to treat depressed patients. Other MAOIs were developed, but because of their toxicity, several (including iproniazid) were withdrawn from the market. At present, two are widely sold in the United States: phenelzine and tranylcypromine. A third, isocarboxazid, is also available. Pargyline is approved only as an antihypertensive.

There seem to be at least two types of MAO enzyme and the three drugs in clinical use inhibit both of them. Several selective MAOIs, including deprenyl and clorgyline, are investigational drugs now being assessed for clinical efficacy. They are not yet approved by the FDA for the treatment of depression. If they are established as safe and effective, they may be preferable to the nonselective MAOIs since they cause fewer side effects.

Risks and Risk Management

The use of the first MAOI, iproniazid, was often complicated by liver toxicity, and the drug was withdrawn from the market. Modifications were introduced, resulting in the development of phenelzine. The other widely used MAOI, tranylcypromine, initially was associated with several hypertensive fatalities and also was withdrawn. Once it was learned that dietary restriction of tyramine successfully prevents the development of hypertensive crises, the drug was reintroduced and is now considered safe as long as a tyramine-free diet is maintained. At present, all patients who take MAOIs must follow a tyramine-free diet throughout the duration of this treatment. In addition, they should be taught to recognize early signs of hypertensive crisis such as sudden onset of severe hypertension with palpitations, chest pain, sweating, headache, and related signs. If such symptoms occur, patients are instructed to get immediate medical attention, at an emergency room if necessary. Treatment of hypertensive crises depends on the height of the blood pressure. Blood pressure above 170/110 should be treated with either intravenous phentolamine or intramuscular chlorpromazine.

Apart from precipitation of hypertensive crises associated with dietary violations, which are best dealt with prophylactically, other side effects of MAOIs include dizziness, orthostatic hypotension, headache, and sometimes impaired sexual function. Weight gain is a fairly common complaint. As Blackwell[23] noted in a comprehensive review of antidepressant adverse effects, "Apart from their interaction with foods and other drugs, the MAOIs have relatively fewer specific side effects and appear somewhat safer in overdose than the tricyclic antidepressants" (p. 206). He cautioned, however, that no good epidemiologic data are available to provide equivalent rates for the two drug classes.

MAOIs interfere with various enzymes in addition to MAO, thereby intensifying the effects of other drugs taken simultaneously. This is particularly dangerous in relation to central depressants such as general anesthetics and analgesics. These drugs should be avoided whenever possible in patients receiving MAOIs. Other drugs such as sedatives, antihistamines, and alcohol should be used cautiously. A good rule of thumb is to use half the dose of these drugs. Accordingly, patients treated with MAOIs must be warned against the use of concomitant medication without explicit clearance by their treating physician. Certain drugs routinely used by patients should be reviewed before the initiation of treatment with MAOIs and approved or disapproved. For example, low doses of antihistamine can be used by patients with allergies, but sympathomimetics cannot be. Patients who are not reliable, conscientious, or who for some other reason may not meticulously follow dietary, drug, and alcohol restrictions, are not good candidates for MAOI treatment. Before dental procedures, the type of anesthesia should be reviewed. Local anesthetics are safe; sympathomimetics are not. Frequently, epinephrine is combined with local analgesics, and the combination is dangerous for patients on MAOIs. In addition, some authorities[22] do not recommend their use by patients with cardiac disease or hypotension or who are over age 60, although the grounds for these judgments are not clear and they can only be considered relative contraindications.

Treatment Applications

Pretreatment evaluation A complete physical examination and psychiatric and medical history are necessary. Patients currently receiving antihypertensive medication are not suitable candidates. Other criteria for exclusion on medical grounds follow from the drug interaction risks noted above.

Patients with severe allergies for whom adrenalin may be required in emergency situations constitute another risk category. The issue is complicated because the interaction of MAOI and direct and indirect actions of sympathomimetics differs. Elis and associates[24] suggest that the chief function of MAOIs at adrenergic nerve endings is to metabolize norepinephrine that escapes reentry into the granules. The major mechanism for disposing of norepinephrine released as a neurotransmitter is limited by reuptake and metabolism by catechol-O-methyltransferase. Therefore, an MAOI should not interfere with the usual mechanisms for disposing of released norepinephrine if these amounts are not increased. This prediction has been confirmed by Boakes and associates,[25] who found that a direct-acting sympathomimetic such as norepinephrine was not potentiated by phenelzine, but indirect-acting sympathomimetics such as phenylephrine were.

Asthma is probably the most common condition in which there is a potential toxic interaction between MAOIs and sympathomimetic agents. In such cases, the risk can be avoided by treating the asthma with agents which are not sympathomimetic, such as aminophylline. For other allergic conditions where direct-acting sympathomimetics such as norepinephrine or epinephrine might be life saving, the alternatives are not as obvious. Available evidence suggests that such agents given intravenously should not be potentiated by MAOIs. However, puzzling inconsistencies still exist concerning the method of action of hypertensive crises. We therefore think that there should be extremely potent indications for prescribing MAOIs in patients who might have to resort to the use of sympathomimetic agents in the event of an emergency.

Prescription of MAOIs The usual starting dose of phenelzine is 15 mg daily, gradually increasing every three or four days until a maximum of 90 mg daily is reached, unless a therapeutic response is achieved or toxic side effects occur at a lower level. Some clinicians use a starting dose of 45 mg daily. Tranylcypromine is prescribed in similar graduated fashion, beginning with 10 mg daily and increasing to 40–60 mg. A six-week trial is considered adequate if the maximum dose level has been given for at least 10 days. The antidepressant effect may take two to three weeks to become apparent once a therapeutic dose level is reached.

Choice of MAOI Phenelzine is sometimes preferred, since some clinical reports suggest it is less toxic. One the other hand, some anecdotal evidence suggests that phenelzine is more likely than tranylcypromine to cause weight gain and may thus be unacceptable to some patients. If a patient is taking phenelzine and a change to tranylcypromine is contemplated, a washout period of one week is necessary to prevent negative interactions.

Management of Side Effects

In addition to the rare and medically serious risk of hypertensive crisis associated with tyramine ingestion discussed above, patients often experience nonserious but subjectively distressing side effects of MAOI. These require judicious management to maintain the patient on medication. In general, distressing side effects are handled by one or more of the following methods: education and reassurance, increased surveillance, lowering of dose, change of dose schedule, ancillary medication, and ultimately drug discontinuation. We will briefly refer to remedies for the side effects often reported, and refer the reader to the excellent paper of Sheehan et al[26] for a more comprehensive review.

Common troubling side effects of MAOIs are orthostatic hypotension, sleep disturbances, anorgasmia, and weight gain. Orthostatic hypotension, also commonly associated with TCAs, can be addressed by reassurance, advice to avoid sudden postural changes, and use of surgical elastic stockings. If these conservative measures are insufficient, fludrocortisone, a mineral corticoid, may be used adjunctively at 0.1 mg one to three times a day. Since this drug itself can cause major side effects, the patient's serum potassium levels should be checked regularly, and he or she should be advised to drink orange juice regularly. In many cases, the severity of orthostatic hypotension gradually diminishes over time.

Sleep disturbance usually consists of shortened nocturnal sleep time. When this causes distress, adjunctive, short-acting hypnotic benzodiazepines such as lorazepam and alprazolam may be prescribed.

Weight gain can be controlled by restriction of caloric intake, although this prescription is not always effective. Sexual dysfunctions are not easily altered; the best one can do is offer reassurance and note that these side effects sometimes go away over time. If the patient finds these or other side effects unacceptable, a change to another MAOI may be helpful. In our clinical experience, for example, weight gain is less commonly observed with tranylcypromine.

Continuation treatment The same rationale and procedures described with respect to TCAs apply here. Six months of continuation treatment is considered standard.

Patients for Whom MAOIs May Be the Treatment of Choice

In the past, TCAs were routinely prescribed as the treatment of choice for all patients with depressive symptoms, and MAOIs were prescribed as the second step after nonresponse to TCAs of different kinds. In the last several years, however, MAOIs have become more widely used in clinical practice as fears about adverse reactions have been allayed by cumulative favorable research and clinical reports. Equally important for this change in prescribing practice is increasing recognition that MAOIs may be more effective than TCAs for a particular subtype of depressed patient whose illness has been described variously as "neurotic" or "atypical" depression.

Atypical depression is a term first used by British investigators in the late 1950s or early 1960s to refer to patients without endogenous symptoms. The term has been extended and refined by our group to refer to patients whose symptoms meet RDC criteria for major, minor, or intermittent depressive disorder and who have the essential or core characteristic of mood reactivity. This refers to temporary improvement in mood, ideation, or interest or pleasure associated with positive environmental events and is the converse of mood autonomy associated with endogenicity. In this context we have found it useful to differentiate between two general categories: anticipatory pleasure and consummatory pleasure. The former refers to mood associated with a planned future event (eg, having dinner in a fine restaurant), whereas the latter refers to the experience of the event itself (actually eating the good food). Patients with endogenous depression lose the capacity for both anticipatory and consummatory pleasure; their mood remains autonomous and unrelated to environmental events. In contrast, only the ability to anticipate pleasure is impaired in atypical patients. Although they have a generally apathetic, uninterested approach to impending events, they do retain the capacity to enjoy the events themselves when they actually occur. Thus, a patient with atypical depressive disorder may try to avoid and resist participation in formerly pleasurable events such as attending a party, but if others insist that he go, he will enjoy himself during the event even though the effect is transient. We find this distinction between anticipatory and consummatory pleasures effective in identifying patients with atypical depressive disorder who are likely to respond to MAOI treatment.

Associated features of atypical depression include oversleeping, increased appetite and overeating, loss of energy to the extent that the patient perceives a sense of leaden paralysis, and pathological rejection sensitivity. This term refers to the distress engendered by perceived or actual rebuff by other people, especially in the context of a romantic relationship. Atypical depressed patients resemble those referred to as neurotic depressives. They are often described as anxious and emotionally expressive and sometimes have hysterical features. The syndrome of hysteroid dysphoria described by Klein et al[17] is a subtype of atypical depressive disorder.

In the Depression Evaluation Service of New York State Psychiatric Institute, we are currently conducting a double-blind, randomized clinical trial of imipramine, phenelzine, and placebo with patients who have atypical depressive disorder. Preliminary results based on the first

50 patients who have completed the study indicate a statistically significant preferential response to phenelzine over placebo, whereas there is no difference in rate of response to imipramine compared with placebo. If these results continue to hold up, this will be the first clear-cut demonstration of the superior efficacy of phenelzine over imipramine for a subtype of depressive patients. These data will provide justification for increased use of MAOIs in clinical practice for atypical depressive patients, who have been estimated to comprise about 30% of depressed outpatients and who are not notably responsive to TCAs.

ELECTROCONVULSIVE THERAPY

History and Description

Convulsive therapy was first developed as a treatment for mental disorders in 1934 by the Hungarian, L. Meduna. It was modified to use electricity for induction by the Italians, Cerletti and Bini, and by 1939 was accepted in the United States. Initially used as a treatment for schizophrenia, its apparent efficacy led to trials with almost all types of psychiatric disorder. Over time, its effectiveness for depression became widely recognized, whereas for schizophrenia the results came to be seen as less compelling. At present, severe depressive disorder, almost regardless of subtype, is the principal indication for ECT.[27]

When first introduced, ECT was associated with many medical complications including fractures, cyanosis, panic, and cardiovascular problems. During the 1940s, refinements were introduced to ameliorate these effects. Barbiturate premedication, anesthesia, hyperoxygenation, and muscle relaxants greatly improved the safety of the procedure so that these complications are now very rare. The popularity and use of ECT declined with introduction of psychotropic drugs in the 1950s, and many ECT facilities were closed. By the mid-1970s, however, as the limitations of antidepressants became recognized, interest in ECT revived.[28] At the same time, both public and professional concern about patients' rights, safety, and efficacy led to the establishment of commissions, conferences, legislative regulation, and increased interest in well-designed research. Investigators are now seeking to assess the comparative efficacy of ECT and to develop procedural modifications and improved techniques to augment its safety and to clarify indications for its use.

Today's modified ECT consists of a series of treatments, usually scheduled two or three times a week for a total of six to ten treatments for depressed patients.[29] In each treatment, a major seizure lasting at least 25 seconds is induced by passage of an electrical current between two electrodes situated either bilaterally (bitemporally) or, less commonly, both on the same side as the dominant hand. According to current safety standards, an anesthetic agent, muscle relaxant, and oxygen supplementation are introduced before seizure induction. To assure efficacy, muscle convulsive activity or electroencephalographic monitoring should be used to ascertain that a therapeutically adequate seizure has been induced.

During the course of treatment, patients may manifest an organic brain syndrome, are hesitant and slowed in response, and have problems in speech and memory. These characteristic transient accompaniments to ECT are seen even in optimal treatment conditions.

Risks and Risk Management

With the use of modified ECT, measurable long-term complications are relatively infrequent; adverse reactions are usually limited to transient impairment of memory and new learning ability. Deaths resulting from ECT are very rare and are far outnumbered by suicides among treatment-refractory or untreated depressed patients who do not receive ECT.[17] Minor side effects such as postseizure confusion and headaches and skin burns at electrode sites are not uncommon.

A major source of risk in unanesthetized patients, now rare, is the phenomenon called a "missed" or "incomplete" seizure in which a current passes between the scalp electrodes without inducing a seizure and its associated amnesia. Patients consequently experience pain, panic, fear, and are often unwilling to continue treatment. The use of anesthesia is an effective prophylactic for this complication. In anesthetized patients, a missed or incomplete seizure may occur and may go unrecognized unless the seizure is monitored. When recognized, the treatment should be repeated.

Transient recent memory loss is a routine consequence of bilateral ECT, although far less common with right unilateral electrode placement. Those memories acquired during the days preceding a course of ECT may be lost permanently, but others are recovered, usually within a few weeks. Some patients complain about their memory months and even years later, but pretreatment measures are not available to show that the ECT was the cause.[30] Although investigators have not observed permanent cognitive deficits after ECT, it is conceivable that subtle brain damage may occur, but it is impossible to prove a negative of this sort. Other physiological effects of ECT, such as electroencephalograph changes, redundancy in speech, and changes in language use and performances of psychomotor tasks, improve gradually after the last treatment and are substantially normal after six months.[29]

The risk for long-lasting or permanent impairment of memory and other cognitive functions increases with extended use of ECT. Patients who have received more than 50 treatments have been found to show long-term memory loss and other cognitive impairments. It is difficult to attribute these deficits specifically to ECT, however, since these patients are ill for longer periods, are more severely ill than patients who did not get as much ECT, are refractory to other treatments, and in many cases have received cingulotomy as well as ECT.

Risk of memory loss can be reduced by use of unilateral ECT. Although controlled studies have not found significant differences in clinical response to unilateral and bilateral ECT, some authorities (eg, Kalinowsky) regard the unilateral procedure as less effective and suggest that more treatments may be necessary to achieve equivalent clinical results.[31]

Spontaneous seizure activity after ECT occasionally has been reported, with an estimated prevalence of 0.5%; this is similar to that of the general population. It is difficult to reconcile the notion that ECT lowers the cerebral threshold for an epileptic focus with the observations that progressively more current is often needed to induce ECT seizures during the course of treatment. A causal relationship between ECT and subsequent seizures has not been demonstrated.

In general, risk management consists of keeping the number and length of treatments to the minimum necessary for clinical improvement. The American Psychiatric Association (APA) Task Force on ECT recommends that no more than 15 ECT treatments be given to depressed patients in a given series, and that "care, judgment and restraint be exercised before prescribing a second course of ECT within a 12-month period."[29] Another approach to risk management is further refinement of current techniques such as use of pulsed rather than continuous current. More controlled studies of the relationship between treatment intensity, duration and efficacy are needed.

Informed consent ECT is widely known and often feared by members of the general public, including patients and their families. For clinical, ethical, and legal reasons, patients and their relatives should be told about the treatment course in some detail. This discussion should include the nature and severity of the patient's illness; a description of the procedure; the nature, degree, duration, and probability of side effects; reasonable alternative treatments and why ECT is being recommended instead; the cost; and the right of the patient to refuse treatment or discontinue it at any time. The APA Task Force recommends that the patient and/or close relative or guardian sign a consent form for the procedure in which the duration of the treatment course is specified.

Treatment Applications

Pretreatment evaluation Medical and psychiatric histories should be obtained, and patients should be given a complete physical examination with laboratory tests as indicated. The histories should include previous response to anesthesia, orthopedic disease, head trauma, indications of organic brain syndrome, and prior ECT treatments (including the dates). The physical examination should include special attention to cardiovascular, neurologic, and orthopedic disorders and the presence of dentures. The major risk is cardiovascular, both from the anesthesia and the seizure itself. Laboratory procedures often include x-rays, which are useful to demonstrate radiographic abnormalities manifested before the proposed ECT.

Guidelines for prescription Once a decision has been reached to use ECT, the major issues concern the choice of bilateral or unilateral electrode placement, the number of treatments to administer, whether outpatient treatment should be undertaken, and subsequent management. Proponents of bilateral treatment such as Abrams and Kalinowsky[31] argue that unilateral electrode placement is less effective and that more treatments may be required which increase the dangers and cost more money. The APA Task Force on ECT, on the other hand, favors the use of unilateral treatment, as its members have been persuaded of its therapeutic equivalence to bilateral treatment and the clear advantages in causing far less memory loss and confusion. For most patients, other things being equal, unilateral treatment is considered the preferable strategy.[32] Further research is under way to resolve this question.

The number of treatments depends both on the patient's age and clinical response. The guidelines established by the APA Task Force, noted above, are recommended.[29] With respect to site of treatment, hospitalization is sometimes indicated, although for patients with available family members to look after them and a history of successful prior ECT, outpatient treatment is feasible.

Maintenance therapy with antidepressant medication is usually prescribed for six months after ECT to prevent recurrence of depression.[17] Some authorities regard this as a reason not to use ECT for any but medication-refractory patients. Otherwise, it may be argued, the patient will be getting two treatments with different sets of potentially serious side effects, doubling their exposure to risk. Other authorities do not regard this as a valid reason to withhold ECT, especially for severely depressed and delusional patients.

Patients for Whom ECT Is Indicated

As noted, severe depressive disorder is the principal indication for ECT. As noted by Baldessarini,[22] "ECT remains the most rapid and effective treatment for severe acute depression and is sometimes lifesaving for acutely suicidal patients." Efficacy is believed greatest for patients with the most extreme depressions and greatest number of symptoms, particularly those referred to as endogenous (nonresponsivity of mood, terminal insomnia, and weight loss). Another indicator for ECT as the first treatment to be considered is a prior history of good response to ECT, assuming that there has been no organic deterioration in the interval since such treatment.

In customary practice, ECT is considered when severely depressed patients are refractory to or cannot tolerate the side effects of antidepressant medication. After adequate trials of TCAs and MAOIs, to which the patient fails to respond, a course of ECT is indicated. At present, there is no consensus about whether to introduce additional pharmacological strategies such as combined MAOI-TCA treatment before ECT is scheduled. Our own preference is to institute ECT for severely ill endogenous patients at this point. For patients with features of atypical depression, pronounced anxiety, and panic attacks, we recommend a trial of combined treatment before ECT.

Neither age nor medical condition is necessarily a contraindication for ECT. In fact, ECT is particularly useful for older patients without preexisting organic impairment whose cardiac status mitigates against use of TCAs. ECT may also be preferred to psychotropic drugs for depressed patients with cardiovascular disease, recent myocardial infarction, renal disease, or recent surgery.[27]

Patients with prominent "neurotic" and anxiety symptoms do not respond well to ECT. Diagnostic contraindications include the categories of anxiety, factitious, somatoform, dissociative, and adjustment disorders, and those of impulse control. Patients with somatoform disorders are particularly unsuitable for ECT.

NONSTANDARD TREATMENTS FOR REFRACTORY PATIENTS

A certain number of endogenous patients fail to improve after a trial of TCAs lasting five to six weeks at an adequate dose level. There are also patients with atypical depression who do not improve with MAOIs or for whom the effect is transient. Some show signs of partial response, whereas others are completely refractory. In such cases, it should first be ascertained by detailed questioning of the patient as well as family members that the prescribed number of pills were taken the specified number of times daily. If medication compliance is confirmed, the clinician may find it useful to review the diagnosis and physical status of the refractory patients. Various medical disorders such as thyroid disease may masquerade as depressive illness. Hall's[33] recent work in this area has led to identification of at least 25 diseases which may cause or appear as depression (see Table 3-1). In addition, concurrent medications should be reviewed to make sure that the patient is not taking a drug for another disorder or condition such as antihypertensive medication or birth control pills that may contribute to the depression. Finally, relatives should be asked about affective changes and improved functional capacity since some patients fail to mention improvements that do in fact occur.

Table 3-1
Medical Illnesses That Frequently Induce Depression[33]

Pernicious anemia	Hyperaldosteronism
Folic acid deficiency	Addison's disease
Multiple sclerosis	Hyperparathyroidism
Influenza	Hypoparathyroidism
Viral hepatitis	Hyperthyroidism
Cirrhosis	Hypothyroidism
Uremia	Acromegaly
Disseminate carcinomatosis	Systemic lupus erythematosus
Oat-cell carcinoma of the lung	Ulcerative colitis
Lymphomas	Regional enteritis
Chronic myelogenous leukemia	Whipple's disease
Carcinoma of the pancreas	Amyloidosis
Cushing's disease	

Another recommended step is to determine drug plasma level if the patient is taking TCA. Although evidence for a direct corespondence between drug plasma level and clinical outcome has not been established decisively, a number of studies of imipramine plasma levels have shown such an association.[17] In view of the considerable variation in metabolism rates of drugs, plasma levels may fall below that associated with therapeutic efficacy even if the patient is taking 250 or 300 mg of TCAs per day. Available data suggest a linear relationship between drug plasma level and efficacy for imipramine, with best results associated with plasma levels over 300 ng/mL. With nortriptyline, there is some evidence of a therapeutic window, where dose levels can be either too high or too low to achieve a therapeutic effect.

Plasma levels for MAOIs have not yet been established. Several studies suggest a relationship between degree of platelet MAO inhibition and clinical response to MAOIs. The greater the amount of platelet MAO inhibition, the more likely it is to find a drug response. MAO inhibition of 80% is suggested as the lower limit for the achievement of therapeutic response to phenelzine; other drugs have not yet been studied. When further research has been conducted, measures of platelet MAO inhibition may serve a function equivalent to that of TCA plasma level measurement: to monitor drug compliance and to guide dose adjustment in the rare patient who has received the usual maximum dose and is showing only slight benefits. At present, the method is not recommended for routine clinical practice.

Some patients remain partially or completely unresponsive to adequate drug trials of standard medications. Others experience severe or distressing side effects at low doses so that the dose cannot be increased enough to achieve a therapeutic effect. In all of these cases, other treatment strategies should be instituted. In selecting the next step, we consider whether the patient has been partially or completely refractory to the first treatment, whether his depression is severe and incapacitating, and whether he has unipolar or bipolar affective disorder. The implications of each of these determinations is reviewed in turn (Figure 3-1). We wish to emphasize that this sequence is not intended as a fixed hierarchy. At present, not enough is known to make such specific recommendations. Instead, we present alternatives with the expectation that the practitioner will decide on sequence.

Figure 3-1 Alternative treatment strategies for partial or transient responders.

*TCA Partial Responders**
1. High dose
2. (Another TCA)
3. Amphetamine supplement
4. Thyroid supplement
5. Lithium supplement

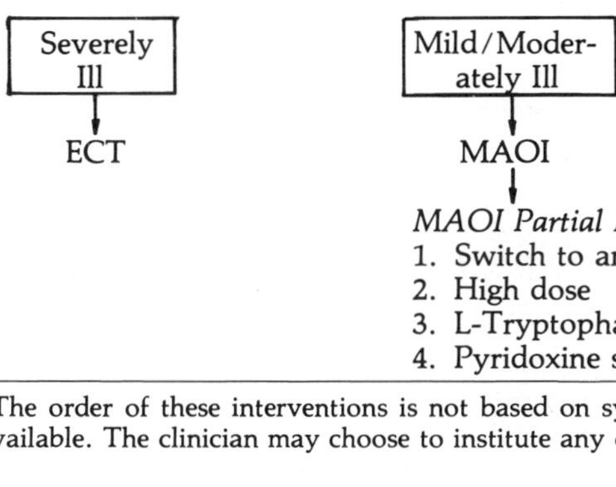

MAOI Partial Responders
1. Switch to another MAOI
2. High dose
3. L-Tryptophan supplement
4. Pyridoxine supplement

*The order of these interventions is not based on systematic evidence since none is yet available. The clinician may choose to institute any of these treatments.

Partial Responders to TCAs

No systematic research has been designed to compare alternative strategies for patients who show mild but not significant signs of improvement after medication trials of up to 300 mg of TCAs per day. Clinical experience points to several possibilities, including high doses of standard antidepressants, trials of another TCA, or the addition of another drug that may potentiate the antidepressant effect of the standard drug. As we have noted, no research evidence exists regarding the order in which these strategies should be tried; it remains a matter of individual preference at this time. We do wish to note, however, that we have seldom seen any of them lead to clinical improvement *after* two weeks if improvement is not apparent within that time. Accordingly, we suggest a maximum of two weeks' trial for each, or less as noted in the following discussions.

High doses Some patients who show only partial response to 300 mg of TCAs per day do very well on doses of 350 to 450 mg/day. Before prescribing these high doses, it is essential to ascertain that the patient has neither heart block nor serious orthostatic hypotension. Serial electrocardiograms are recommended at approximately weekly intervals. This is an arbitrary estimate since there are no standard guidelines. For elderly patients and those with significant side effects, they probably should be done more frequently. If patients do not respond within two weeks to doses of 450 mg of imipramine or the equivalent, the trial should be discontinued and another strategy should be employed.

Change to another TCA For patients only partially responsive to an adequate trial of a TCA, the usual procedure has been to switch to another TCA with the most dissimilar mode of action. That is, if the first drug is a serotonin-reuptake blocker (eg, imipramine, amitriptyline), the second would be a norepinephrine-reuptake blocker (desmethylimipramine, nortriptyline). This sequence is recommended in standard texts about treatment procedure such as those of Shopsin and Waters,[34] Berger,[35] and Baldessarini.[22] This strategy is based on the deductive belief that there are two different kinds of depression related to deficits in brain serotonin or norepinephrine rather than on the outcome of controlled clinical trials.

Over time, it has been our experience and that of others such as Ayd[36] that a more effective strategy for the patient who fails to respond to an adequate trial of a TCA is to forego trials of other TCAs and instead follow one of the treatment options described below. We have found that, beyond extending treatment for an additional six weeks, another TCA trial has less likelihood of efficacy than the use of an adjunctive drug supplement or change of drug class. There are exceptions to this policy of not trying a second TCA. For example, if treatment nonresponse is attributable to either noncompliance because of intolerable side effects, another TCA without those particular objectionable side effects (eg, sedation) may be appropriately substituted. Similarly, if the dose cannot be raised to a therapeutic level because of side effects, another TCA may be more suitable. In other cases, we proceed with one of the options presented below.

Amphetamine supplement to TCAs For a long time it has been recognized that amphetamines alleviate some dysphoric moods, and indeed a number of patients with chronic or recurrent depression report a prior history of amphetamine use and, occasionally, abuse. Since amphetamine is less effective than standard antidepressants and has addictive potential, it is not generally prescribed for depression as a first strategy. However, it has been observed that in addition to a TCA an adjunctive dose of 5 to 20 mg of amphetamine per day can convert a partial response to a complete response. Used in this way, one may begin with a daily dose of 5 mg which can be adjusted up to 20 mg during the next week. If no effect is achieved within 10 days, the trial should be discontinued. If it is successful, we recommend that it be prescribed at a fixed dose for four to six weeks and then slowly withdrawn. If symptoms recur, the ancillary medication can be reinstituted for another four to six weeks.

Thyroid supplement to TCA Research evidence is limited but supports the utility of L-triiodothyronine (T_3) supplements to standard antidepressants for those patients who do not respond satisfactorily to the antidepressant alone. Five uncontrolled studies found that between 64% and 90% of patients unresponsive to TCAs did respond after supplemental T_3 administration. Most recently, Goodwin and colleagues[37] assessed the efficacy of T_3 supplements in 12 patients who responded minimally or not at all to trials of imipramine or amitriptyline and whose TCA blood levels were all in the range considered therapeutic. After the addition of 25 μg/day (10 patients) or 50 μg/day (2 patients), two-thirds showed a marked improvement and one other patient showed mild improvement. This improvement generally began within three days; side effects were minimal. The authors concluded that "a trial of tricyclic antidepressant in a depressed patient should not be considered a failure until T_3 potentiation has been tried."

These research findings, together with clinical experience, suggest the utility of adding a thyroid supplement (T_3) to a TCA in patients who show only a minimal clinical response to the TCA alone. Doses of 25 to 40 μg/day should be added to the daily TCA regimen of 300 mg. As in the case of adjunctive amphetamine, a 10-day trial is recommended. If effective, it should be continued for four to six weeks.

Lithium supplement to TCA If the foregoing high-dose strategy and supplements have not proved beneficial, another option would be to add a supplement of lithium to 300 mg of TCA. This is a new treatment strategy developed by de Montigny and associates.[38] It is based on the observation in animal studies that short-term lithium treatment increases the efficacy of the serotonin system. In patients, lithium would be expected to increase the sensitization of serotonin receptors and thus enhance antidepressant response.[36]

de Montigny has reported using 900 mg of lithium per day added to the daily dose of TCA to which the patient failed to respond after three weeks of treatment. Within 24 hours, all eight patients studied reported a marked alleviation of symptoms and sustained this improvement as long as lithium was taken during a three- to nine-month followup. Although this method has been used with only a small number of patients, it is worth mentioning because it appears to be safe, low risk, and fast as well as possibly effective. Common clinical experience, however, has not so far borne out the early enthusiastic reports. In any case, if a lithium supplement is prescribed, results should occur within a few days. If improvement is not observed by then, another treatment strategy is recommended.

If at this point a patient has shown only partial response to a TCA and to all of the appropriate additional treatment strategies noted, we would assess the current severity of his or her clinical condition. If the patient is still severely depressed, we recommend ECT. If the patient is mildly or moderately ill, we initiate a trial of MAOI, as described above.

Partial Responders to MAOIs

The following discussion concerns alternative strategies for patients whose response to MAOI is either partial or temporary.

Switch to another MAOI This is recommended if the side effects of one MAOI are unacceptable to the patient. For example, phenelzine may be experienced as too sedating or may cause dramatic weight gain in some patients who find tranylcypromine less objectionable in these respects.

High doses For partial responders whose side effects are not severe, we consider raising the dose of phenelzine as high as 120 mg/day or of tranylcypromine to 75 mg/day. The risks and benefits of this dose schedule have not been assessed in randomized clinical trials, nor is there an extensive clinical literature regarding the efficacy of this procedure.

L-Tryptophan supplement to MAOI L-Tryptophan, a naturally occurring amino acid, is the immediate precursor to 5-hydroxytryptophan (5HTP), which is converted to serotonin (5HT). Scientists have reasoned that, since depression is believed related to insufficient amounts of 5HT in the hypothalamus, the disorder might be ameliorated by supplying additional amounts of the precursor amine from which it is derived. Presumably, this will increase the concentration of neurotransmitter at the postsynaptic receptor.

Based on this thinking, L-tryptophan alone or in conjunction with antidepressants has been studied by several groups of investigators as a therapeutic agent.[39] The results are not entirely consistent and furnish suggestive but not conclusive evidence that L-tryptophan is a useful adjunctive treatment. It seems to enhance the efficacy of MAOIs,[40] but not TCAs, with the apparent exception of clomipramine, which itself is an especially potent inhibitor of serotonin reuptake.[41]

L-Tryptophan is hydroxylated to 5HTP before being converted to 5HT. 5HTP does cross the blood-brain barrier, but 5HT does not. Thus, 5HTP has been used as a precursor load. A preliminary study by Van Hiele[42] suggests that 5HTP may be used as an adjunct in patients unresponsive to antidepressants alone. Further studies of the use of 5HTP in refractory patients are needed. Neither tryptophan nor 5HTP is approved by the FDA, and patients should be so informed.

Although L-tryptophan has the appeal of being a "natural" remedy, it can cause disagreeable side effects, including nausea and drowsiness. It is clearly in need of further systematic assessment, but the available evidence suggests that it may be useful in combination with an MAOI for patients with only partial response to MAOI alone.

Pyridoxine supplement to MAOI Several small studies reviewed by Klein et al[17] found that women taking oral contraceptives who reported depression benefited from pyridoxine. Furthermore, depressed patients have been found, in preliminary studies, to have lower pyridoxine levels than normal controls. Among depressed patients, those with evidence of vitamin B_6 deficiency have a particularly good response to a therapeutic trial of pyridoxine. Although this is still an unproven therapeutic strategy, it appears to be without risk. We suggest that patients with only partial response to MAOI who have low B_6 levels be given an adjunctive trial of pyridoxine.

Refractory Patients

If these techniques fail to elicit an adequate treatment response, there remain three options to be considered. For patients who are moderately or severely depressed, we recommend ECT, lithium, or combined TCA plus MAOI therapy. For mildly ill patients who have failed to respond to all of the foregoing methods, we recommend consideration of a nonsomatic therapy such as cognitive therapy or behavioral treatment (Figure 3-2).

Lithium For refractory bipolar patients or for refractory unipolar patients with a family history of bipolar illness, a trial of lithium is indicated. Lithium clearly has antidepressant effects (see literature review by Klein et al[17]). Although not yet approved for the treatment of depressive episodes by the FDA, lithium has been found effective in this context. It has the additional advantage of not precipitating a sudden switch to mania or hypomania as sometimes happens with TCAs. On the other hand, since the difference between the therapeutic and toxic range is so much narrower for lithium than for TCAs, lithium is not usually the first drug tried.

Before lithium is prescribed, it is necessary to assess the patient's thyroid and renal functioning.[43] In general, lithium is prescribed for

Figure 3-2 Patients refractory to both TCAs and MAOIs.

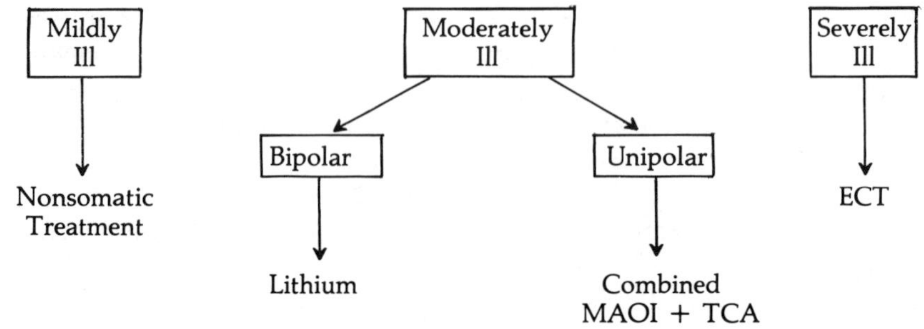

medically healthy adults and adolescents, although exceptions are made when circumstances warrant. Patients using diuretics or those with heart disease require special monitoring. However, these are merely relative contraindications.

When lithium is effective in the treatment of acute depression, standard practice is to continue medication at a lower dose for another six months. Because of the increased risk of mania from TCAs, it is sometimes recommended that lithium be used for continuation treatment of *all* bipolar patients even if TCAs were used to treat the acute episode.

Combined TCA-MAOI therapy The combined use of MAOIs and TCAs has been reported to be both highly toxic and highly effective. Publication of about 40 case reports, most appearing in the early 1960s, led to widespread concern about the hazards of this approach and probably serve as the basis for the current caution[21] against combined treatment because of safety considerations. According to Ayd,[44] however, during the last 20 years "several thousand" patients here and particularly in England have been treated with this method with good results. Accumulating evidence from three controlled studies and clinical experience suggests that the combination is both useful and feasible in limited situations with careful medical surveillance after nonresponse to other treatments.[45]

The risk of dangerous adverse reactions, including convulsions, cerebral hemorrhage, and death are greatest if a TCA is introduced *after* an MAOI already has been administered. For unknown reasons (perhaps the TCA blockage of tyramine uptake), simultaneous initiation beginning at very low doses of both drugs after a drug-free interval of at least one week is considerably less hazardous. In such combinations, imipramine, amitriptyline, or doxepin is recommended. Ayd[44] also described combined use of MAOI with maprotiline in about 10 patients with good results.

As a rule, combined treatment is reserved for patients who fail to respond to either drug separately and for whom ECT is either unsuccessful or unacceptable. Clinicians with limited psychopharmacological experience may choose to refrain from undertaking this form of treatment. We recommend starting with TCAs such as imipramine (50 mg/day) and after one or two days adding 15 mg of phenelzine. The dose of each drug is increased by 1 pill every two to three days until a maximum of 200 mg of imipramine and 60 mg of phenelzine is reached. Obviously, dose increments should be discontinued in patients who develop side effects.

Second-Generation Antidepressants

Since the introduction of imipramine nearly 25 years ago, many other antidepressants have been marketed here and abroad. To date, less than a dozen non-MAOI antidepressants have been approved by the FDA in the United States, whereas there are at least 40 available for prescription in England,[46] many of which are in various stages of clinical trials in this country.

With the exception of trimipramine, which was approved here in 1979, the "new" antidepressants are called second generation because they differ in chemical molecular structure from the standard TCAs, show differences in pharmacological profile, and vary widely in their mechanisms of action. Leonard[47] has suggested that antidepressants be considered "second generation" if they meet at least two of the following criteria: (1) introduction as antidepressants in the past decade, (2) greater selectivity of action on either the serotonergic or noradrenergic system than the TCAs, (3) few anticholinergic effects and less cardiotoxicity than TCAs, and (4) have a structure other than that of a derivative.

No new antidepressant surpasses the prototype imipramine in efficacy. Each is reported to offer one or more of the following advantages, as Ayd[46] has noted: more rapid onset of action, fewer anticholinergic side effects, less cardiotoxicity, less hazard in overdose, and greater compatibility with other medicines for coexisting medical or psychiatric disorders. We do not believe that all of these claims have been substantiated. We are particularly skeptical about claims of rapid onset of action. These characteristics, if in fact true, meaningfully widen the spectrum of patients whose depression could be treated effectively. As in the case of standard TCAs, the new antidepressants were tested with predominantly endogenous patient samples, and it is for these patients that they are characteristically recommended. Although none of the new drugs is a standard first-choice treatment for depression, each might be an appropriate choice for patients who do not respond to or cannot tolerate standard TCAs or may be selected in specific circumstances.

At present, there are more than 30 new antidepressants undergoing clinical trials, and other compounds have been identified as potential antidepressants. Quite certainly, options for the drug treatment of depression are increasing steadily; these new developments warrant careful study. In the following review, we have selected six drugs representative of the second-generation antidepressants. We note their origins and structure, probable mechanisms of action, and clinical and side effects when they differ from those of standard TCAs.

Trimipramine (Surmontil)

This drug is really not "second generation" since it is a tertiary TCA. However, it is new, since FDA approval was granted only in 1979, although it has been used clinically in other countries for 20 years.[46]

The absorption rate and metabolism of trimipramine closely resemble those of imipramine, as does its level of therapeutic efficacy and effective dose range. Side effects resemble those of other tertiary TCAs, are dose related, and decrease over time. Some investigators (eg, Rifkin et al[48]) report fewer adverse reactions in comparison with imipramine. Sedation is the most commonly reported side effect.

The most distinctive characteristic of trimipramine is the claim that, unlike other antidepressants, it does not alter sleep architecture or suppress REM sleep.

Amoxapine (Asendin)

A TCA variant, amoxapine closely resembles both loxapine and clozapine, two effective antipsychotics with very different pharmacologic and clinical effects. As described by Hollister,[49] amoxapine has many of the pharmacological properties of antidepressants, but retains some of the postsynaptic dopamine receptor-blocking action of antipsychotics.

Given in doses approximately double those of imipramine, amoxapine has been established as therapeutic both in comparison to placebo and standard TCAs and was approved for clinical use by the FDA in 1980. Its most conspicuous asset is the claim of early onset of action; it may begin to exert its antidepressant effect within four to seven days, and 80% of responders show significant improvement within two weeks. The FDA has approved a package insert bearing this statement. However, similar claims of more rapid onset of action, made with other antidepressants, have not been supported after they have had more extensive study and use. It remains to be seen whether in this case the claim is justifiable.

The side effects of amoxapine resemble those of imipramine and are predominantly anticholinergic. Their incidence and severity, like those of imipramine, are dose related, as are the toxic effects of overdose. Based on his review of clinical trial data, Ayd[50] suggests that anticholinergic and cardiotoxic effects may be fewer and less troublesome than those of standard TCAs.

In view of the fact that amoxapine is an analog to the antipsychotic loxapine, the question has been raised whether it has the clinical and pharmacological effects of an antipsychotic drug. Donlon,[51] reviewing the available evidence, concludes that neither point has been established. To date, incidence of extrapyramidal symptoms is reported less than 1% (although we have observed their occurrence). No adequate studies of the efficacy of amoxapine in psychotic depression have been published.

Maprotiline (Ludiomil)

Maprotiline is the only tetracyclic antidepressant currently marketed in the United States, having received FDA approval in 1980. It has been studied widely abroad since 1966 and has been marketed in most European countries for a considerable time period, so that it is scarcely a "new" drug, despite the recency of its FDA approval. In other countries, it has been administered to many thousands of patients.

Maprotiline is structurally more similar to the demethylated metabolites of imipramine and amitriptyline (desipramine and nortriptyline) than to the tertiary drugs themselves. As noted by Settle,[52] the most distinctive pharmacologic characteristic of maprotiline is its almost complete lack of effect on the serotonin systems. Its most obvious effect is in the inhibition of noradrenaline uptake in both peripheral and central neurones.

Maprotiline's therapeutic effect is comparable to that of imipramine, as is its dose range. Faster onset of action sometimes has been reported, but is not clearly established. Side effects, including anticholinergic side effects, are similar to those of other antidepressants, but may be less intense at comparable doses.[53] Most commonly reported are drowsiness and dry mouth. Drug rashes may occur more often than with other antidepressants, whereas evidence suggests that postural hypotension and tachycardia occur less frequently. Based on a critique of the clinical data, Ananth and Ayd[54] concluded that the drug is less toxic than most other antidepressants, has anxiolytic effects, and only minor anticholinergic and cardiovascular effects. Its compatibility with many other drugs makes it particularly useful for cardiac, geriatric, and medically ill depressed patients. Drawing contrary conclusions, Blackwell[55] states that "despite the structural and biochemical differences between maprotiline and the TCAs, its adverse effects are similar to and more serious than the older compounds and it possesses no clear advantages over them." He was particularly concerned about recent data released by the British Committee on Safety of Medicines revealing a disproportionate risk of seizures associated with maprotiline.

An interesting characteristic of maprotiline, shared with other second-generation antidepressants such as nomifensine and trazodone, is the general equivalence of oral and parenteral administration. It is well absorbed in either form and can be administered intravenously without serious side effects. This development has led to the increasing popularity of antidepressant infusion therapy in Europe, although there is no substantial evidence for its superiority. No intravenous formulations of this drug are available in the United States at this time.

Mianserin

Mianserin, like maprotiline, is a tetracyclic compound, although its geometric structure is rather different. It was synthesized in 1966 and has been marketed in Europe for a decade, but is not yet approved by the FDA at the time of this writing (November 1982).

The mechanism of action of mianserin remains unclear. It has little effect on the reuptake of either serotonin or norepinephrine, and has no central anticholinergic action. This distinctive pharmacology raises some interesting questions about the explanatory comprehensiveness of the biogenic amine theory of depression.[49]

Compared to both placebo and standard TCAs, mianserin has been shown clinically effective in acute treatment of both endogenous and reactive depression, in our own trials and those of others in this country and abroad. The drug's distinctive assets include a striking paucity of anticholinergic and cardiovascular side effects, compatibility with concomitant medications such as antihypertensives and other psychotropic drugs,[56] and a high ratio of therapeutic to toxic dose. It appears to lack cardiotoxic properties, even in cases of overdose. A study of 100 consecutive cases of mianserin overdose found that, when mianserin was taken alone, only mild symptoms developed.[57] These results suggest less toxicity than that of the standard TCAs. Feighner[53] refers to its "main side effects as being drowsiness, lethargy, and weight gain," but other investigators are impressed with the rarity of any side effects. Our own study of 150 patients leads us to agree with the latter view, although as Blackwell[55] notes, the question remains unresolved pending further data.

Trazodone (Desyrel)

Trazodone, a phenylpiperazine derivative, was approved by the FDA in 1982, although it has been used widely in Europe for many years. It has a unique molecular structure and is inactive in the standard laboratory tests for antidepressants. As Shopsin and colleagues[56] note, it does not antagonize reserpine, it does not potentiate levodopa, it is not an MAOI, and it displays no anticholinergic activity. Like other antidepressants, it does suppress REM sleep. It also shows some pharmacological properties of both antipsychotics and anxiolytics, while having characteristics which distinguish it from any of these drug classes.[58]

Neurochemically, trazodone's most potent effect is inhibition of synaptic serotonin reuptake. It also exhibits some peripheral alpha-adrenergic blocking.[53] It is devoid of any muscarinic receptor affinity, which accounts for the absence of anticholinergic side effects.

In numerous clinical trials here and in Europe, trazodone's efficacy has been found to be 60% to 70% with endogenous patients, comparable to that of standard antidepressants. Risch and Janowsky,[58] reviewing the available research data, conclude that trazodone appears effective in both endogenous and neurotic (anxious) depression. Gershon et al[59] participated in a 10-center study of endogenous patients and also found the drug effective. In addition to its antidepressant effects, trazodone has been used to treat anxiety states and alcohol withdrawal syndrome.

One of trazodone's distinctive assets is the low reported incidence of anticholinergic side effects. It also has a unique profile of cardiac effects that may make it useful for depressed patients with cardiac disease, not an uncommon combination among elderly patients. Although further study is needed to document this claim, it is said to be safer in overdose than standard TCAs. Trazodone does tend to cause significant sedation and drowsiness, which is a setback to utilization in certain cases. Other reported, if rare, side effects include an increased number of neurologic complaints: tingling, numbness, dizziness, and loss of balance. Shopsin et al[56] reported that "a subtle but rather unmistakable toxic-confusional state was consistently observed in most patients who were given trazodone" (p 229). This effect has not been reported by other senior investigators who have studied this drug such as Gershon, Davis, Rickels and Feighner. Overall, based on available evidence, the risk-benefit ratio of trazodone is sufficiently persuasive to warrant its clinical use.

The *Journal of Clinical Psychopharmacology* has published a 93-page supplement in November 1981 entirely devoted to studies of trazodone. Safety, efficacy, and pharmacological characteristics of trazodone are presented in 15 separate papers. The interested reader will find this issue a comprehensive review and summary of the available literature on trazodone.

Nomifensine (Merital)

Nomifensine is a tetrahydroisoquinoline compound and differs structurally from both TCAs and MAOIs. At this time, FDA approval for routine clinical use is pending. Its mechanism of action consists principally of blocking uptake of norepinephrine and dopamine, like amphetamine, with virtually no effect on serotonin and little anticholinergic action.[49] Other antidepressants have noradrenergic effects, and amphetamine also has a dopaminergic effect, but nomifensine does both and is thus pharmacologically distinctive among antidepressants.

Both European studies and investigational trials conducted here since 1973 show nomifensine's efficacy to exceed that of placebo and equal that of the standard TCAs. At the time of this writing, it still remains an experimental drug.

Nomifensine has minimal anticholinergic effects, minimal or no clinically significant cardiovascular side effects, and a lack of serious cardiotoxicity in overdose.[60] It causes little or no sedation or weight gain and does not appear to affect psychomotor performance. It may, in fact, have a mild stimulating effect. It also does not seem to lower the seizure threshold as TCAs do, nor are convulsions associated with overdose. The most commonly reported side effects are sleep disturbance, restlessness, paranoid symptoms, nausea, and tachycardia, all of which are characteristically mild and either less frequent or less severe than TCA side effects.[60]

The novel pharmacology and distinctive side effects profile of nomifensine suggest that it may be clinically useful particularly for patients who are sensitive to sedative side effects or whose work would be significantly disrupted by some degree of sedation, and those who are unable to tolerate anticholinergic side effects. It may also be a safer drug than the standard antidepressants in cases of overdose.

We believe that the utility of a variety of antidepressants has been clearly established. This has kindled an interest in better definition of depressive subtypes. Particularly relevant at this time are treatment trials with subgroups of depressives which would identify specific clinical and/or biological characteristics associated with a higher rate of response to the different types of antidepressants. This is an area in which little work has been done. Further work is also needed in improving strategies of treating patients refractory to a first trial of antidepressants. Studies of treatment-refractory patients are time consuming and costly and probably can only be done effectively with several research centers cooperating in joint protocols.

REFERENCES

1. Shapiro R, Keller M: Initial 6-month follow-up of patients with major depressive disorder. *J Affective Disord* 1981;3:205–220.
2. American Psychiatric Association: *Diagnostic and Statistical Manual of*

Mental Disorders: DSM-III. Washington, DC, 1980.

3. Feighner JP, Robins E, Guze S, et al: Diagnostic criteria for use in psychiatric research. *Arch Gen Psychiatry* 1972;26:57–63.
4. Spitzer R, Endicott J, Robins E: *Research Diagnostic Criteria (RDC) for a Selected Group of Functional Disorders.* New York, New York State Psychiatric Institute, 1978.
5. Huapaya L, Ananth J: Depression associated with hypertension: A review. *Psychiatr J Univ Ottawa* 1980;5:58–62.
6. Leckman JF, Merikangas KR, Pauls D, et al: Anxiety disorders associated with episodes of depression: Family study data contradict DSM III convention. Submitted for publication (1983).
7. Schlesser M, Winokur G, Sherman B: Hypothalamic-pituitary-adrenal axis activity in depressive illness. *Arch Gen Psychiatry* 1980;37:737–743.
8. Frazer A: Biological aspects of mania and depression, in Frazer A, Winokur A (eds): *Biological Bases of Psychiatric Disorders.* New York, Spectrum, 1977, p 219.
9. Carroll BJ: Clinical applications of the dexamethasone suppression test. *Int Drug Therapy Newsl* 1981;16:1–4.
10. Gold MS, Potash AL, Ryan N, et al: TRH-induced TSH response in unipolar, bipolar and secondary depressions. *Psychoneuroendocrinology* 1980;5:147–155.
11. Loosen PT, Prange AJ: TRH test in psychiatric patients. *N Engl J Med* 1980;303:224–225.
12. Kupfer D, Foster FG, Coble P, et al: The application of EEG sleep for the differential diagnosis of affective disorders. *Am J Psychiatry* 1978;135:69–74.
13. Guze S, Robins E: Suicide and primary affective disorder. *Br J Psychiatry* 1970;117:437–438.
14. Beck AT: *Cognitive Therapy and the Emotional Disorders.* New York, International Universities Press, 1976.
15. DeMascio A, Neu C, Klerman G, et al: *Manual for Short Term Interpersonal Psychotherapy (IPT) of Depression.* Mimeograph, August, 1978.
16. Lewinsohn P, Arconad M: Behavioral treatment of depression: A social learning approach, in Clarkin J, Glazer H (eds): *Depression: Behavioral and Directive Intervention Strategies.* New York, Garland STPM Press, 1981, pp 33–67.
17. Klein DF, Gittelman R, Quitkin F, and Rifkin A: *Diagnosis and Drug Treatment of Psychiatric Disorders.* ed 2. Baltimore, The Williams & Wilkins Co, 1980.
18. Kantor S, Glassman A, Bigger J, et al: The cardiac effects of therapeutic plasma concentrations of imipramine. *Am J Psychiatry* 1978;135:534–537.
19. Lewis J, Winokur G: The induction of mania. *Arch Gen Psychiatry* 1982;39: 303–306.
20. Jackson J, Bressler R: Prescribing tricyclic antidepressants. Part III: Management of overdose. *Drug Therapy* 1982;12:49–63.
21. *Physician's Desk Reference.* ed 37. Oradell, NJ, Medical Economics Co, 1983.
22. Baldessarini RJ: Drugs and the treatment of psychiatric disorders, in Goodman LS, Gilman A (eds): *The Pharmacological Basis of Therapeutics.* ed 6. New York, Macmillan, 1980, pp 391–447.
23. Blackwell B: Adverse effects of antidepressant drugs. Part 1: Monoamine oxidase inhibitors and tricyclics. *Drugs* 1981;21:201–219.
24. Elis J, Laurence D, Mattice H, et al: Modification by MAOI of the effect of some sympathomimetics on blood pressure. *Br Med J* 1967;2:75–78.

25. Boakes A, Laurence DR, Teoh PC, et al: Interactions between sympathomimetic amines and antidepressant agents in man. *Br Med J* 1973;1: 311–315.
26. Sheehan D, Claycomb JB, Kouretas N: Monoamine oxidase inhibitors: Prescription and patient management. *Int J Psychiatry Med* 1980–81;10: 99–121.
27. Fink M: *Convulsive Therapy: Theory and Practice.* New York, Raven Press, 1979.
28. Comeback for shock therapy? *Time,* Nov 19, 1979, p 76.
29. American Psychiatric Association Task Force on Electroconvulsive Therapy: *Electroconvulsive Therapy.* Task Force Report 14. Washington DC, American Psychiatric Assoc, Sept 1978.
30. Freeman CP, Kendell RE: ECT: I. Patients' experiences and attitudes. *Br J Psychiatry* 1980;137:8–16.
31. McDonald M: ECT: Lothar Kalinowsky remembers. *Psychiatr News* May 5, 1978;13:8–11.
32. Kendell RE: The present status of electroconvulsive therapy. *Br J Psychiatry* 1981;139:265–283.
33. Hall RC (ed): *Psychiatric Presentations of Medical Illness.* New York, SP Medical and Scientific Books, 1980, p 38.
34. Shopsin B, Waters B: The pharmacotherapy of major depressive syndrome. I. Treatment of acute depression. *Psychosomatics* 1980;21:542–553.
35. Berger PA: Antidepressant medications and the treatment of depressions, in Barchas JD, Berger P, Ciaranello R, et al: *Psychopharmacology: From Theory to Practice.* New York, Oxford University Press, 1977, pp 174–207.
36. Ayd F: New hope for tricyclic refractory unipolar depressives? *Int Drug Therapy Newsl* 1981;16:25–27.
37. Goodwin F, Prange A, Post R, et al: Potentiation of antidepressant effects by L-triiodothyronine in tricyclic nonresponders. *Am J Psychiatry* 1982;139: 34–38.
38. de Montigny C, Grunberg F, Mayer A, et al: Lithium induces rapid relief of depression in tricyclic antidepressant drug non-responders. *Br J Psychiatry* 1981;138:252–256.
39. Coppen A, Shaw DM, Herzberg G, et al: Tryptophan in the treatment of depression. *Lancet* 1967;2:1178–1180.
40. Cole JO, Hartmann E, Brigham P: L-Tryptophan: Clinical studies, in Cole JO (ed): *Psychopharmacology Update.* Lexington, MA: D. C. Heath and Co, 1980, pp 119–148.
41. Stern S, Mendels J: Drug combinations in the treatment of refractory depression: A review. *J Clin Psychiatry* 1981;42:368–373.
42. Van Hiele LJ: L-5-Hydroxytryptophan in depression: The first substitution therapy in psychiatry? *Neuropsychobiology* 1980;6:230–240.
43. *AMA Drug Evaluations,* ed 3. Littleton, MA, Publishing Sciences Group, Inc, 1977.
44. Ayd F: Combined TCA-MAOI treatment for partial responders to maprotiline. *Int Drug Therapy Newsl* 1982;17:4.
45. White K, Simpson G: Combined MAOI-tricyclic antidepressant treatment: A reevaluation. *J Clin Psychopharmacol* 1981;1:264–282.
46. Ayd F: New antidepressant drugs. *Psychiatr Ann* 1981:11:370–374.
47. Leonard BE: Second generation of antidepressants, in Mendlewicz J, Coppen A, van Praag HM (eds): *Advances in Biological Psychiatry,* vol 7. Basel, S. Karger, 1981, pp 174–187.

48. Rifkin A, Saraf K, Kane J, et al: A comparison of trimipramine and imipramine: A controlled study. *J Clin Psychiatry* 1980;41:124–129.
49. Hollister L: "Second generation" antidepressants. *Psychosomatics* 1981;22: 872–879.
50. Ayd F: Amoxapine: A new tricyclic antidepressant. *Int Drug Therapy Newsl* 1980;15:33–40.
51. Donlon PT: Amoxapine: A newly marketed tricyclic antidepressant. *Psychiatr Ann* 1981;11:379–383.
52. Settle EC: Maprotiline: Update 1981. *Psychiatr Ann* 1981;11:384–390.
53. Feighner J: Clinical efficacy of the newer antidepressants. *J Clin Psychopharmacol* 1981;1:23S–26S.
54. Ananth J, Ayd F: Maprotiline therapy: Update 1980, in Ayd F (ed): *Clinical Depressions.* Baltimore, Ayd Medical Communications, 1980.
55. Blackwell B: Adverse effects of antidepressant drugs. II. Second generation antidepressants and rational decision making in antidepressant therapy. *Drugs* 1981;21:273–282.
56. Shopsin B, Cassano G, Conti L: An overview of new "second generation" antidepressant compounds: Research and treatment implications, in Enna SJ, et al (eds): *Antidepressants: Neurochemical, Behavioral and Clinical Perspectives.* New York, Raven Press, 1981.
57. Chand S, Crome P, Dowling S: One hundred cases of acute intoxication with mianserin hydrochloride. *Pharmakopsychiatria* 1981;14:15–17.
58. Risch SC, Janowsky DS: Trazodone. *Psychiatr Ann* 1981;11:396–401.
59. Gershon S, Mann J, Newton R, et al: Evaluation of trazadone in the treatment of endogenous depression: Results of a multi-center double-blind study. *J Clin Psychopharmacol* (Suppl) 1981;1:39S–44S.
60. Pohl R, Gershon S: Nomifensine: A new antidepressant. *Psychiatr Ann* 1981;11:391–395.

CHAPTER 4

DRUG TREATMENT OF MANIA

ARTHUR RIFKIN
SAMUEL G. SIRIS

Drug treatment of mania is one of the great successes of psychopharmacology. Few disorders have such severe symptoms requiring rapid amelioration. Schizophrenia may cause equally severe symptoms but the person with mania is often paradoxically healthier, ie, in a social and vocational position that is higher than most persons with schizophrenia, so that the eruption of severe symptoms may have a more devastating effect. The successful businessman may ruin himself financially by using grossly poor judgment; persons may behave when manic in a sexual manner far removed from their usual actions, with terrible consequences. On inpatient services few patients cause such difficult problems of management because of their anger and boisterousness. Consequently, few patients are medicated so vigorously with heightened danger of adverse reactions.

Despite the introduction of lithium as an antimanic drug in 1949[1] and phenothiazines in the early 1950s, methodologically adequate controlled clinical trials were not done in manic patients until years later.

PLACEBO-CONTROLLED STUDIES

Schou[2] did the first placebo-controlled trial, by alternating two-week periods of lithium and placebo in 30 patients with "typical" mania and eight with "atypical" manic symptoms (non-mood congruent delusions, persistent hallucinations, excitement commingled with periods of withdrawal, or marked histrionic symptoms). Of the "typical" patients 14 of 30 had a clearly positive response; 18 others had a "possible" response. The results were somewhat less encouraging for the few "atypical" patients. More sophisticated studies would follow, but this early trial was encouraging.

The next study was by Maggs,[3] who randomly assigned 28 patients to lithium or placebo for two weeks, followed by two weeks of treatment with the alternate drug. While on lithium the patients were calmer to a statistically significant extent.

Goodwin and co-workers,[4] using multiple cross-overs of lithium and placebo, found that 8 of 12 patients had a complete response, 1 had an incomplete response, and 3 actually worsened. Most responsive patients relapsed when switched to placebo. This study is not a "pure" drug-placebo comparison, which would be either a parallel design (ie, randomly assigning patients to either treatment concomitantly) or an intensive design, in which each patient is his own control and randomly there are several cross-overs. The study by Goodwin and associates cannot test adequately the probability of their results occurring by chance, although their anecdotal experience remains impressive. If a patient with mania improves while on lithium and worsens when switched to placebo, this is strongly suggestive of a lithium effect, especially in a disorder such as mania, which is known not to respond often to placebo.

Stokes and co-workers[5] compared lithium with placebo in 28 manic patients. Each treatment was alternated for 10 days. Complete remission during the first treatment period occurred in 5 lithium-treated subjects and in none of those given placebo — not a statistically significant finding, but suggestive. There was improvement in 75% of the 56 lithium periods and in 42.5% of the 42 placebo periods, a difference the authors report as statistically significant. However, this design, alternate treatment periods, is not a bona fide test of the null hypothesis that no difference exists between treatments as it combines within and between group comparisons, and if treatments were alternated they were not assigned randomly. However, it is suggestive.

The only other placebo-controlled study of mania was done by Klein,[6] who compared 1200 mg of chlorpromazine per day with placebo for six weeks in 13 manic inpatients. Despite the small number of subjects, chlorpromazine was superior to a statistically significant extent; indicating a large clinical effect.

All of the remaining double-blind controlled studies compared two or more active drugs. Thus, we see that there are few good trials of lithium or an antipsychotic tested against placebo. This undoubtedly is due to the disinclination to treat manic patients with placebo and the conviction among clinicians that lithium and antipsychotics work. We have no doubt that this conviction is based on truth, and we strongly advocate drug treatment of mania; yet, the uncomfortable fact is that such treatment is not supported by much data.

LITHIUM-ANTIPSYCHOTIC COMPARISONS

The comparison of lithium with an antipsychotic has much stronger experimental support. The largest and therefore most convincing study was done by Prien and co-workers[7] in a multi-hospital study with 255 patients. The antipsychotic used was chlorpromazine (200–3000 mg per day; mean dose was 1000 mg per day). Patients were assigned on the basis of their clinical symptomatology into highly or mildly active groups and randomized separately. Among the mildly active patients, both treatments were equal. For highly active patients, there was an advantage for chlorpromazine to a statistically significant extent for symptoms of grandiosity, psychotic disorganization, and conceptual disorganization. Also, chlorpromazine acted faster. The lithium-treated group had much more difficulty with adverse reactions as the treating psychiatrists pushed the dose to its limit, no doubt because of the severe symptomatology of these patients.

Other controlled comparisons between lithium and chlorpromazine used small samples and did not demonstrate any statistically significant differences,[8,9] although such studies, because of the small sample sizes, were not powerful tests of any differences.

Two other studies with rather small samples claimed an advantage for lithium over an antipsychotic. In one, with only 11 patients, the authors concluded that those on lithium did better. But on only 1 item of 19 was the difference between the groups statistically significant, a finding easily attributed to chance, especially since that item ("using mannerisms") is peripheral to the syndrome and not often seen.[10]

Another study by Shopsin and co-workers[11] compared lithium with chlorpromazine and haloperidol in a small number of inpatients with mania. The rating scale data showed little difference among the three drugs. The investigators concluded, however, that lithium was the superior treatment because the quality of improvement in patients treated with lithium was superior to that seen in those given either of the antipsychotics. They cite as evidence the more rapid discharge of those given lithium. It is difficult to evaluate their conclusion, which goes against the findings of the rating scale data, although it is our impression as well that lithium is usually preferred to antipsychotics by patients because of fewer, or less bothersome, adverse reactions.

In Japan, Takahashi and associates,[12] in 80 patients with mania, compared lithium with chlorpromazine and found lithium to be superior on several measures. They used rather low doses of both drugs; the average for chlorpromazine was 256 mg per day, and the average blood level of lithium was only 0.57 mmol/L. The authors say that Japanese patients with mania do not need or tolerate high doses. This may be true. Lower doses of many psychotropic drugs are used in many ethnic groups, not only Japanese, than is common in the United States and Europe, but we are not aware of any controlled trials that show that these differences are due to true differences in tolerance and dose needed for equal efficacy or whether it is due to different practices of prescribing. We notice that prescribing practices have altered, sometimes markedly, within the United States during the past 25 years, eg, the dose of antipsychotics commonly used appears to be much higher now than formerly. Whether this represents an advance in treatment or not, ie, whether such changes are rational or due to impatience, cannot be answered in the case of mania because of the paucity of dose-response studies, but we can be sure that the change is not due to biological alterations in patients making them less sensitive to drugs. We therefore view with some skepticism the assertion that some ethnic groups have differing dosage requirements until it has been established by clinical research.

This leaves us uncertain how to interpret the findings of Takahashi and co-workers.

What we conclude from this review of the double-blind controlled studies of drug treatment of mania is that both lithium and antipsychotics are most likely effective. We say this with less than absolute conviction because neither has been tested often against placebo, but we really do not doubt that both are effective.

SCHIZO-AFFECTIVE EXCITED STATES

As the years progress since the diagnosis of schizo-affective schizophrenia was first introduced, its place in the diagnostic schema appears to be less clear. For many years it was considered a variant of schizophrenia, to be treated as that; then, with the widespread use of the Research Diagnostic Criteria,[13] it was treated as a separate entity whose final place would be determined by research; and finally, in the present age of DMS-III (in the United States) it is widely thought of as a variant of affective disorder. The last position has been ably presented by Pope and Lipinsky.[14] The designers of DSM-III were, of all the diagnostic categories in the schema, unable only for schizo-affective disorder to agree on operational criteria. The user of DSM-III is left with the rather vague advice to use the term if so inclined, if the patient seems somewhat between schizophrenia and affective disorder. Given the fact that all of the other diagnoses have solid identification, and one need not ever have to resort to the vaguely defined schizo-affective disorder, ie, any person who would fit previous definitions of schizo-affective disorder would fit some other DSM-III category such as schizophrenia, mania, major depression, bipolar depression, atypical psychosis, atypical depression, etc, the implicit message of DSM-III is clear, at least to us: stay away from the term.

Our preference is for the more agnostic position of the Research Diagnostic Criteria, which is that it is too early to close the door on the issue. If we define it out of existence we lose the opportunity of discovering whether it is a useful diagnosis. We grant that the definition in the

Research Diagnostic Criteria is fairly arbitrary; ie, not supported by much data that this category is distinguishable from its neighbors by family history, treatment response, and course, yet it is clear and specific. It takes the criteria for mania and adds the presence of any symptom commonly thought to be more characteristic of schizophrenia, especially those considered by Schneider to be first-rank symptoms of schizophrenia, such as voices conversing with each other, thought broadcasting, delusions of control, etc. At least for clinical research we hope that the category of schizo-affective will be preserved. This is discussed further in the chapter on drug treatment of acute schizophrenia.

In this light we should address the question of how drugs work in schizo-affective excited states. The relevant literature is even smaller than that for mania. The largest and most definitive study was done by Prien and associates[15] as a companion project to their previously described study of mania.[7] The design was the same. Patients from several Veterans Administration hospitals were randomly assigned to lithium carbonate or chlorpromazine and stratified separately into more and less active. The results were the same as for those with mania: both drugs were equally effective in the mildly active patients and chlorpromazine was better for the highly active patients, because of more adverse reactions to lithium as the dose was elevated to control symptoms. The impression of these two studies in mania and excited schizo-affective disorder is that in highly excited patients chlorpromazine is superior because it has a wider margin of safety. During treatment with lithium, going past 1.4 mmol/L seems to bring no further benefit, but a lot more side effects whereas the therapeutic range with chlorpromazine is much wider. This would be even more true, we hazard, if a high-potency antipsychotic was used, because the higher dose ranges are better tolerated than with low-potency drugs. Once one goes past about 1000 mg of chlorpromazine per day there is a high likelihood of bothersome adverse reactions, and it is not usually possible to go past 3000 mg per day, even very excited patients with mania become oversedated and occasionally stuporous. Yet comparable doses, say, of haloperidol, can be given past that point; it is not difficult in most patients to go past 60 mg per day.

In a small study of only 14 patients diagnosed as "schizophrenic," lithium was compared with chlorpromazine. Most patients on both treatments improved. The number of subjects is too small to permit an adequate test of the hypothesis that the treatments were equivalent.[16]

Another relevant study of the treatment of excited schizo-affective disorder is that of Biederman and co-workers.[17] They addressed the question of whether combining lithium and an antipsychotic, haloperidol in this instance, was superior to standard treatment of haloperidol alone. They used as their sample patients referred to one ward that served a catchment area in Jerusalem. The defined "pure" schizophrenia as "1" and "pure" mania as "6"; then, they defined "2" through "5" as states between depending upon the degree of excitement and "schizophrenic" symptoms. To patients in groups 2 through 5 they randomly gave haloperidol with or without lithium under double-blind conditions. In all groups, combined treatment was superior to a statistically significant degree, and there was no difference in this superiority according to diagnostic category. They did not find any unexpected or severe adverse reactions from the combination.

Before stating our opinion about how mania should be treated based on the drug trials and our experience, we should review the controversial issue of the danger of combining lithium and an antipsychotic.

The storm broke when Cohen and Cohen[18] reported on four patients treated with lithium and haloperidol who developed serious neurological toxicity, consisting mainly of symptoms of encephalitis, irreversible in some instances. Ayd[19] reviewed the case histories carefully and concluded that they were instances, most likely, of lithium toxicity. Further, Baastrup and co-workers[20] reported that they had treated over 400 patients with just that combination without any instances of the severe toxicity described by Cohen and Cohen. Strayhorn and Nash,[21] on the other hand, described nine cases of neurotoxicity from the combination of lithium and an antipsychotic despite careful attention to keeping the blood level of lithium within the usual therapeutic range.

Spring[22] also reported cases (six) of neurotoxicity from lithium and thioridazine (five) or fluphenazine (one), and divided the neurotoxicity into two forms:[23] a "lithium" type with delirium, seizures, highly abnormal electroencephalographs, and no extrapyramidal symptoms; and an "antipsychotic" type with hyperpyrexia, coma, and marked extrapyramidal symptoms—ie, the malignant syndrome.[24]

The most recent and well-described instance of neurotoxicity is by Spring and Frankel.[25] It resembles those reported by Cohen and Cohen,[18] but is without question not due to excessive dosage of lithium. The patient, 53 years old with a long history of bipolar disorder, was treated for mania with lithium and chlorpromazine, which was changed to haloperidol after four days (40 mg per day). His peak lithium level was 1.5 mmol/L. He developed symptoms of rigidity and a parkinsonian gait and was given benztropine and diphenhydramine, and the haloperidol was stopped. The symptoms of toxicity progressed to marked rigidity, festinating gait, cogwheeling, paresis, and difficulty swallowing. His lithium level was 1.15 mmol/L. He developed a fever, almost fatal paralysis, and stupor. A blood level of haloperidol was only 5 ng/mL. Despite intensive evaluation no other cause of his symptoms was found. He never recovered fully—requiring assistance to walk and still showing extrapyramidal symptoms and truncal dyskinesia. The authors cite this as an example of the malignant syndrome and suggest that the lithium predisposed the patient to it by enhancing the dopamine receptor blockade of the antipsychotic. West and Meltzer[26] suggest that during mania, persons have heightened metabolism, which makes them more vulnerable to drug toxicity. This would explain why acutely ill manics have toxic reactions despite dosages and blood levels not usually associated with adverse reactions. West and Meltzer make the important observation that severe neurotoxicity from the combination of lithium and an antipsychotic has only been observed during the acute phase of the disorder.

We remain skeptical that the case has been proven that lithium and antipsychotics produce neurotoxicity as a combination to an extent greater than what can be due to the drugs taken alone. The case reports show that patients do develop symptoms of toxicity from the combination, but these symptoms may be seen as well when the drugs are used separately. Spring[22,23] argues convincingly that the cases of neurotoxicity may be divided into the malignant syndrome, rarely seen with antipsychotics, and lithium toxicity, rarely seen when blood levels are not excessive.[27] The crucial question then is not whether neurotoxicity may occur during treatment with lithium and an antipsychotic, but whether the risk is greater than what it would be if either treatment had been used separately. The literature is unable to provide data about this. Case reports cannot answer the question; only a study that has the denominator as well as the numerator while comparing treatments could definitively answer the question.

Yet, we must act without definitive knowledge. Considering all the foregoing we make the following recommendation for treatment of mania.

TREATMENT OF MANIA

A person who is manic requires vigorous treatment. The symptoms are usually painful; it is not often true that people with mania are so elated that they are enjoying themselves. Perhaps in the impossible world where each person with mania could have what he wishes, he would be only elated; but, inevitably the person cannot have his demands met, which leads to anger and frustration. This is particularly true when the patient is hospitalized and his expansive desires are curtailed. It is clear that lithium does not ameliorate symptoms immediately; it takes, usually, at least a week for improvement to begin and several weeks for it to be maximum.

It is not reasonable to wait a week for symptoms to improve unless the mania is mild or is hypomania. A patient who is not sleeping, is disturbing those around him with his loud boisterousness, is threatening violence perhaps, or may be violent, requires rapid relief—as do the people around him. If the patient is treated as an outpatient, a difficult procedure that is usually regretted, there is even more reason to reduce symptoms rapidly. The only drug that appears to work rapidly is an antipsychotic, and we recommend that it be used promptly and in fairly high dosage.

Since diminished need for sleep is characteristic of mania it might be thought attractive to use a low-potency antipsychotic to take advantage of its marked sedative side effects. We find this usually inadvisable for two reasons. Sedation does not usually calm mania. Sedatives such as barbiturates are not helpful. Second, the sedative adverse reactions of the low-potency drugs limit the dose that can be given. Even a very excited person may be oversedated by high doses of low-potency drugs. It appears that parenteral antipsychotics given every half hour do rapidly reduce symptoms, but this has been demonstrated only for the first 24 hours. We doubt if the route of administration is crucial in the treatment of mania. The more important point is to raise the dose rapidly, even if it means using doses around 5.0 g per day in chlorpromazine equivalent units, in order to get some relief of symptoms promptly. The dreaded dangers of treatment with antipsychotics such as the malignant syndrome are not known to be associated with dose. The common adverse reactions are associated with dose, but can be monitored and reversed if necessary by lowering the dose. These common adverse reactions, which rarely pose a serious threat to the patient's health, include sedation, anticholinergic symptoms (dry mouth, constipation, blurred vision, and delayed micturition), postural hypotension, and extrapyramidal symptoms. The latter can usually be controlled with anti-parkinson drugs, which should be given prophylactically when treatment with the antipsychotic is started because with high dosages of high-potency antipsychotics the chance of more than mild extrapyramidal symptoms must be close to 100%.

Should lithium be started with the antipsychotic at onset of treatment? Many clinicians do this, hoping to use the antipsychotic for initial treatment and withdraw it once the lithium takes hold; using the lithium at once means that it will take effect sooner than if its use is delayed. Why use lithium at all? There seem to be two cogent reasons. Although the evidence from controlled studies is far from conclusive, it is believed by many that once the worst of the excited stage is over, lithium provides better relief of symptoms at a lower cost of adverse reactions. Second, lithium is the drug of choice for long-term treatment or prophylaxis, and since it will be used eventually, why not use it earlier for the acute episode?

We support the use of lithium to treat mania, but do not think it best to use it as initial treatment or as combined treatment with an antipsychotic during the acute phase. The reason not to use lithium alone as initial treatment is that it works too slowly. One might not object to the week or so delay in action if the mania is mild, as was shown in the studies by Prien et al,[7,15] in which patients with mild mania did equally well with chlorpromazine as with lithium, but this equality is outweighed, we feel, by the risk of mania becoming severe—rapidly. The main difficulty in the treatment of mania is not, usually, knowing what drug treatment to use or deciding how to treat patients who have not responded to standard treatment, because most patients do quite well on standard treatment. The problem is mainly how to administer standard treatment to a patient who is uncooperative. One of the most difficult situations in psychiatry is trying to "catch up" with a patient with mania who is running around the community—or the world— causing terrible social and financial harm to himself and others by overspending, using atrocious judgment about business and personal matters, while not being so obviously disordered as, say, someone with schizophrenia might be, making it difficult to convince yourself and others that involuntary treatment is indicated. When your patient is making an impassioned speech to the board of directors exhorting them to expand operations to the Philippines, it is not easy to drag him away to a hospital; or, if you are convinced that he is sick enough to be committed, it is often very difficult to locate him and arrange an admission because he moves around so quickly. Even if these horrible experiences are not common, they occur sufficiently frequently to make their prevention a high priority in deciding what treatment to use.

Therefore, the major reason to initiate treatment of mania with an antipsychotic is to ameliorate symptoms rapidly. The adverse reactions of antipsychotics are often more severe than those of lithium, if the antipsychotic is pushed to a high dose and the lithium is given within the usual therapeutic range of 0.6 to 1.4 mmol/L. However, in most instances these adverse reactions are a price worth paying for the relief of manic symptoms. Dry mouth, drowsiness, extrapyramidal symptoms not alleviated by an anti-parkinson drug, postural hypotension, and so on are bothersome, but minor, usually, compared with the difficulty that continued manic symptoms can cause. The more worrisome problem of tardive dyskinesia is not a serious worry if antipsychotic drug treatment is kept short term.

Why not use lithium with the antipsychotic as initial treatment? This is commonly done, but we are against it for several reasons.

First, giving sufficient antipsychotic during the initial, most severe phase of mania often requires large doses which causes troublesome side effects. Concomitant lithium would add further side effects and reduce the reservoir of tolerance the patient has for adverse reactions, thus to some extent limiting the dose of antipsychotic that could be used.

Second, it might be difficult to distinguish which adverse reactions come from which drug. If the patient develops slurred speech, mental confusion, and unsteadiness, which drug is doing it, and which drug should be changed?

Third, if there is increased risk of neurotoxicity from the combination of lithium and an antipsychotic it seems to be confined to the initial, acute phase.[26]

Considering that the lithium is not initially contributing to the amelioration of symptoms, these three drawbacks of concomitant treatment during acute mania seem compelling to us. We prefer to calm the patient with antipsychotics alone, using high dosage if necessary, and once the patient has almost reached remission, use lithium and gradually withdraw the antipsychotic.

As the mania breaks, the dose of antipsychotic often produces more adverse reactions and should be reduced. Similarly, if lithium is used for acute treatment, lithium clearance seems to change, going from severe symptoms to mild. Commonly, the blood level goes up as manic symptoms clear, if the dose is kept constant. This may cause lithium toxicity. When the symptoms improve, blood levels should be watched carefully. Usually the dose requires reduction at that point to maintain blood levels within the therapeutic range.

If an antipsychotic is used without lithium during acute treatment, we recommend that once these symptoms ameliorate the dose of antipsychotic be reduced and lithium begun. This combined treatment is then continued for several weeks, during which the patient should continue to improve. Then we stop the antipsychotic (and the antiparkinson drug two weeks later) and rely upon lithium for continuating treatment.

Although drug treatment of mania is usually quite successful, there is a range of response. It would be nice to know which patient will rapidly respond to moderate doses and who will not, so the latter patient could be treated more vigorously. Unfortunately, we are not able to predict course. Taylor and Abrams[28] have made the most valiant attempt. They followed 111 patients with mania, using as predictors demographic data, clinical symptoms, family history of mental disorders, and electroencephalographic and other neuropsychological measures. Of all these factors, only one, an abnormal electroencephalogram, was related to outcome, a result that could well be due to chance. The best predictor, in a sense, was early termination from treatment. Such patients did poorly, no doubt due to the absence of treatment that is usually effective, although another explanation might be that less cooperative patients have a more severe form of the illness with a worse prognosis. This study looked at overall course and was not a treatment study, which means it could not have helped us determine optimum treatment; yet the absence of any strong predictor (other than dropping out of treatment) tends to support the notion that we cannot predict response to treatment based on available clinical information. The most serious drawback of this ignorance is that we cannot tell which patient who has recently become hypomanic or somewhat worse is going to quickly worsen considerably and be extremely difficult to treat outside of a hospital. The psychiatrist faces a difficult decision in treating the manic patient: who may safely be treated as an outpatient? It probably is too drastic to hospitalize everyone with mania, although we wish often that we had the courage of our convictions to do so, especially after the experience of trying to keep up with a patient with mania who is not hospitalized, or having a patient cause considerable harm to himself, or others, by his excitement, aggressiveness, and poor judgment. The best predictor of future behavior during mania is probably past manic behavior. The psychiatrist should treat a manic patient outside of a hospital only with great caution.

Some manic patients are only tenuously involved in treatment, yet the psychiatrist does not think the disorder is sufficiently severe to require involuntary hospitalization. A useful tactic in this situation is to capitalize on the patient's modicum of cooperativeness during the session and administer a depot antipsychotic, which in the United States at present means fluphenazine decanoate or enanthate.

Use of Lithium

We offer these practical pointers concerning the use of lithium. The following questions are relevant: dose, frequency of dosage, frequency and timing of blood levels, different preparations, and adverse reactions.

As mentioned previously, we do not know what blood level is optimal for the treatment of mania, or even if it matters where within the usual therapeutic range the patient lies; ie, if the blood level is at 0.8 mmol/L and the patient is still excited, should the dosage be increased? Until clear data are available we recommend that the level be kept between 0.8 and 1.2 mmol/L and leave it where it falls within that range for several weeks before considering a higher level.

Cooper and Simpson[29] have shown that the correspondence of dose to blood level during steady state can be determined accurately by the blood level at 24 hours after a 600-mg single dose of lithium carbonate. That is, 24 hours after the first dose, the proper dose can be determined. This is a useful tactic that has not been used by many psychiatrists. Its value would be particularly cogent if lithium was being used to treat acute severe symptoms. In that situation a delay in reaching adequate dosage would be very unfortunate. It takes about five days for a steady level of lithium to be reached; therefore, it would require five-day intervals to adjust dosage. If lithium is not begun for controlling severe symptoms, but for second-stage treatment, which is our recommendation, it is less important to rapidly determine optimal dose.

How frequently should lithium be given? With regular lithium carbonate preparations, the less frequently the dose is divided the larger the fluctuation of the blood level. Amdisen,[30] using computer-stimulated concentration curves, compared the effect of once, twice, or three times daily dosage, assuming that the total dose per 24 hours is the same, that the half-life is 13 hours, and that the absorption rate is constant and equal to that observed from conventional tablets. The 12-hour blood levels for twice or three times per day were almost identical (around 1.00 and 1.07 mmol/L), and the blood level for once daily dosage was 1.37 mmol/L. The large difference was seen in peak blood levels: almost 3.0 mmol/L for once daily, around 2.1 mmol/L for twice daily, and around 1.9 mmol/L for three times daily. The worry about once daily dosage is that the peak level falls within the toxic range. The disadvantage of frequent daily dosage is that compliance diminishes. We recommend twice or three times daily dosage.

Sustained release preparations are available. Although not all studies are in agreement, most show that sustained-release preparations produce fewer side effects.[31–33] Our usual practice is to use a sustained-release drug twice daily especially if adverse reactions are a problem.

Adverse reactions Common side effects of lithium are nausea, diarrhea, metallic taste, difficulty concentrating, ataxia, tremor, polydipsia, lethargy, and several types of skin reactions. The list is much longer if uncommon adverse reactions are included. Most patients tolerate the drug well. The difference between the toxic and therapeutic dose is small, but in practice the likelihood of getting into serious difficulty is small because the relatively innocuous side effects appear before the more serious ones, with occasional exceptions. That is, before lithium would cause renal shutdown and stupor the patient would likely have very bothersome nausea or diarrhea which should be a clue to evaluate the blood level. Several side effects are most worrisome.

Thyroid Taking all surveys together, the mean incidence of hypothyroidism in lithium-treated patients is 3.28%, although in the United States it is only 1%.[34,35] The usual way of determining it is through laboratory tests of thyroid function. The most sensitive indicatory is measurement of thyroid-stimulating hormone, especially the thyrotropin-releasing hormone-induced thyroid-stimulating hormone response. The symptoms of hypothyroidism most commonly are fatigue, weight gain, loss of hair, sensitivity to cold, pretibial edema, hoarseness of voice, and coarseness of skin. Several of these symptoms are seen in depression. The danger for the psychiatrist, who is more used to diagnosing depression than hypothyroidism, is to mistake the latter for the former.

Renal Lithium's renal effects are separable into tubular and glomerular functions. Lithium causes a nephrogenic diabetes insipidus, ie, the kidney becomes insensitive to the effect of antidiuretic hormone (ADH). Almost all patients have some degree of increased urine excretion. About 10% develop actual diabetes insipidus. Loss of concentrating ability is not life threatening, but it is a terrible bother to the patient who is forever thirsty and cannot venture too far from a toilet. It also renders the patient vulnerable to dehydration, especially during hot weather or exertion. Fortunately, thiazide diuretics are effective in reducing the polyuria. Such diuretics also reduce lithium clearance and elevate blood levels, so blood levels must be watched carefully when thiazides are begun.

Whether lithium affects glomerular function is a more serious matter. Loss of the ability to clear wastes is life threatening. The recent concern that lithium may injure the kidney's glomerular function has cast a pall upon lithium treatment, and has threatened to tip the risk-benefit ratio adversely. The report by Hestbech and co-workers[36] in 1977 ignited the fuse. They did renal biopsies on 14 patients treated with lithium who had previously had lithium poisoning. They found sclerotic glomeruli and tubular atrophy increased by several times compared with age-matched controls.

Other studies found similar changes and found that glomerular filtration rates were diminished in some patients. But when compared with patients with affective disorder not treated with lithium, surprisingly, there were no differences in glomerular filtration rate or, in one study, in renal biopsy findings between biopsies taken before and after lithium treatment. The latest review of the matter by Schou and Vestergaard[37] indicates that the scare that lithium was nephrotoxic is not supported by the data. Psychiatrists should still watch for indicators of reduced glomerular filtration rate such as levels of creatinine and blood levels of lithium rising despite a constant dose. Should a decline in glomerular filtration rate be found, do not assume that it is due to lithium, but assiduously look for some other cause.

Cardiovascular side effects By and large, lithium is quite innocuous to the cardiovascular system. Reversible T-wave flattening or even inversion is commonly seen, but is without obvious clinical relevance, frequently disappears under continued treatment, and is reversible when lithium treatment is stopped.[38] Of more concern are disorders of impulse generation and conduction. Uncommonly, lithium treatment is associated with sinus mode abnormalities, sinoatrial blocks, atrioventribular blocks, as well as ventricular and atrial premature contractions.

There are no absolute contraindications to the use of lithium in persons with heart disease, as long as the psychiatrist works closely with a cardiologist in questionable cases. The danger of cardiotoxicity from lithium appears to increase with age. Patients over 40 should probably have electrocardiograms taken once or twice yearly if they are taking lithium, which is probably true even if they are not taking lithium.

Summary of adverse reactions The foregoing has been a brief overview of the major adverse reactions to lithium which the psychiatrist should keep in mind during lithium treatment of mania. How bothersome are they? In our experience very few patients have sufficient side effects to require discontinuation of lithium during the acute episode. It is later, when the mental symptoms have abated, that the patient is less likely to tolerate constant minor side effects. It is then that the metallic taste, mild nausea, and diarrhea that are common lead a fair minority of patients to refuse further lithium treatment.

Electroconvulsive treatment of mania Some clinicians assert that electroconvulsive therapy (ECT) is an effective treatment and should be used if drug treatment is not effective, or even as initial treatment if symptoms are severe. A review of the literature is not encouraging to these claims. There are no true controlled studies. The best ones use retrospective control groups that were not assigned treatment randomly. McCabe[39] compared the course of 28 manic patients treated with ECT as inpatients between 1945 and 1949 with other manic patients admitted during the same period, not treated with ECT, but matched for age and sex. The group given ECT was more improved at discharge, had a shorter hospital stay, and had a better social recovery—all to a statistically significant degree. Of those given ECT, 96% were discharged to their homes compared with 44% of the control group.

McCabe and Norris,[40] in a similar manner, compared ECT with chlorpromazine and no somatic treatment and found that the drug and ECT were similar and both superior to the no treatment group in measures of duration of hospitalization, symptoms at discharge, and, interestingly, mortality rate during long-term follow-up.

These studies are suggestive that ECT is an effective treatment of mania, but no more than that, since they are retrospective and cannot adequately test an hypothesis. Our opinion is that ECT should be used in the treatment of mania only if vigorous drug treatment has failed. In our experience, that is a rare event.

Overall conclusion We recommend initial treatment of mania with an antipsychotic. Once the severe symptoms have subsided we would add lithium and gradually withdraw the antipsychotic. With vigorous use of the antipsychotic almost all patients' symptoms can be ameliorated. The response to treatment is usually excellent. In rare instances in which drug treatment is ineffective, we recommend ECT.

REFERENCES

1. Cade JFS: Lithium salts in the treatment of psychotic excitement. *Med J Aust*

1949;2:349–352.
2. Schou M: Lithium in psychiatric therapy. Stock-taking after ten years. *Psychopharmacologia* 1959;1:65–78.
3. Maggs R: Treatment of manic illness with lithium carbonate. *Br J Psychiatry* 1963;109:56–65.
4. Goodwin FK, Murphy DL, Bunney WE: Lithium carbonate treatment in depression and mania. *Arch Gen Psychiatry* 1969;21:486–496.
5. Stokes PE, Stohl PM, Shamoian CH, et al: Efficacy of lithium as acute treatment of manic-depressive illness. *Lancet* 1971;1:1319–1325.
6. Klein DF: Importance of psychiatric diagnosis in prediction of clinical drug effects. *Arch Gen Psychiatry* 1967;16:118–126.
7. Prien RF, Caffey EM, Klett CJ: Comparison of lithium carbonate and chlorpromazine in the treatment of mania. *Arch Gen Psychiatry* 1972;21:146–153.
8. Spring G, Schweid D, Gray C, et al: A double-blind comparison of lithium and chlorpromazine in the treatment of manic states. *Am J Psychiatry* 1970;126:140–144.
9. Platman SR: A comparison of lithium and chlorpromazine in mania. *Am J Psychiatry* 1970;127:351–353.
10. Johnson G, Gershon S, Burdock E, et al: Comparative effects of lithium and chlorpromazine in the treatment of acute manic states. *Br J Psychiatry* 1971;119:267–276.
11. Shopsin B, Gershon S, Thompson H, et al: Psychoactive drugs in mania. *Arch Gen Psychiatry* 1975;32:34–35.
12. Takahashi R, Sakuma A, Hoh K: Comparison of efficacy of lithium carbonate and chlorpromazine in mania. *Arch Gen Psychiatry* 1975;32:1310–1318.
13. Spitzer R, Endicott J, Robins E: *Research Diagnostic Criteria (RDC) for a Selected Group of Functional Disorders.* New York, Biometrics Division, New York State Psychiatric Institute, 1978.
14. Pope HG Jr, Lipinski JF Jr: Diagnosis in schizophrenia and manic depressive illness. *Arch Gen Psychiatry* 1978;35:811–828.
15. Prien RF, Caffey EM, Klett CJ: A comparison of lithium carbonate and chlorpromazine in the treatment of excited schizoaffectives. *Arch Gen Psychiatry* 1972;27:182–189.
16. Brockington IF, Kendell RE, Kellett JM, et al: Trials of lithium chlorpromazine and amitriptyline in schizoaffective patients. *Br J Psychiatry* 1978;133:162–168.
17. Biederman J, Lerner Y, Belmaker RH: Combination of lithium plus haloperidol in schizoaffective disorder: A controlled study. Presented at Psychiatric Research Society, San Francisco, CA, Sept 22–24, 1978.
18. Cohen WJ, Cohen NH: Lithium carbonate, haloperidol, and irreversible brain damage. *JAMA* 1974;230:1283–1287.
19. Ayd FJ: Lithium-haloperidol for mania—is it safe or hazardous? *Int Drug Therapy Newsl* 1975;10:29–36.
20. Baastrup PC, Hollnagel P, Sorensen R, et al: Adverse reactions in treatment with lithium carbonate and haloperidol. JAMA 1976;236:2645–2646.
21. Strayhorn JM, Nash JL: Severe neurotoxicity despite "therapeutic" serum lithium levels. *Dis Nerv Sys* 1977;38:107–110.
22. Spring GK: Neurotoxicity with combined use of lithium and thioridazine. *J Clin Psychiatry* 1979;40:135–138.
23. Spring GK: EEG observations in confirming neurotoxicity (letter to editor). *Am J Psychiatry* 1979;136:1099–1100.
24. Caroff SN: The neuroleptic malignant syndrome. *J Clin Psychiatry* 1980;41:79–83.

25. Spring GK, Frankel M: New data on lithium and haloperidol incompatibility. *Am J Psychiatry* 1981;138:818–821.
26. West AP, Meltzer HY: Paradoxical lithium neurotoxicity. *Am J Psychiatry* 1979;136:963–966.
27. Rifkin A, Quitkin F, Klein DF: Organic brain syndrome during lithium carbonate treatment. *Compr Psychiatry* 1973;14:251–254.
28. Taylor MA, Abrams R: Prediction of treatment response in mania. *Arch Gen Psychiatry* 1981;38:800–803.
29. Cooper TM, Simpson GM: The 24-hour lithium level as a prognosticator of dosage requirements: A 2 year follow-up study. *Am J Psychiatry* 1976;133:440–443.
30. Amdisen A: Serum level monitoring and clinical pharmaeokinetics of lithium. *Clin Pharmacokin* 1977;2:73–92.
31. Amdisen A: Variations of serum lithium concentrations during the day in relation to treatment control, absorptive side effects and the use of slow-release tablets. *Acta Psychiatr Scand Suppl* 1969;207:55–57.
32. Consbruch U, Koufen H: Zur Pharmaeokinetik von Lithiumpalzen beim akuten Belastungsversuchen Gesunder. *Pharmakopsych Neuropsychiatr* 1972;5:3–11.
33. Matussek N, Von Hessling P: Vergleich von Lithium-Nebenwirkungen zwischen einem Kurzzeit (Quilonum) und einem Depotpraparat (Lithium Duriles). *Nervenarzt* 1971;42:376–378.
34. Mannisto PT: Endocrine side-effects of lithium, in Johnson FN (ed): *Handbook of Lithium Therapy.* Lancaster, England, MTP Press Ltd, 1980, p 311.
35. Piziak VK, Sellman JE, Othmer K: Lithium and hypothyroidism. *J Clin Psychiatry* 1978;39:709–711.
36. Hestbach J, Hansen HE, Amdisen A, et al: Chronic renal lesions following long-term treatment with lithium. *Kidney Int* 1977;12:205–213.
37. Shou M, Vestergaard P: Lithium and the kidney scare. *Psychosomatics* 1981;22:92–94.
38. Albrecht JW, Muller-Oerlinghausen B: Cardiovascular side-effects of lithium, in Johnson FN (ed): *Handbook of Lithium Therapy,* Lancaster, England, MTP Press Ltd, 1980, pp 323–337.
39. McCabe MS: ECT in the treatment of mania. A controlled study. *Am J Psychiatry* 1976;133:688–691.
40. McCabe MS, Norris B: ECT versus chlorpromazine in mania. *Biol Psychiatry* 1977;12:245–254.

CHAPTER 5

LONG-TERM MAINTENANCE THERAPY IN AFFECTIVE DISORDERS

ROBERT F. PRIEN

Most clinical studies of the pharmacotherapy of affective disorders focus on the acute episode and are limited to a three- to eight-week period. Antidepressants, lithium, and electroconvulsive therapy are of proven efficacy in controlling symptomatology during this acute phase of treatment. Maintenance pharmacologic treatment aimed at preventing the reemergence of symptoms and the occurrence of new episodes has been less well studied. As a result, there are many critical gaps in our knowledge as to how to treat affective disorders after the initial control of acute symptomatology.

It is vital that the longitudinal nature of affective disorders be considered in treatment and research planning. Two basic problems need to be addressed. First, affective episodes do not necessarily end with the drug-induced control of acute symptomatology. Continued administration of drugs may be required for months after the initial suppression of symptoms. This form of maintenance therapy is termed "continuation therapy." Continuation therapy is based upon the assumption that antidepressant drugs may suppress the manifest symptoms of depression without immediately correcting the biological process underlying the disorder. There may be a gap of several weeks or months between control of symptoms and the end of the episode. It is not known whether antidepressants actually shorten the episode or merely suppress symptoms until the episode runs its natural course. In any event, if medication is withdrawn before the underlying illness is resolved, the patient will relapse. A major problem is that when continuation therapy is effective, it may be extremely difficult to determine when the episode is completed. This may cause the clinician to either withdraw the drug prematurely or unnecessarily prolong treatment.

A second problem concerns the recurrent or chronic nature of affective illness. It is estimated that 50% to 80% of patients with an initial episode of mania or major depression will have one or more new episodes during the following 10 years.[1] A new episode is more likely for bipolar rather than unipolar disorders.[2] The recurrences tend to occur more frequently with each successive episode. These recurring episodes not only cause great disruption in social, occupational and family functioning, but also may be fatal, as about 15 in 100 depressed persons commit suicide.[3] In a significant number of patients, affective illness is both episodic and chronic. As many as one-third of patients with a major depressive disorder or mania have a chronic course between episodes characterized by persistent symptomatology and/or significant social impairment.

Pharmacologic treatment administered over long periods for the purpose of preventing the occurrence of further episodes, or reducing their severity and duration, is termed "long-term preventive therapy." Most of the research on long-term preventive therapy has been conducted with lithium, imipramine, or amitriptyline in patients with a history of frequent and severe episodes of primary major depression or mania.

This chapter will deal with research findings, issues, and strategies pertaining to the continuation and long-term preventive therapy of affective disorders.

CONTINUATION MAINTENANCE THERAPY

There are two critical questions that may be asked about continuation therapy: (1) After drug-induced remission of symptomatology, is continuation therapy really required? (2) Assuming that continuation therapy is required, how long should it continue and at what dosage?

Is Continuation Therapy Required?

Research findings strongly support the need for continuation therapy. A number of studies[4–9] demonstrate that patients often relapse when treatment is discontinued as soon as apparent remission is obtained. Table 5-1 shows the results of placebo-controlled studies of continuation therapy. In each of these studies, an antidepressant was used to control acute symptomatology. After symptomatology was successfully controlled, approximately half of the patients were switched to placebo and the other half continued to receive active medication. Patients were observed for three to eight months. The high relapse rate for patients receiving placebo illustrates their continued vulnerability for months after apparent recovery. Most relapses on placebo occurred relatively

Table 5-1
Continuation Therapy Studies

Investigators	Treatments	N	Relapse Rate (%)
Seagar and Bird[4]	Imipramine	12	17
	Placebo	16	69*
Mindham et al[5]	Amitriptyline or Imipramine	50	22
	Placebo	42	50*
Prien et al[6]	Lithium	45	27
	Imipramine	38	37*†
	Placebo	39	67
Klerman et al[7]	Amitriptyline	50	12
	Placebo/No Pill	49	29*
Coppen et al[8]	Amitriptyline	13	0
	Placebo	16	31*
Stein et al[9]	Amitriptyline	29	28
	Placebo	26	69*
Total	Active Drug	237	22
	Placebo/No Pill	188	50*

*$P < 0.05$ by Fisher's exact probability test.
†Lithium vs. Placebo $P < 0.05$.
Imipramine vs. Placebo $P < 0.05$.
Lithium vs. Imipramine P = N.S.

soon after withdrawal of active medication, usually within two to three months.

Studies also support the need for continuation pharmacotherapy after treatment with electroconvulsive therapy. Both antidepressants[4,10,11] and lithium[11,12] are reported to be effective in reducing the incidence of relapse after electroconvulsive therapy-induced recovery.

It is possible that patients who relapse after discontinuation of antidepressants or electroconvulsive therapy may be manifesting a new episode rather than a continuation of the old episode. However, this is probably not the case with most patients. Most relapses occur relatively rapidly after withdrawal of medication, generally within a few weeks. Also, reemergence of symptoms after withdrawal of medication seems to be independent of the patient's prior course of illness. Patients with long intervals between episodes relapse as quickly as patients with relatively short intervening periods of recovery.[13]

Duration of Continuation Therapy

Ideally, continuation therapy should be maintained for as long as the episode is expected to last. However, as mentioned previously, if continuation therapy is effective in suppressing symptomatology, it may be difficult to determine when the episode is over.

The timing of withdrawal of medication is of no small importance. Antidepressant drugs may produce uncomfortable and potentially dangerous cardiovascular or anticholinergic side effects. Lithium therapy may lead to a variety of adverse reactions, including fine hand tremor, weight gain, and renal complications. The teratogenic effects of lithium necessitate extreme caution in treatment of women of child-bearing age.

The literature is of only limited help in estimating length of episodes. Studies of the natural course of depressive illness[14] indicate that the duration of episodes tends to remain constant or lengthen slightly with each new episode. Thus, the length of the prior episode may serve as the lower estimate of the length of the next episode. There is one problem: effective drug treatment of the prior episode may make the episode appear shorter than it was.

Work with biological variables such as rapid eye movement sleep activity,[15] level of cortisol secretion,[16] dexamethasone suppression,[17,18] thyroid-stimulating hormone (TSH) blunting,[19] and other measures of neuroendocrine secretory patterns ultimately may provide the clinician with a biological marker of episode length. The most promising work has been done with the dexamethasone suppression test (DST). In many depressed patients, the daily secretion of cortisol is significantly elevated, and the usual pattern of diurnal variation is altered. The DST is an easily applied test for this aberrant pattern of secretion. Abnormal "early escape" from cortisol suppression after an overnight DST may appear in 25% to 67% of patients with primary major depression.[16,18,20] This abnormal dexamethasone suppression continues throughout the episode. As the patient recovers, the DST tends to revert to normal. In patients receiving antidepressant drugs, the DST may be a better indicator of episode length than clinical symptomatology. Several small sample uncontrolled trials[18,21–25] report that return of a normal dexamethasone suppression pattern indicates that it is safe to discontinue antidepressant drug therapy. This finding requires confirmation. Abnormal dexamethasone suppression is also reported to be specific to endogenous or melancholic depression,[17,18] a finding that has led some clinicians to suggest that the DST be used during continuation therapy to differentiate between patients whose remaining symptoms reflect situational or psychosocial problems and those with a continuing endogenous process.[24]

TSH blunting is another promising indicator of episode length. A blunted TSH response to thyrotropin-releasing hormone (TRH) infusion is reported in 25% to 64% of patients with endogenous depression.[19,26–28] Kirkegaard and co-workers[29,30] claim that in patients being treated with antidepressants TSH response to TRH infusion is a better indicator of episode length than overt clinical symptomatology. These investigators report that changes in growth hormone and prolactin response to TRH infusion also may be accurate markers of episode length in selected patients.[31] A recent report[32] indicates that upward of 80% of patients with primary unipolar depression may show either an abnormal DST or TSH blunting, suggesting that a combination of the two tests may cover the majority of patients with major depression.

Another clue for determining when continuation therapy can be withdrawn is provided by preliminary results from a five-hospital collaborative study on maintenance drug therapy in depression coordinated at the National Institute of Mental Health (NIMH).[13] Patients were admitted to the study during a major depressive episode which was treated by the physician's choice. Once acute symptomatology was controlled, patients received continuation therapy with imipramine plus lithium. After at least 10 weeks of clinical stability on the drug combination, patients were randomly assigned to long-term treatment with one of several regimens, including placebo and continuation of imipramine plus lithium. During the first three months of long-term treatment, 39% of the placebo-treated patients relapsed, compared with only 6% of the patients who continued to receive imipramine plus lithium. In the placebo-treated group, the probability of relapse was related to the length of time the patient had been symptom free before discontinuation of active medication (Table 5-2).

Table 5-2
NIMH Collaborative Study

		Weeks Symptom Free*				
Treatment Group		*1–5*	*6–10*	*11–15*	*Over 15*	*Total*
Placebo	N	10	7	8	8	33
	Relapsed†	80%	43%	13%	13%	39%
Lithium +	N	10	8	11	6	35
Imipramine	Relapsed	0%	0%	9%	17%	6%

*Based on Raskin severity of depression scale[33] and global assessment scale.[34]
†Relapse rate: By treatment group and length of symptom-free period preceding withdrawal of continuation therapy.

Sixty-five percent of the placebo-treated patients who had been symptom free for less than 10 weeks relapsed, compared with only 13% who had been symptom free for more than 10 weeks ($P < 0.05$ by Fisher's exact probability test). Corresponding figures for the group that continued to receive active medication were 0% and 12%, respectively, ($P > 0.05$). Most of the patients who manifested symptomatology during the 10 weeks preceding drug withdrawal had only mildly severe symptoms on clinical rating scales.

The preliminary findings from the NIMH study suggest that every attempt should be made to continue treatment until symptoms have been absent for two or three months. The often-cited practice of routinely maintaining patients on continuation therapy for six to nine months may unnecessarily prolong treatment for many patients. The results also indicate the need for focusing upon mild as well as moderate and severe symptomatology in determining continued need for medication.

Findings from the NIMH study correspond to those reported from a multihospital study conducted by the Medical Research Council in England.[5] Patients with residual symptomatology at the time of withdrawal of continuation therapy had a significantly higher relapse rate than patients who showed no symptomatology before withdrawal. The study report did not specify the nature of the residual symptomatology other than to state that it was present only on patient self-assessment scales. Depressive pathology recorded on psychiatric interview scales did not differentiate between relapsed and nonrelapsed patients.

Dosage of Continuation Therapy

There is considerable variability among clinicians in dosage strategies employed during continuation therapy. There are three general strategies: (a) dosage is maintained at the therapeutic level (ie, the level used during acute treatment) throughout the continuation phase; (b) dosage is reduced to a fixed level (often to 50% of the therapeutic level) that is maintained for the duration of continuation therapy; and (c) dosage is reduced in graduated steps over a period of months, with a rapid dosage buildup at the first sign of symptomatology. A key issue is whether patients require the full therapeutic dose to maintain control over the episode or can remain stable with lower maintenance levels. Some clinicians argue that the dose employed during continuation treatment is not as critical as the ability of the physician to recognize and identify signs of reemerging depression. They contend that relapses that occur at reduced dose levels of a previously effective regimen are reversed within a few days when the dose is increased – in contrast to the two to four weeks required for therapeutic effect when the drugs are first administered.[35] However, a review of maintenance drug therapy by Coppen and Peet[36] argues that there is no evidence for using low doses during continuation therapy and that the maintenance dose should be similar to that employed during acute treatment. Clearly, there is need for further research on these strategies.

LONG-TERM PREVENTIVE MAINTENANCE THERAPY

There are six critical questions that may be asked about long-term preventive therapy: (1) Who should receive treatment? (2) What drug should be used? (3) What dosage should be employed? (4) How long should treatment be administered? (5) What is the role of maintenance treatment in chronic depression? (6) Are there alternatives to continuous drug treatment?

Who Should Receive Treatment?

In clinical practice, the physician must consider four factors in determining whether to treat a patient with long-term preventive drug therapy: (a) the likelihood of a recurrence in the near future; (b) the potential impact of the recurrence on the patient, family, job, and therapeutic relationship; (c) the patient's willingness to commit himself or herself to a program of indefinite maintenance treatment; and (d) the presence of possible medical contraindications to long-term treatment.

Most clinicians feel that there should be at least two or three well-defined episodes requiring psychiatric treatment before a patient is treated with long-term preventive therapy. Patients who have had only a single attack, mild attacks, or a long interval between episodes (eg, over five years) should probably not receive long-term treatment. The exception is the patient for whom a second episode would be life threatening or highly disruptive to career or family functioning. There are supportive data for using long-term preventive treatment after two episodes. Surveys on the natural course of depressive illness[37-39] clearly demonstrates the relationship between episode frequency and risk of recurrence. Cycle length (the period between the onset of one episode and the onset of the next) tends to decrease with successive episodes through the first four or five episodes (Table 5-3). The average cycle length ranges from 33–37 months for the first cycle to 20–22 months for the second, and 11–13 months for

Table 5-3
Relationship Between Number of Episodes and Mean Cycle Length

Number of Episodes	Mean Cycle Length (Mos.)	
	Unipolar	*Bipolar*
1	37	33
2	22	20
3	18	16
4	13	13
5	13	11
6	12	11
7	11	10
8	11	11
9	9	9
10	9	8

Adapted from Angst J, Baastrup P, Hippius W, et al: The course of monopolar depression and bipolar psychoses. *Psychiatr Neurol Neurochir* 1973;76:489–500.

the fifth. The progressive decrease in cycle length is attributed to a shortening of the period between episodes rather than to a decrease in the duration of the episode. These findings suggest that patients with two or more episodes are at high risk for an early recurrence and might be suitable candidates for preventive pharmacotherapy.

In an interesting utilization of survey data, Grof and co-workers[40] examined the relationship between frequency of prior episodes and risk of recurrence for patients not treated with maintenance medication. The purpose was to use the survey data to develop guidelines for the selection of appropriate patients for long-term preventive therapy. Whenever a patient met the criterion of two episodes within two years, the number of episodes in the successive two years was counted. The number of episodes was also tabulated for a random sample of patients who did not meet the criterion. Patients were considered a good choice for long-term maintenance treatment if they had one or more recurrences during the successive two years. Using a bipolar sample, the investigators found a specificity of 65% and a sensitivity of 40% (specificity is the percentage of patients who met the criterion and had a recurrence; sensitivity is the percentage who did not meet the criterion and did not have a recurrence). With a unipolar sample, specificity was 47% and sensitivity was 74%. The moderately low sensitivity with bipolar patients and low specificity with unipolar patients indicate the problem in translating findings from surveys to the individual patient. Nonetheless, this approach for developing more precise patient selection criteria is promising. The investigators are developing a "combined selection procedure" that will incorporate other history factors that are significantly correlated with risk of recurrence (eg, age at onset of first episode and length of the prior free interval). The inclusion of the additional factors may increase the specificity and selectivity of the selection procedure.

Choice of Drug

Thus far, the choice of a drug for long-term preventive therapy is limited to lithium or a tricyclic antidepressant. Other drugs have not been adequately evaluated in this capacity. Studies evaluating the effectiveness of lithium and the antidepressants are summarized in Table 5-4.

Lithium is the recommended long-term treatment for bipolar disorder. Studies indicate that lithium is significantly superior to placebo in treating the bipolar patient.[6,41–45] Imipramine, the only antidepressant to be evaluated in bipolar illness, has demonstrated little effectiveness against manic attacks.[44] Two multihospital collaborative studies[6,46] report that lithium, imipramine, and amitriptyline are equally effective with unipolar patients and that all three treatments are more effective than placebo. Other studies

Table 5-4
Long-Term Maintenance Therapy Studies

		Unipolar		Bipolar	
Investigators	Treatment	*N*	*Relapse Rate (%)*	*N*	*Relapse Rate (%)*
Baastrup et al[41]	Lithium	17	0	28	0
	Placebo	17	53*	22	55*
Coppen et al[42]	Lithium	11	9	17	18
	Placebo	15	80*	21	100*
Cundall et al[43]	Lithium	4	75	12	33
	Placebo	4	50	12	83*
Prien et al[44]	Lithium			101	43
	Placebo			104	80*
Prien et al[6]	Lithium	27	48	18	28
	Imipramine	25	48*	13	77
	Placebo	26	92	13	77
Fieve et al[45]	Lithium	14	57	17	59
	Placebo	14	64	18	94*
Coppen et al[47]	Lithium	12	25		
	Maprotiline	8	75*		
Coppen et al[48]	Lithium	15	0		
	Mianserin	13	54*		
Kane et al[49]	Lithium			38	21
	Lithium + Imipramine			37	32
Quitkin et al[50]	Lithium	11	27		
	Imipramine	11	73		
	Lithium + Imipramine	14	14*		
	Placebo	13	85		
Glen et al[46]	Lithium†	12	33		
	Amitriptyline†	7	57*		
	Placebo†	9	89		
	Lithium‡	56	64		
	Amitriptyline‡	47	65		

*$P < 0.05$ by Fisher's exact probability test.
†Patients had one prior episode.
‡Patients had two or more prior episodes.

report that lithium is more effective than imipramine,[47] maprotiline,[43] and mianserin.[44] Neither lithium nor the antidepressants are presently approved by the Food and Drug Administration for the long-term preventive treatment of unipolar illness.

The issue of the effectiveness of lithium and the tricyclic antidepressants for the long-term preventive treatment of affective disorders is a subject of debate. Neither lithium nor the antidepressants are approved for this indication by the FDA. The FDA contends there is a need for further systematic study. Some clinicians disagree, at least with respect to lithium, and argue that available evidence is sufficient to justify the use of lithium for the long-term preventive treatment of unipolar disorder. An interesting discussion of this issue is provided in back-to-back articles by Schou,[47a] who recommends the preventive use of lithium for unipolar illness, and by this author,[47b] who contends that the issue is far from settled.

There is obvious need for evaluating the long-term efficacy of drugs other than lithium and the tricyclic antidepressants. There are no controlled studies of long-term maintenance therapy with monoamine oxidase inhibitors, even in populations that are known to respond therapeutically to the drugs. Carbamazepine, which is reported to produce good results in bipolar patients who fail to respond to lithium,[51] has not yet been studied on a long-term basis. Newer antidepressants such as amoxapine, buproprion, maprotiline, mianserin, and trazodone also require careful evaluation of their effectiveness as long-term preventive treatments. Reports of reduced risk of cardiovascular and anticholinergic side effects and lowered risk of lethal effects from overdosage with some of the newer antidepressants[52–54] may make them particularly attractive alternatives to the standard tricyclic antidepressants for long-term administration.

In choosing a drug for long-term maintenance treatment, there should be realistic expectations about what the medication can achieve. Neither lithium nor the tricyclic antidepressants are panaceas for recurrent affective disorders. Failure rates for lithium in bipolar populations and for lithium and imipramine in unipolar populations average 30% to 40%. The failure rate tends to increase significantly where there is a history of rapid cycling, poor compliance in taking medication, or atypical features such a formal thought disorder, mood incongruent delusions or hallucinations, and depressive withdrawn personality.[55–58] Even with responsive patients, there is question as to whether lithium and the antidepressants actually prevent the occurrence of major episodes or merely dampen the episode sufficiently to prevent a full attack. Research findings[59,60] suggest that the drugs may act in both ways, depending upon the individual case. Also, studies on lithium and the antidepressants have focused primarily on patients with histories of severe and frequent episodes. The "typical" study patient has a history of at least two episodes of major depression or mania during the two to three years preceding the study and a lifetime incidence of five or more episodes. The effectiveness of long-term preventive drug therapy with patients who have less frequent and severe episodes has not been adequately studied.

Side effects may also influence choice of drug for long-term maintenance treatment. Most studies of maintenance antidepressant drug therapy do not report the frequency of side effects or their impact on the course of treatment. Two studies that report on the incidence of side effects during maintenance treatment with antidepressants indicate that adverse reactions may persist during long-term treatment. Coppen et al[47] reported that 6 of 18 patients treated with maprotiline were dropped from the study within an average of 12 weeks because of side effects. Prien et al[6] reported that 53% of imipramine-treated unipolar patients experienced side effects during long-term maintenance therapy; the most common adverse reactions were dry mouth, muscle weakness, constipation, and somnolence. Constipation was a particular problem with older patients, resulting in a number of patients withdrawing from the study.

Studies with lithium report frequent and persistent adverse reactions during long-term treatment. The most frequent are fine hand tremor, polyuria and polydipsia, and weight gain; 30% to 60% of patients treated with lithium on a long-term basis experience one or more of these reactions.[61-63] Occasionally, there may be dermatologic reactions such as acne, allergic skin reactions, or aggravation of psoriasis. A small proportion of patients may develop hypothyroidism with or without goiter. Occasional patients may also experience difficulties in concentration and memory.

Within recent years, studies reporting possible renal complications with lithium have generated considerable interest in the long- term effects of lithium treatment on kidney structure and function. Microscopy of kidney samples has revealed structural changes in some lithium-treated patients.[64-67] The significance and frequency of these changes are not known. Although a number of recent studies have failed to demonstrate a relationship between lithium treatment and renal damage,[68-70] the issue is unlikely to be settled until the results of ongoing prospective studies are available. Reports also suggest that lithium-induced nephrogenic diabetes insipidus may persist for many months (perhaps indefinitely) after cessation of lithium treatment.[71-73] However, the incidence of a persistent defect in renal concentrating ability is unknown; existing studies have not ruled out the possible contributions of other factors to the disorder (eg, other psychopharmacologic agents and concurrent medical illness), nor is it certain that the defect is truly irreversible. Since the studies available to date are not definitive and, at worst, suggest that only a small minority of patients develop renal insufficiency, fear of renal effects should not deter the clinician from employing lithium for appropriate clinical indications.

Dosage

There is no well-defined dosage strategy for long-term preventive therapy. Lithium is the best studied of the long-term drug treatments.

The maintenance dose guidelines specified in the lithium package insert (0.6 to 1.2 mEq/L)[74] are based mainly on the trial and error experiences of individual investigators. Some sources recommend a higher minimum level (0.7 to 0.8 mEq/L),[75-77] whereas others advocate more conservative levels (0.4 to 0.6 mEq/L).[78-80] The reports of structural renal damage in lithium-treated patients have contributed to the movement toward lower maintenance doses.

In a provocative trial designed to determine minimum effective plasma levels for long-term maintenance therapy, Jerram and McDonald[79] found that levels below 0.5 mEq/L were just as effective as levels exceeding 0.7 mEq/L. A follow-up study indicated that the relapse rate does not increase until plasma levels fall below 0.4 mEq/L.[81] Although these findings require confirmation, they have implications for long-term management of lithium-treated patients. The need for a minimum effective dose will be even more critical if morphological renal changes or seriously impaired renal function is found to be related to total lithium dosage.

It is difficult to ascertain what doses of lithium are used by practitioners. There are no published survey data on the dosage schedules employed in clinical practice. Informal inquiries by the author to several "lithium clinics" and "affective disorders units" in the United States suggest that the majority of clinicians use target levels of 0.6 to 0.8 mEq/L for maintenance treatment. Lower levels are usually reserved for elderly patients, patients with compromised renal or cardiovascular function and patients who have a history of troublesome side effects at levels as high as 0.6 mEq/L. Higher levels are generally used with patients who have a documented history of failure at lower levels.

There are even more uncertainties with dosage for the tricyclic antidepressants. There are no established dosage guidelines or plasma level ranges for long-term preventive therapy with the tricyclic-antidepressants. Most experienced clinicians usually maintain patients on a dose equivalent to 75 to 150 mg of imipramine per day. Clinicians who maintain patients on lower levels (eg, 25 to 50 mg per day) often do so with the expectation of rapidly increasing dosage at the first sign of symptomatology. The value of this strategy has not been adequately studied.

Plasma level measures of antidepressant drugs may be useful during maintenance treatment to evaluate patient compliance in taking medication. Loo and co-workers[82] obtained the plasma levels of several tricyclic antidepressants over a 3- to 26-month period and found that good response was associated with small fluctuations in plasma levels over time, whereas poor outcome was associated with large fluctuations (usually due to poor patient compliance). Thus, the variability of plasma levels over time may be of use in identifying patients who are at high risk for poor response due to noncompliance in taking medication.

Duration of Treatment

A critical decision facing the practitioner is how long to continue long-term maintenance treatment with pharmacologic treatments. There is evidence that recurrences may cease spontaneously after a number of years of illness. A survey by Angst[83] indicates that one of three unipolar patients and one of eight bipolar patients over 65 years of age stop having episodes. This suggests that patients with a long duration of illness who have been free of abnormal mood swings for several years may no longer require medication. However, the only way to determine whether the patient still needs long-term preventive therapy is to discontinue treatment. In determining whether to discontinue treatment, the physician and patient should consider the likelihood and potential consequences of a new episode and balance this against the risks involved in continuing medication. Patients with a history of attacks characterized by suicide attempts, need for hospitalization, or serious disruption of career or family life should be taken off medication only if there is reasonable assurance that subsequent episodes can be detected early enough to prevent development of serious symptomatology. Schou[84] recommends an arrangement in which patient and physician agree to continue drug treatment for a specific period (eg, four or five years). After this period, they discuss whether treatment should be stopped, taking into account the course of illness before and during treatment.

Chronic Depression

Most of the studies on long-term maintenance therapy have used patients who have a history of well-defined episodes with intervening periods of good recovery. There has been no well-controlled maintenance drug therapy study directed specifically at patients who have a history of chronic depression or frequent subacute mood swings (depressive or cyclothymic). This is not an insignificant population. It is estimated that 20% to 35% of patients who have major depressive episodes have a chronic course with mild or moderate symptomatology and social impairment.[85-87] Keller and Shapiro[86] have coined the term "double depression" to represent the state in which a major depressive episode is superimposed upon an underlying chronic depression. Some chronic depressions have an early onset (in adolescence or childhood) and develop in the context of significant neurotic or characterological pathology.[88] Other patients may develop a chronic course after an acute major depression; this chronicity may represent either an incomplete remission of the episode or a previously unrecognized chronic condition that worsened during the acute depression.

Research on the treatment of chronic disorders has been relatively neglected in the preoccupation with the treatment and prevention of acute episodes, despite evidence that patients with the disorders are highly vulnerable to episodes of major depression. About 75% develop a major depression at some point in their lives.[88] Also, patients with a superimposed major depression tend to relapse at a significantly higher rate after recovery from the acute episode than do patients without superimposed depression.[86] A few studies report symptomatic improvement in chronic depression during short-term antidepressant drug therapy,[89–91] but provide little information on the effectiveness of maintenance treatment in modifying the long-term course of the illness. Some investigators[92–94] report that the combination of pharmacotherapy and psychotherapy is effective in reducing both symptomatology and social impairment in chronic disorders. However, the combination has not been evaluated in systematic fashion over a prolonged period. There is need for carefully controlled studies to evaluate the responsiveness of both the acute and chronic components of the illness to various modalities of treatment in comparison with the response of patients with only episodic or only chronic depressive disorders.

Alternatives to Continuous Drug Treatment

The reports of structural renal damage, teratogenic effects, and other complications associated with lithium therapy have rekindled interest in an old alternative to continuous maintenance treatment. Over the past decade, several investigators[95–98] have suggested that depressive recurrences can be prevented or attenuated by carefully observing the untreated patient and rapidly initiating treatment at the first sign of an emerging episode. This procedure is being utilized in several clinics in the United States and Europe. Thus far, there is little feedback on the success of these efforts.

There are obvious limitations to an approach that substitutes continuous surveillance for continuous medication. One limitation is that it requires well-motivated patients, preferably ones with well-motivated and observant families who can be relied upon to contact the clinician at the first sign of symptomatology. Ancillary family education geared toward prevention of recurrence is an important aid to the program. Another limitation is that the episode may develop too quickly for the clinician to initiate an effective medication program. Also, it may require several weeks for the medication to achieve its full effect, whereas an increase in dosage of an ongoing maintenance regimen might be effective in a much shorter period. The latter consideration, if true, would suggest that a homeopathic dose that can be built up quickly in event of a recurrence might be a viable treatment strategy.

On the positive side, there are several reasons for considering alternatives to continuous drug treatment. First, there is the ever-present risk of adverse reactions and medical complications with prolonged use of psychopharmacological agents. Second, continuous drug therapy, especially with antidepressants, can be quite expensive. Third, in the absence of guidelines on how long treatment should be continued, many clinicians keep patients on medication indefinitely, even though some patients eventually stop having recurrences. There is no way of identifying these patients while they are still on maintenance medication.

IMPLICATIONS FOR RESEARCH

There has been relatively little systematic evaluation of strategies for maintenance drug therapy. There is need for carefully controlled studies to establish meaningful guidelines for selection of patients and choice of drug, dosage, and duration of treatment. There is particular need to identify patients who might benefit from long-term preventive drug therapy. It is clear that lithium and antidepressants can reduce the morbidity associated with recurrent affective disorders. However, there are questions about who should receive long-term treatment, what dosage should be employed, and when, if ever, long-term treatment can be discontinued. Alternatives to continuous medication should be evaluated to determine what patients might benefit from these programs. The dosage and duration of continuation therapy also requires careful study to assure that patients receive adequate but not excessive treatment. The possible use of measures such as escape from dexamethasone suppression, TSH blunting, and shift in rapid eye movement activity in determining length of continuation therapy is a particularly promising area of study. Another promising lead comes from preliminary findings from an NIMH collaborative study on maintenance drug therapy which indicates that it is safe to withdraw continuation treatment after two to three months of symptom-free behavior.

Studies of long-term preventive therapy have focused primarily on the effectiveness of drugs in preventing or attenuating major recurrences. Little attention has been paid to the functioning of patients between major episodes. The effect of lithium and the antidepressants on the chronic mood disturbance, frequent mood swings, and impairment of social functioning manifested by many patients with recurrent major affective disorders has not been adequately assessed. There should be greater emphasis on measures of social, vocational, and family adjustment, personality functioning, and psychosocial stress to complement the measures of psychopathology heavily emphasized in most studies. The value of combining psychotherapeutic approaches with drug therapy should also be explored. Claims that psychotherapy is more effective than pharmacotherapy in treating "characterologic depressions" and impairment in social functioning, whereas drugs are more effective in preventing or attenuating major recurrences,[90,93,99] require verification in long-term trials.

Finally, we need to know more about how drug maintenance therapies are used in clinical practice. We know very little about what types of patients are treated with maintenance pharmacotherapy, what dosage schedules are used, how long treatment is maintained, and what proportion of patients stop treatment. There is little available information on the decision-making process involved in assigning and withdrawing patients from maintenance drug programs. This information would be valuable, not only in defining relevant research areas, but also in establishing guidelines for the proper use of antidepressants and lithium in maintenance therapy. If nothing else, an adequate survey would help delineate problems that may not be receiving adequate attention in the psychopharmacologic literature.

REFERENCES

1. Nystrom S: Depressions: Factors related to 10 year prognosis. *Acta Psychiatr Scand* 1979;60:225–238.
2. Winokur G, Clayton P, Reich T: *Manic-Depressive Disease.* St. Louis, CV Mosby Co, 1969.
3. Murphy CE: Clinical identification of suicidal risk. *Arch Gen Psychiatry* 1972;27:356–359.
4. Seager CP, Bird RL: Imipramine with electrical treatment in depression—a controlled trial. *J Ment Sci* 1962;108:704–707.
5. Mindham RH, Howland C, Shepherd M: An evaluation of continuation therapy with tricyclic antidepressants in depressive illness. *Psychol Med* 1973;3:5–17.
6. Prien RF, Klett CH, Caffey EM: Lithium carbonate and imipramine in prevention of affective episodes. *Arch Gen Psychiatry* 1973;29:420–425.
7. Klerman GL, DiMascio A, Weissman M, et al: Treatment of depression by drugs and psychotherapy. *Am J Psychiatry* 1974;131:186–191.
8. Coppen A, Montgomery S, Rao V, et al: Continuation therapy with amitriptyline in depression. *Br J Psychiatry* 1978;133:28–33.
9. Stein MK, Rickels K, Weisse C: Maintenance therapy with amitriptyline: A controlled trial. *Am J Psychiatry* 1980;137:370–371.
10. Imlah NW, Ryan E, Harrington J: The influence of antidepressant drugs in the response to electroconvulsive therapy and subsequent response rates. *J Neuropsychopharmacol* 1965;4:439–442.
11. Perry A, Tsuang MT: Treatment of unipolar depression following electroconvulsive therapy. *J Affective Discord* 1979;1:123–129.
12. Coppen A, Abou-Saleh MT, Milliv P, et al: Lithium continuation therapy following electroconvulsive therapy. *Br J Psychiatry* 1981;139:284–287.
13. Prien RF, Kupfer DJ, Mansky PM, et al: Continuation therapy in depression: Preliminary findings from the National Institute of Mental Health-Pharmacologic and Somatic Treatments Research Branch Collaborative Study of Long-Term Maintenance Drug Therapy in Affective Illness.

Presented at the 19th Annual Meeting of the American College of Neuropsychopharmacology. San Juan, December 16–18, 1980.
14. Grof P, Angst J, Haines T: The clinical course of depression: Practical issues, in Angst J (ed): *Classification and Prediction of Outcome in Depression.* Berlin, Springer Verlag, 1974, pp 141–147.
15. Kupfer DJ: Sleep and neuroendocrine abnormalities in affective disorders: New findings. Presented at the 19th Annual Meeting of the American College of Neuropsychopharmacology, San Juan, December 16–18, 1980.
16. Carroll BJ: Neuroendocrine function in psychiatric disorders, in Lipton MA, DiMascio A, Killam KF (eds): *Psychopharmacology: A Generation of Progress.* New York, Raven Press, 1978, pp 487–497.
17. Brown W: The 24-hour dexamethasone suppression test in a clinical setting: Relationship in diagnosis, symptoms and response to treatment. *Am J Psychiatry* 1979;136:413–423.
18. Carroll BJ: The dexamethasone suppression test for melancholia. *Br J Psychiatry,* in press.
19. Kirkegaard C, Smith E: Continuation therapy in endogenous depression controlled by changes in the TRH stimulation test. *Psychol Med* 1978;8:501–503.
20. Schlesser MA, Winokur G, Sherman BM: Genetic subtypes of unipolar primary depressive illness distinguished by hypothalamic pituitary-adrenal axis activity. *Lancet* 1979;1:739–741.
21. Amsterdam JD, Winokur A, Caroff S: Dexamethasone suppression test as a prognostic tool: Two case reports. *Am J Psychiatry* 1981;138:979–980.
22. Gold MS, Pottash ALC, Extein I, et al: Dexamethasone suppression tests in depression and response to treatment (letter to editor). *Lancet* 1980;1:1190.
23. Goldberg IK: Dexamethasone suppression test as indicator of safe withdrawal of antidepressant therapy (letter to editor). *Lancet* 1980;2:376.
24. Greden TF, Albala AA, Haskett RF, et al: Normalization of dexamethasone test: A laboratory index of recovery from endogenous depression. *Biol Psychiatry* 1980;15:449–458.
25. Greden JF, DeVigne JP, Kronfol A, et al: Dexamethasone suppression test classifications and prediction of treatment response. Presented at the 3rd World Congress of Biological Psychiatry. Stockholm, June 1981.
26. Extein I, Pottash AC, Gold MS: TRH test in depression. *N Engl J Med* 1980;302:923–924.
27. Prange AJ, Wilson IC, Lara OO, et al: Effects of thyrotropin-releasing hormone in depression. *Lancet* 1972;2:999–1002.
28. Whybrow PC, Prange AJ: A hypothesis of thyroid-catecholamine receptor interaction: Its relevance to affective illness. *Arch Gen Psychiatry* 1981;38: 106–113.
29. Kirkegaard C: The thyrotropin response to thyrotropin-releasing hormone in endogenous depression. *Psychoneuroendocrinology* 1981;6:189–212.
30. Kirkegaard C, Norlem N, Birk-Lauridsen U, et al: Prognostic value of thyrotropin-releasing hormone stimulation test in endogenous depression. *Acta Psychiatr Scand* 1975;52:170–177.
31. Kirkegaard C, Eskildsen PC, Bjorum N: Parallel changes of the responses of thyrotropin growth hormone and prolactin to thyrotropin-releasing hormone in endogenous depression. *Psychoneuroendocrinology* 1981;6: 253–259.
32. Gold MS, Pottash AC, Extein I, et al: Diagnosis of depression in the 1980's. *JAMA* 1981;245:1562–1564.
33. Raskin A, Schulterbrandt J, Reatig N, et al: Replication of factors of psychopathology in interview, ward behavior and self-report ratings of

hospitalized depressives. *J Nerv Ment Dis* 1969;148:87–98.
34. Endicott J, Spitzer RL, Fleiss JL, et al: The global assessment scale: A procedure for measuring overall severity of psychiatric disturbance. *Arch Gen Psychiatry* 1976;33:766–771.
35. Hollister LE: *Clinical Pharmacology of Psychotherapeutic Drugs.* New York, Churchill Livingstone, 1978.
36. Coppen A, Peet M: The long-term management of patients with affective disorders, in Paykel ES, Coppen A (eds): *Psychopharmacology of Affective Disorders.* New York, Oxford University Press, 1979, pp 248–256.
37. Angst J, Baastrup P, Hippius W, et al: The course of monopolar depression and bipolar psychoses. *Psychiatr Neurol Neurochir* 1973;76:489–500.
38. Perris C: The course of depressive psychoses. *Acta Psychiatr Scand* 1968;44: 238–248.
39. Zis AP, Goodwin FK: Major affective disorder as a recurrent illness: A critical review. *Arch Gen Psychiatry* 1979;36:835–839.
40. Grof P, Angst J, Karasek M, et al: Patient selection for long-term lithium treatment in clinical practice. *Arch Gen Psychiatry* 1979;894–897.
41. Baastrup PC, Poulson JC, Schou M, et al: Prophylactic lithium: Double-blind discontinuation in manic-depressive and recurrent disorders. *Lancet* 1970;2:326–330.
42. Coppen A, Noguera R, Bailey J, et al: Prophylactic lithium in affective disorders. *Lancet* 1971;2:275–279.
43. Cundall RL, Brooks PW, Murray LG: Controlled evaluation of lithium prophylaxis in affective disorders. *Psychol Med* 1972;3:308–311.
44. Prien RF, Caffey EM, Klett CF: Prophylactic efficacy of lithium carbonate in manic-depressive illness. *Arch Gen Psychiatry* 1973;28:337–341.
45. Fieve RR, Kumbarachi T, Dunner DL: Lithium prophylaxis of depression in bipolar I, bipolar II and unipolar patients. *Am J Psychiatry* 1976;133: 925–929.
46. Glen AIM, Johnson AL, Shepherd M: Continuation therapy with lithium and amitriptyline in unipolar depressive illness: A controlled clinical trial. *Psychol Med* 1981;11:409–416.
47. Coppen A, Montgomery SA, Gupta RK, et al: A double-blind comparison of lithium carbonate and maprotiline in the prophylaxis of the affective disorders. *Br J Psychiatry* 1976;128:479–485.
47a. Schou M: Lithium as a prophylactic agent in unipolar affective illness. *Arch Gen Psychiatry* 1979;36:849–851.
47b. Prien RF: Lithium in the prophylactic treatment of affective disorders. *Arch Gen Psychiatry* 1979;36:847–848.
48. Coppen A, Chose K, Rao R: Mianserin and lithium in the prophylaxis of depression. *Br J Psychiatry* 1978;133:206–210.
49. Kane JM, Quitkin FM, Rifkin A, et al: Prophylactic lithium with and without imipramine for bipolar I patients: A double-blind study. *Psychopharmacol Bull* 1981;17:144–145.
50. Quitkin FM, Kane JM, Rifkin A, et al: Lithium and imipramine in the prophylaxis of unipolar and bipolar II depression: A prospective placebo-controlled comparison. *Psychopharmacol Bull* 1981;17:142–144.
51. Post RM: Efficacy of carbamazepine in manic-depressive illness: Implications for underlying mechanisms, in Post RM, Ballenger JC (eds): *Neurobiology of Mood Disorders.* Baltimore, The Williams & Wilkins Co, 1982.
52. Hollister LE: Second generation antidepressant drugs. *Psychosomatics* 1981; 22:872–879.
53. Feighner JP: Clinical efficacy of the newer antidepressants. *J Clin Psychiatry*

1981;1(Suppl):23–26.
54. Prien RF: A synopsis of the status of the new antidepressants. *Psychopharmacol Bull* 1981;17:10–11.
55. Ananth J: Predicting response to antidepressants: Demographic and personal history variables. *Psychosomatics* 1980;21:24–31.
56. Carroll BJ: Predictors of treatment outcome with lithium. *Arch Gen Psychiatry* 1979;36:870–878.
57. Kocsis JH, Stokes PE: Lithium maintenance factors affecting outcome. *Am J Psychiatry* 1979;136:563–566.
58. Prien RF, Caffey EM, Klett CJ: Factors associated with treatment success in lithium carbonate prophylaxis. *Arch Gen Psychiatry* 1974;31:189–192.
59. Kukopulos A, Reginaldi D, Giraldi P, et al: Course of manic-depressive recurrences under lithium. *Compr Psychiatry* 1975;16:517–524.
60. Schou M, Thomsen K: Prophylaxis of recurrent endogenous affective disorders, in Johnson FN (ed): *Lithium Research and Therapy.* London, Academic Press, 1975, pp 63–84.
61. Brown WT: The pattern of lithium side-effects and toxic reactions in the course of lithium therapy, in Johnson FN (ed): *Handbook of Lithium Therapy.* Lancaster, England, MTP Press Ltd, 1980, pp 279–288.
62. Schou M, Baastrup PC, Grof P, et al: Pharmacological and clinical problems of lithium prophylaxis. *Br J Psychiatry* 1970;116:615–619.
63. Vacaflor L: Lithium side effects and toxicity: The clinical picture, in Johnson FN (ed): *Lithium Research and Therapy.* London, Academic Press, 1975, pp 211–225.
64. Burrows GD, Davies B, Kincaid-Smith P: Unique tubular lesion after lithium. *Lancet* 1978;1:1310–1311.
65. Hestbech J, Hansen HE, Amdisen A, et al: Chronic renal lesions following long-term treatment with lithium. *Kidney Int* 1977;12:205–213.
66. Jenner FA: Lithium and the kidney, in Cooper TB, Gershon S, Kline NS (eds): *Lithium: Controversies and Unresolved Issues.* Amsterdam, Princeton, NJ, Excerpta Medica, 1979, pp 567–577.
67. Vestergaard P: Renal side effects of lithium, in Johnson FN (ed): *Handbook of Lithium Therapy.* Lancaster, England, MTP Press Ltd, 1980, pp 345–357.
68. Braden G, Amsterdam J, Gehab M, et al: A prospective study of lithium-induced neuropathy: Preliminary results, in Abstracts of the 14th Annual Meeting of the American Society of Nephrology. Thorofare, NJ, American Society of Nephrology 1981.
69. Lithium and the kidney: Grounds for cautious optimism (editorial). *Lancet* 1979;2:1056–1057.
70. Ramsey AT, Cox M: Lithium and the kidney. *Am J Psychiatry* 1982;139: 443–449.
71. Bucht G, Wahlin A: Renal concentrating capacity in long-term lithium treatment and after withdrawal of lithium. *Acta Med Scand* 1980;207:309–314.
72. Forrest JN: Lithium-induced polyuria: Cellular mechanisms and response to diuretics, in Cooper TB, Gershon S, Kline NS (eds): *Lithium: Controversies and Unresolved Issues.* Amsterdam, Princeton, NJ, Excerpta Medica, 1979, pp 632–641.
73. Rabin EZ, Garston RG, Weir RV, et al: Persistent nephrogenic diabetes insipidus associated with long-term lithium carbonate treatment. *Can Med Assoc J* 1979;121:194–198.
74. Lithium Carbonate Package Insert Prescribing Information for Eskalith (Smith, Kline and French Laboratories), Lithium Carbonate Capsules and Tablets (Phillips Roxane), and Pfi-Lith (Pfipharmecs), 1981.

75. Fieve RR: *Physician's Guide to Depression.* New York, PW Communications Inc, 1975.
76. Kerry RJ: Management of patients receiving lithium treatment, in Johnson FN (ed): *Lithium Research and Therapy.* London, Academic Press, 1975, pp 143–163.
77. Prien RF, Caffey EM: The relationship between dosage and response to prophylaxis. *Am J Psychiatry* 1976;133:567–570.
78. Brown W: The use of lithium carbonate in the treatment of mood disorders. *Can Med Assoc J* 1973;108:742–752.
79. Jerram TC, McDonald R: Plasma lithium control with particular reference to minimum effective levels, in Johnson FN, Johnson S (eds): *Lithium in Medical Practice.* Baltimore, University Park Press, 1978, pp 407–414.
80. Maletzky B, Blachly PH: *The Use of Lithium in Psychiatry.* Cleveland, Cleveland Rubber Company Press, 1971.
81. Hullin RP: Minimum serum lithium levels for effective prophylaxis, in Johnson FN (ed): *Handbook of Lithium Therapy.* Lancaster, England, MTP Press Ltd, 1980, pp 243–247.
82. Loo H, Benyacoub AK, Rovei V, et al: Long-term monitoring of tricyclic antidepressant plasma concentrations. *Br J Psychiatry* 1980;137:444–451.
83. Angst J: The course of affective disorders: II. Typology of bipolar manic-depressive illness. *Arch Psychiatr Nervenkr* 1978;226:65–73.
84. Schou M: *Lithium Treatment of Manic-Depressive Illness: A Practical Guide.* New York, S. Karger, 1980.
85. *Diagnostic and Statistical Manual of Mental Disorders.* ed 3. Washington, DC, American Psychiatric Association, 1980, p 216.
86. Keller MB, Shapiro RW: Double depression: Superimposition of acute depressive episodes on chronic depressive disorders. *Am J Psychiatry* 1982; 139:438–442.
87. Klerman GL: Other specific affective disorders, in Freedman AM, Kaplan HI, Adock BJ (eds): *Comprehensive Textbook of Psychiatry.* ed 3, vol 2. Baltimore, The Williams & Wilkins Co, 1980.
88. Weissman MM: Acute and chronic depressions and depressive personality. Presented at the Conference on Clinical Depressions: Diagnostic and Therapeutic Challenges. San Juan, December 10, 1979.
89. Akiskal HS, Rosenthal TL, Haykal RF, et al: Characterological depressions—clinical and sleep EEG findings separating subaffective dysthymias from character spectrum disorders. *Arch Gen Psychiatry* 1980;37:777–783.
90. Rounsaville BJ, Sholomskas D, Pruskoff BA: Chronic mood disorders in depressed outpatients. *J Affective Discord* 1980;2:73–88.
91. Ward, NG, Bloom VL, Friedel RO: The effectiveness of tricyclic antidepressants in chronic depression. *J Clin Psychiatry* 1979;40:49–52.
92. Akiskal HS, King D, Rosenthal TL, et al: Chronic depressions. Part I. Clinical and familial characteristics in 137 probands. *J Affective Discord* 1981;3:297–315.
93. DiMascio A, Weissman MM, Prusoff BA, et al: Differential symptom reduction by drugs and psychotherapy in acute depression. *Arch Gen Psychiatry* 1979;36:1450–1456.
94. Blackburn IM, Biship S, Glen AIM, et al: The efficacy of cognitive therapy in depression: A treatment trial using cognitive therapy and pharmacotherapy, each alone and in combination. *Br J Psychiatry* 1981;139:181–189.
95. Ayd FJ: Drug holidays during maintenance tricyclic antidepressant drug therapy. *Int Drug Ther Newsl* 1974;9:18–20.
96. Bech P, Vendsborg PB, Rafaelsen OJ: Lithium maintenance treatment: Its

role in the daily routine. *Acta Psychiatr Scand* 1976;53:70–81.

97. Fieve RR, Platman SR, Plutchik RR: The use of lithium in affective disorders. I. Prophylaxis of depression in chronic recurrent affective disorders. *Am J Psychiatry* 1968;125:492–498.
98. Quitkin F, Rifkin A, Klein DF: Prophylaxis of affective disorders. *Arch Gen Psychiatry* 1976;33:337–346.
99. Weissman MM: Psychotherapy and its relevance to the pharmacotherapy of affective disorders, in Lipton MA, DiMascio A, Killam KF (eds): *Psychopharmacology: A Generation of Progress.* New York, Raven Press, 1978, pp 1313–1321.

CHAPTER 6

SIDE EFFECTS OF DRUGS USED IN THE TREATMENT OF AFFECTIVE DISORDERS

SAMUEL G. SIRIS
ARTHUR RIFKIN

Side effects are pharmacological actions of drugs being used to treat a disorder. What makes them "side effects" is that they are unwanted effects. Generally these are not toxic effects—effects related to disproportionately elevated amounts of drug in the patient's system, or grossly exaggerated sensitivity of the patient's system to some aspect of the drug's action—although these two sets of effects are lumped together for purposes of discussion. Some side effects can be a danger to patients, but those most frequently encountered are merely annoying. Nevertheless, even annoying side effects may jeopardize the patient by undermining medication compliance and/or interfering with the patient's relationship with his or her physician, as well as creating morbidity in their own right.

Many side effects of drugs under consideration here may also be manifestations of depression. These include gastrointestinal symptoms (dry mouth, irregularities of swallowing, "nervous stomach" of various sorts, constipation), sleep disturbances (restless sleep, hypersomnolence, daytime fatigue), and symptoms associated with anxiety (abnormal perspiration, palpitations). Under these circumstances it can be difficult to determine clinically which symptoms are disease effects and which are drug effects. Scientifically, these issues may be resolved through the use of double-blind placebo trials. Clinically, the practitioner will regulate treatment best through a thorough knowledge of the patient's baseline clinical state, knowledge of the side effects of the drug in question, and knowledge of relevant aspects of the patient's personality (suggestibility, tendency toward hypochondriasis, etc). The clinician will also take advantage of known drug effects to be employed in a favorable manner in relationship to the patient's clinical state (ie, a nighttime dosage of an antidepressant with sedative properties for a depressed patient troubled by insomnia), so that in such a situation "side" effects are not undesirable effects at all, but useful adjuncts to the patient's overall management.

TRICYCLIC ANTIDEPRESSANTS

Most of the side effects of tricyclic antidepressant medications are due to their anticholinergic and adrenergic effects.[1-3] Individuals may vary considerably in their vulnerability to these side effects, in the ability of their autonomic nervous system to adapt to the changes, and in their general level of tolerance to the annoying nature of these effects. Usually the effects are most bothersome during the initial week or two of treatment. After that, many patients seem to adapt, either biologically or psychologically, and the side effects become less troublesome. Older patients do seem to be more vulnerable to these sorts of side effects, however, in part because they may metabolize the drugs more slowly and consequently have higher levels of antidepressants in their systems at a given dose, and in part because their autonomic nervous systems and physiology in general may lack the degree of plasticity and adaptive reserve of a younger individual.

Dry mouth is perhaps the most frequent complaint to be voiced by patients on tricyclic antidepressants, with estimates of its incidence ranging up to 50%.[3] Dental caries is a potential complication of reduced saliva, as is oral monaliasis and parotitis. These complications may be further promoted by the patient's tendency to keep a hard candy constantly in his mouth to counteract the dryness. Patients should be advised to chew sugarless gum instead, or synthetic saliva substitutes may be tried. Bethanechol chloride (25 mg orally three times daily) may be used for this as well as for other anticholinergic effects, if they are so bothersome as to require the addition of another pharmacological agent. Oral pilocarpine has also been used in cases of severe dry mouth unresponsive to other treatments. It is possible that increased fluid intake could lead to some degree of amelioration of this symptom, but this attempted remedy itself could lead to too many undersirable effects to be worthwhile.

Blurry vision is the other most common anticholinergic complaint associated with tricyclic antidepressant usage. There is interference with the proper cholinergic stimulation of the ciliary muscle of the lens, which is the cause of this problem. Frequently, adaptation occurs over the course of a few weeks, and this problem disappears. Patients should be advised not to spend money on new glasses in the meantime. They should also be cautioned about driving if their vision is blurry, although near vision is more often seriously affected than distant vision. Local cholinergic compounds, such as 1% pilocarpine eye drops, may be of some benefit.

A less frequent but potentially more serious ophthalmological complication of tricyclic antidepressants is aggravation of narrow-angle glaucoma. Here the issue is interference with cholinergic stimulation of the sphincter muscle of the iris. The resulting mydriasis can then physically impede proper fluid outflow. Patients with narrow-angle glaucoma can probably still be safely treated with tricyclic antidepressants if they are maintained on their antiglaucoma medications, but close ophthalmological collaboration and frequent tonometry are indicated. In open-angle glaucoma (the more common form of glaucoma), pupil size is not the relevant factor it is in narrow-angle glaucoma, so there is less danger from the anticholinergic effects of tricyclic antidepressants. However, once again, ophthalmological consultation is prudent before initiating therapy.

Constipation is another symptom which may result from the anticholinergic activity of tricyclic agents. Increased norepinephrine availability at peripheral receptor sites may further compromise intestinal motility. The danger of constipation is fecal impaction or, worst of all, adynamic ileus. Fortunately, paralytic ileus is a very rare event, but when it does occur it is life threatening, and hospitalization is required. The clinician should be aware that it may occur in the presence of a scant diarrhea rather than complete constipation. The most severe side effects of this sort are most likely to occur in the elderly and/or in patients receiving combinations of strongly anticholinergic drugs that may include a tricyclic antidepressant. Ordinarily, constipation can be managed, if it occurs, by conservative measures such as by the administration of milk of magnesia or other water-retaining laxatives.

The remaining important peripheral anticholinergic tricyclic antidepressant side effects are urologic. Inhibition of the action of acetylcholine at the neuromuscular junction of the detrussor muscle can result in the urinary retention syndrome. This is more likely to happen in older patients, particularly men who have enlargement of the prostate. In mild cases, a lowering of antidepressant dosage may relieve the problem. Bethanechol chloride may at times also be helpful, and patients may be maintained on this adjunctive medication, if necessary, throughout a needed course of tricyclic antidepressant treatment. Urologic consultation should be sought, however, in cases of possible significant urinary retention to rule out urinary tract obstruction. With obstruction, the danger of bladder rupture would exist with the use of bethanechol.

Difficulties with erection may also be encountered occasionally with tricyclic antidepressants, on an anticholinergic basis, because the achieving and maintaining of an erection is dependent on a cholinergic mechanism.

Central anticholinergic effects can lead to sedation or drowsiness. Patients may naturally experience this as less disagreeable if they take their daily medication allotment as a single bedtime dose. Often, the majority of the sedative effect wears off over six to eight hours so that patients will not be troubled during their waking hours, although this is not invariably the case. Patients should be advised accordingly with regard to driving or operating machinery if sedative effects linger.

Patients prone to seek pharmacologic relief from symptoms should also be cautioned about the use of "uppers" while on tricyclic antidepressants, although the caffeine in an occasional cup of coffee may provide a useful lift.

There is a more serious central anticholinergic syndrome about which the clinician needs to be aware. This is anticholinergic psychosis. In its full-blown state, it is a toxic organic delirium with disorientation, stupor, agitation, anxiety, and hallucinations. Hyperpyrexia, myoclonus, convulsions, and coma may occur. Vulnerability to this side effect increases with age. Anticholinergic psychosis most typically occurs when patients are being treated with a combination of medications (such as neuroleptics, antiparkinsonian agents, and antidepressants), each of which is anticholinergic. Stopping medications, of course, is an important component of treating this emergency. Physostigmine salicylate may also be judiciously employed as a cholinesterase inhibitor which crosses the blood-brain barrier.

Drowsiness and sedation may also occur in the course of tricyclic antidepressant treatment through the mechanism of inhibition of the histamine H_1 receptor.[4] An additional effect thought to be mediated through the inhibition of the histamine H_1 receptor is the increase in appetite with resultant weight gain experienced by a number of patients being treated with tricyclic antidepressants. Patients with a proclivity for corpulence should be advised to manage this side effect by dietary means since over-the-counter appetite suppressants may contain stimulants, the safety of which has been untested in patients receiving concomitant antidepressant medication, and whose efficacy is dubious anyway.

Other effects of the tricyclic antidepressants are thought to be mediated on the basis of their anti-alpha-adrenergic properties. The most common and notable of these effects is orthostatic hypotension (to be considered below under the heading of Cardiovascular Effects). The fact that some antidepressant side effects result from the drugs' anticholinergic properties, whereas others are related to anti-alpha-adrenergic properties, and still others may be due to blockade of the histamine H_1 receptor allows for some degree of dissociation among patterns of side effects for different drugs. Amitriptyline is the most potent muscarinic (cholinergic) receptor blocking agent among tricyclic antidepressants.[5] Desipramine and nortriptyline have this property to the least degree. Doxepin and amitriptyline result in the greatest degree of alpha-adrenergic receptor blockade, with desipramine and protriptyline resulting in the least. Doxepin and amitriptyline have the most histamine H_1 receptor blocking activity, with desipramine having the least. It is not surprising, then, that desipramine results in fewer side effects than amitriptyline and doxepin. Nortriptyline and protriptyline also have a relatively low profile of side effects, particularly when the lower dosage they require is taken into account. The therapeutic window of plasma nortriptyline concentrations allows relatively low doses of this drug to be used to "sneak into the bottom of the window," attaining antidepressant benefit while avoiding side effects.[6] As the most potent tricyclic antidepressant on a milligram basis, protriptyline also requires low doses for antidepressant effect. The value of this drug, however, is offset in any patient with a risk of suicide by the extremely long half-life of protriptyline. This extended half-life (in excess of 50 hours, in comparison with a 14- to 24-hour half-life for most other tricyclic antidepressants) makes protriptyline a particularly difficult drug to manage medically in an overdose situation.

More recently, a "new generation" of antidepressant drugs has been developed. The drugs have chemical structures which are not tricyclic, but their spectrum of clinical efficacy roughly parallels that of tricyclic drugs. Some may possess beneficial treatment features such as, perhaps, a more rapid onset of action, although this has not been proven conclusively. Patterns of side effects parallel those of the tricyclic antidepressants, although each is a variation on the theme and one may be particularly beneficial to the appropriately selected patient. Maprotiline has a tetracyclic structure and is touted as having a low incidence of hypotension, although sedative and anticholinergic effects are present. It also has a relatively long half-life. Amoxapine is a dibenzoxazepine agent with anticholinergic properties in a range that is similar to those of some of the tricyclic drugs. Amoxapine also has dopaminergic blocking properties so that serum prolactin levels rise and galactoria may be a harmless side effect in some patients as it is in the case of neuroleptics. Trazodone is a triazolopyridine derivative antidepressant. It has modest anticholinergic side effects which, however, are within the frequency range of some of the other antidepressant agents as well.

Cardiovascular Side Effects of Tricyclic Antidepressants

The most frequently encountered cardiovascular side effect of tricyclic antidepressants is orthostatic hypotension.[7] These drugs do not seem appreciably to lower the blood pressure of reclining individuals—ie, blood pressure itself is not lowered except for interference with the complex reflex mechanisms involved in postural regulation. This is generally attributed to these drugs' alpha-adrenergic blocking activity.[8] These effects can be of sufficient severity to lead not only to dizziness, but also to falling, and may require alterations in treatment for as many as 10% to 15% of patients. Orthostatic hypotension, and for that matter falling, is not limited to the elderly; it occurs in younger patients as well. But it is of most concern in the elderly, whose balancing reflexes may not be as quick and whose bones are more brittle.

The most intensively studied tricyclic drug in terms of orthostatic hypotension is imipramine.[7,9] One predictor of orthostatic hypotension with imipramine has been found to be the degree of drop in systolic pressure with standing before initiation of drug treatment. In other words, the amount of orthostatic drop in blood pressure before drug treatment is a rough predictor of the additional increment in orthostatic hypotension which the patient will experience with the drug. It has also been noted that the relationship of orthostatic hypotension to blood levels of imipramine does not exactly parallel the relationship of blood levels with clinical response. The generally accepted "threshold" plasma imipramine concentration for clinical efficacy is in the range of 180 ng/mL (combined imipramine and desipramine).[9] The orthostatic hypotensive action of imipramine seems to increase with blood level only up to a concentration of 125 ng/mL (combined imipramine and desipramine), however. Beyond that point, a plateau is reached, and further exacerbation of postural hypotension does not occur. Thus, for example, if a patient is known to have a plasma imipramine concentration of 150 ng/mL and the clinician is concerned about raising the dose to achieve a better therapeutic effect because of fears of worsening that patient's orthostatic hypotension, the clinician can proceed. There is no evidence that the orthostatic hypotension will be any worse at 180 or 200 ng/mL than it was at 150 ng/mL. Another interesting feature that has been noted with regard to orthostatic hypotension is its persistence. In the case of imipramine it has been noted that the orthostatic hypotension continues, even after the subjective sense of dizziness or faintness on standing has gone away. Whatever the pathophysiology of dizziness in this circumstance, it is more complex than just a simple reflection of the degree of orthostatic hypotension. Some adaptation apparently occurs over time. To be sure, this observation should provide a note of caution for clinicians with regard to patients at risk for myocardial or cerebral insufficiency with lowered blood pressure. Dizziness may be lost over time in these patients as a warning sign of tricyclic antidepressant-induced orthostatic hypotension.

Often, of course, it is prudent to change tricyclic antidepressant medication to avoid or minimize orthostatic hypotension. Probably the drug of choice in this situation is nortriptyline—particularly if plasma levels can be monitored so that the plasma concentration can be adjusted into the lower part of this drug's therapeutic window. Studies in the literature have noted a lack of hypotensive effects with nortriptyline[10,11] and in one direct comparison with imipramine, although there was some increment of orthostatic hypotension with nortriptyline, it was approximately half that observed with imipramine.[12]

Fludrocortisone acetate (Florinef acetate) has been employed on occasion as a remedy for tricyclic antidepressant-induced orthostatic hypotension.[13] Although it is true that healthy young patients may have their symptoms relieved to some extent by this treatment, as a salt-retaining steroid, fludrocortisone could present a hazard to older patients or those with a vulnerability to hypertension.

Whatever the other measures taken with regard to orthostatic hypotension, it is very important to educate the patient about the need to change positions slowly, especially to sit on the side of the bed for a few minutes before standing, when arising from a recumbent position. Tight-fitting surgical hose may also reduce venous pooling and thereby ameliorate orthostatic symptoms.

Interference with cardiac conduction is another area for concern with regard to tricyclic antidepressants, although this does not present a danger for patients with healthy hearts being treated with the usual therapeutic plasma levels of antidepressants.[7] Tricyclic antidepressants tend to delay cardiac conduction. This can be revealed on an electrocardiogram as a prolongation of the PR interval or a widening of the QRS complex. A 20% increase in the duration of either the PR interval or the QRS complex presents an indication not to raise the tricyclic antidepressant dose further. First-degree heart block is a contraindication to tricyclic antidepressant treatment in the absence of an indwelling cardiac pacemaker. Once such a pacemaker is in place, however, it is safe to proceed, since higher degrees of heart block would no longer put the patient at risk. In fact, in selected patients who truly need tricyclic antidepressant treatment, the existence of first-degree heart block can be an indication for the insertion of a cardiac pacemaker (a relatively benign procedure) to allow antidepressant treatment. Similarly, bundle branch block puts patients at a substantial degree of risk for developing high grades of atrioventricular block. Such patients may be hospitalized in the early stages of their tricyclic antidepressant treatment to allow for frequent pulse and electrocardiogram monitoring.

All of the tricyclic drugs probably possess at least some activity to increase cardiac conduction times. Doxepin has been touted as having fewer cardiac side effects as a reflection of a clinical trial that was conducted in comparison with nortriptyline.[14] This study was flawed for clinical purposes, however, because the average blood level was much higher for nortriptyline (200 ng/mL) than it was for doxepin (56 ng/mL). In fact, this average blood level for nortriptyline is above the top of this drug's therapeutic window. Certainly, the only fair way to compare the side effects of antidepressant drugs is to compare them at equipotent antidepressant doses. The most studied tricyclic drugs in terms of cardiac effects have been nortriptyline and imipramine. At equally antidepressant concentrations, nortriptyline has been found to impede cardiac conduction less than imipramine—again, at least in part, because lower plasma concentrations of nortriptyline are involved.

Patients with the so-called sick sinus syndrome—a disorder in which the sinus node readily loses its pace-making capability in the face of any one of a number of challenges—are vulnerable to the sinus node depressing effects of tricyclic antidepressants. Again, the risk of aggravation of this defect in electrical functioning of the heart is entirely obviated by the placing of a cardiac pacemaker.

Tachycardia is frequently listed as a tricyclic antidepressant side effect. In a statistical sense, this is certainly valid, as studies with various tricyclic antidepressants have documented statistically significant increases in heart rate, and the data indicate that greater increase in heart rate may occur with amitriptyline or nortriptyline than with imipramine or desipramine. However, in none of the cases is the increase in heart rate very significant clinically.

Tricyclic drugs can have a helpful effect on cardiac arrhythmias. Contrary to the original supposition (which was based on extrapolation from cases of overdose), tricyclic antidepressants seem to have an antiarrhythmic effect. This has been most clearly documented in the case of imipramine, the most-studied drug. Imipramine has a clear and definite arrhythmia-suppressing pharmacological activity in the same range of plasma concentrations at which the antidepressant effect is manifest.[7] Apparently, the antiarrhythmic properties of imipramine have a similarity to those of quinidine, the drug being antiarrhythmic in lower (therapeutic) concentrations and arrhythmogenic in higher (toxic/overdose) concentrations. Consequently, tricyclic antidepressant overdoses should generally be treated like quinidine overdoses from the cardiac point of view, and physicians should be cautious about adding additional quinidine—like drugs when signs of arrhythmia emerge.

The antiarrhythmic capability of imipramine, and perhaps other tricyclic antidepressants, raises a caution in the treatment of patients with chronic atrial fibrillation. Here, tricyclic drugs may correct the atrial fibrillation, and the patient may convert to normal sinus rhythm, creating the risk of embolization. Consequently, it is advisable to give such patients anticoagulants before initiating tricyclic antidepressant therapy.

The effects of tricyclic drugs on the mechanical functioning of the heart are complex and, as yet, not fully understood. Apparently, there is generally some degree of negative inotropic effect. However, considerations of venous return and afterload make predictions tricky with regard to the overall effect of tricyclic drugs on cardiac efficiency and cardiac output when the cardiovascular system is in a state of failure. As in the case of any patient with significant cardiac disease, appropriate cardiological consultation should be sought before initiating or substantially altering a regimen of tricyclic antidepressant treatment.

Miscellaneous Tricyclic Antidepressant Side Effects

There are a variety of rather rare physiological reactions which are possible with tricyclic antidepressants. Skin rashes may occur on an allergic basis. Most often, these subside with a reduction of dosage, although switching to an alternative medication may be necessary. Increased sweating may occur during tricyclic antidepressant treatment, particularly on the face, arms, and upper torso. Cholestatic jaundice in the absence of other abnormal liver function tests has been reported and has been associated with fever, anorexia, and abdominal pain. Most usually it subsides after discontinuation of the antidepressant. Agranulocytosis is a very rare hematological reaction. It should be treated with discontinuation of the offending drug and supportive measures. These side effects occur sufficiently infrequently that routine hematological evaluation or blood chemical studies are not called for. However, the clinician should be alert to their rare occurrence so these tests can be ordered if the patient has otherwise unexplained fever, infection, abdominal pain, or jaundice.

Less infrequent is the side effect of weight gain. In fact, this is quite common with many tricyclic antidepressants and can become a source of significant discomfort to weight-conscious patients. Increased appetite on the basis of the drug's blocking property of the histamine H_1 receptor has been implicated, although changes in carbohydrate metabolism may play a role. This problem should be discussed with patients, and appropriate dietary measures should be encouraged so that this effect does not become a source of noncompliance.

A form of paradoxical agitation has been observed with tricyclic antidepressants—most classically in the case of imipramine, on occasion, when it is being used in the treatment of patients with panic disorder. Patients may complain of a subjective sense of anxiety and have motor restlessness and insomnia. Typically this lasts for several hours after the oral dose is taken. Diazepam is often useful for control of this symptom, and with lowered tricyclic antidepressant dose or a more gradual increase, it may not recur.

The use of tricyclic antidepressants has also been reported to be associated with an increased incidence of mania.[15,16] In a review of the literature, mania or hypomania was observed in 8.6% of 2346 cases of depression after the initiation of tricyclic antidepressant treatment, which has contributed to the hypothesis that tricyclic drugs are capable of activating the biological "switch" mechanism responsible for cycling into mania from depression.[15] Such a switch into mania has been observed in patients with no previous history of bipolarity, although the risk of mania after tricyclic administration is greater in those patients with a previous bipolar history.

An increase in manic episodes during maintenance tricyclic antidepressant treatment has also been observed, under double-blind conditions, among patients previously known to be bipolar.[16] Of course, the risk of mania would also be greater in patients with previous histories of mania than in patients without such histories in the absence of tricyclic antidepressant medication, and mania can occur de novo in previously depressed patients with tricyclic antidepressant exposure. Related to the issue of mania and hypomania is the more recent observation of the occasional induction of "rapid cycling" of affectively disordered patients when exposed to tricyclic antidepressants,[17,18] and it has been suggested that tricyclic antidepressants may, in a general way, accelerate the biological rhythmicity of affective disorders.[18] This rapid cycling hypothesis remains to be confirmed by a prospective trial.

The discontinuation of tricyclic antidepressants, especially if rapidly done, can result in a variety of autonomic side effects that can be experienced by the patient as a flu-like syndrome. Headache, malaise, nausea, vomiting, cramps, diarrhea, chills, cold sweats, restlessness, insomnia, and irritability have been reported with tricyclic antidepressant withdrawal. Such responses, of course, can be avoided by a more gradual tapering of medication over a week or two. The fact that sudden discontinuation of tricyclic antidepressants can lead to some degree of autonomic imbalance and therefore more acute side effects than medication continuation should be a consideration in those circumstances where abrupt tricyclic antidepressant cessation would be contemplated, such as emergency surgery.

MAO INHIBITORS

Monoamine oxidase (MAO) inhibitors have been associated with many of the same side effects that are most commonly thought of as being related to tricyclic antidepressant use. The most frequently troublesome adverse reactions of MAO inhibitors are orthostatic hypotension and sedation. For example, in a double-blind study in which 39 patients received phenelzine (60 mg per day), 44% were found to develop orthostatic hypotension and 49% were troubled by sedation.[19] These percentages were roughly equivalent to the comparison group of patients receiving amitriptyline. The orthostatic hypotension and/or sedation from MAO inhibitors can be as severe as that observed with tricyclic antidepressants and can, at times, require that the drug be discontinued. There have been fewer studies, however, of these effects with MAO inhibitors, so that it is not well-known, for instance, whether switching from one MAO inhibitor to another can retain the therapeutic effect with fewer side effects. If switching from one MAO inhibitor to another is tried, the dose of the first should be slowly tapered. After discontinuation, the dose of the second MAO inhibitor is then gradually raised. Severe reactions have been reported from rapidly switching MAO inhibitors at equipotent doses. As was the case with tricyclic antidepressants, conservative measures can be employed to minimize the nuisance and danger of orthostatic hypotension and sedation.

Other tricyclic antidepressant-like side effects may also be observed with MAO inhibitors.[3] Dry mouth is commonly seen — the incidence being 46% in the previously cited study of phenelzine at a dose of 60 mg per day. Constipation and/or blurred vision are less frequent than with most tricyclic antidepressants, but are certainly observed on occasion with MAO inhibitors. Urinary retention has been reported, and sexual problems including impotence and delayed or absent orgasm have been described. Disorders of perspiration, both decreased sweating and increased sweating, have been noted with MAO inhibitors. Additionally, unlike tricyclic antidepressants, the use of MAO inhibitors has occasionally been associated with hyperthermia — presumably on an autonomic basis.

One reported side effect of the early MAO inhibitor iproniazid which found its way prominently into the early literature was hepatic toxicity.[2] The fatality rate of 25% for this complication was understandably frightening to clinicians, who shied away from its use. The true incidence of severe liver necrosis associated with iproniazid use was most probably in the range of 1 case in 3000 to 10,000. One speculation has been that hydrazine MAO inhibitors may increase susceptibility to clinical hepatitis infection among carriers of the virus. There have also been reports of hepatocellular jaundice occurring during the use of other hydrazine MAO inhibitors such as phenelzine, pheniprazine, isocarboxazid, and nialamide — although the frequency of such a reaction with these drugs may be less than the rate observed with iproniazid, the first hydrazine MAO inhibitor. Pheniprazine, nialamide, and iproniazid, however, are not marketed in the United States. Interestingly, jaundice has not been reported in association with the use of nonhydrazine MAO inhibitors.

Hypertensive crisis is the most frequently occurring dangerous side effect to MAO inhibitors, and it has been estimated that serious hypertensive syndromes occur in approximately 0.3% to 0.5% of patients.[2] The rate of occurrence for less serious hypertensive manifestations, such as paroxysmal headache, has been estimated to be approximately 2%, although there are other estimates that range higher. It is difficult to be certain about these rates because they are sufficiently small that definitive prospective studies have not been done. However, any other approach to the question of side effect incidence leaves the true denominator in doubt. (For example, in questionnaire studies, people who have experienced a troublesome or frightening side effect may be more likely to respond to the questionnaire than patients who have had a trouble-free course.)

One clear precipitant of a hypertensive reaction in patients receiving MAO inhibitors is the ingestion of foodstuffs or medications containing tyramine or other amine pressor agents. This has also been referred to as the "cheese reaction" after the food most frequently implicated. A list of the foods, beverages, and medications to be avoided when patients are on an "MAO inhibitor diet" is shown in Table 6-1.[20]

Table 6-1 should be used as a rough guide only. In general, the most important foods the patient should be told to avoid are cheese (other than cottage, farmers, or cream cheese), pickled meats, chicken liver, chocolate, fava and broad beans, beer, and red wine. Estimates of the concentration of tyramine in foodstuffs vary and are often based on small samples. Factors such as preservation, refrigeration, and age of the product may have dramatic influence on the tyramine concentration. Overripe, spoiled, fermented, or unrefrigerated products are much more likely to contain high concentrations of tyramine. Obviously, the quantity ingested is also directly proportional to the amount of tyramine involved. The variability of these factors can mislead the unwary patient who has "cheated a bit" without apparent ill effect to the erroneous conclusion that he or she may indulge with impunity. The results of this may be disastrous.

It must be remembered that the effects of MAO inhibitors typically continue for 10 days to 2 weeks after the medication has been discontinued. This is because the medications block the synthesis of the enzyme. Thus, when the drug is stopped, it first has to be cleared from the patient's system; then synthesis of the enzyme can resume, which then has to build up to normal physiological concentrations. Patients should be cautioned about the necessary delay in returning to a normal diet or to the use of the medications in Table 6-1 after discontinuation of their MAO inhibitor.

Tricyclic antidepressants are listed in Table 6-1 because there have been reported cases which appear to represent an adverse interaction. This is somewhat controversial, however, and under appropriate supervision properly selected patients benefit from the combination. Nevertheless, tricyclic antidepressants are included in Table 6-1 because it is not prudent to add them to the regimen of a patient who is already taking an MAO inhibitor. If the combination is to be employed, the drugs should be started together or the MAO inhibitor should be added to the tricyclic antidepressant.

Table 6-1
Foods and Drugs to be Avoided When Taking MAO Inhibitors

Foods with high or very high tyramine concentrations	
Boursault cheese	Caviar
Camembert cheese	Pickled herring
Cheddar cheese	Fermented sausages
Emmenthaler cheese	Bologna
Stilton cheese	Pepperoni
Yeast extracts (not a problem in baked goods, however)	Salami
	Summer sausage
Foods with moderate or moderate to high tyramine concentrations	
Blue cheese	Beef liver (unrefrigerated, fermented)
Brick cheese	Chicken liver (unrefrigerated, fermented)
Brie cheese	
Gruyere cheese	Fish (unrefrigerated, fermented)
Mozzarella cheese	Dried fish
Parmesan cheese	Dried salted herring
Romano cheese	Unrefrigerated, fermented meats
Roquefort cheese	
Foods and beverages containing other potential pressor agents	
Fava beans (dopamine)	
Chocolate (phenylethylamine)	
Coffee (caffeine)	
Tea (caffeine)	
Cola drinks (caffeine)	
Other beverages where reactions have been reported	
Imported beer	Drambuie
Chartreuse	Chianti
Sherry	Other red wines
Notable foods and beverages with *little or no* tyramine	
Cottage cheese	
Cream cheese	
White wine	
Drugs that may interact adversely with MAO inhibitors	
Sympathomimetic amines	Levodopa
Amphetamines	Amines which may be present in appetite suppressing drugs and cold and sinus remedies
Dopamine	
Ephedrine	
Epinephrine	Meperidine (hypotension and hyperpyrexia as well as hypertension)
Isoproterenol	
Metaraminol	
Methylphenidate	Hypoglycemics (increased hypoglycemia)
Phenylephrine	
Phenylpropanolamine	Tricyclic antidepressants

Treatment of a hypertensive reaction, should one occur, can be conservative if the blood pressure does not go too high. What is "too high," of course, for any one individual depends on the elasticity and reserve of that individual's cardiovascular system—issues which are only proven with certainty after the fact. Most mild to moderate hypertensive reactions would last between one and three hours, if untreated. Intramuscular chlorpromazine is the drug of choice for treating such episodes. Typically 50 to 100 mg of intramuscular chlorpromazine will satisfactorily reduce the blood pressure in a matter of minutes. Intramuscular phentolamine and intramuscular or oral phenoxybenzamine are alternatives. If the patient is in extreme danger from a fulminant hypertensive crisis, intravenous phentolamine (Regitine) may be employed with a typical starting dose of 5 mg. This will bring down the blood pressure very rapidly, but the patient can easily go into shock. Some psychiatrists recommend that patients carry 100–200 mg of oral chlorpromazine or 100 mg of oral phentolamine with them at all times and take it if they experience sudden throbbing bilateral occipital headache. At any rate, patients should be warned of the potentially serious implications of a sudden throbbing headache when taking an MAO inhibitor, and that it is cause to call his or her psychiatrist immediately or to go to an emergency room and have his blood pressure checked if the psychiatrist is not available.

ADVERSE REACTIONS WITH LITHIUM

The discussion of adverse reactions to lithium will be divided into considerations of toxicity and side effects per se. Toxicity (ie, stigmata of poisoning by virtue of relative overdose, unintentional or otherwise) can occur with any drug, but toxicity becomes a special issue and special caveat with lithium because of lithium's low therapeutic index. That is, the ratio between a toxic dose and an ordinary therapeutic dose is not very great. In the case of lithium, twice an ordinary therapeutic dose in an individual may be a toxic dose. Similarly, with lithium, one patient's therapeutic dose can easily be another patient's toxic dose—or even that same patient's toxic dose at a different point in time or under different conditions (ie, restriction of salt or water intake or addition of a diuretic drug). Occasionally, patients may even experience some symptoms of toxicity with serum levels ordinarily considered to be within the normal therapeutic range. Furthermore, at serum lithium levels consistent with early toxicity, lithium retention via the kidney is enhanced, contributing to a vicious cycle. With toxicity within such easy reach, and with the risk that lithium toxicity can potentially carry serious morbidity or even mortality, the issue of lithium toxicity merits special consideration.

Lithium Toxicity

Although gastrointestinal symptoms such as nausea, vomiting, and/or diarrhea are the most common early manifestations of lithium toxicity, neurological signs and symptoms may follow quickly and become more serious expressions of the toxic state. The presence and sequencing of neurologic symptoms is variable, but a variety of symptoms are usually present. Cerebral symptoms may include confusion, poor concentration, lethargy, subjective sense of weakness, and clouding of consciousness with stupor progressing to coma. Cerebellar dysfunction may be present with poor coordination, ataxia, dysarthria, or nystagmus. Choreiform or parkinsonian movements have been noted as evidence of basal ganglia disturbance in some patients, and other nervous system dysfunctions may be present such as increased muscle tone, tremor, fasciculations, myoclonus, and exaggerated deep tendon reflexes. Not infrequently, with serious lithium toxicity, seizures supervene, and these may progress to status epilepticus. It has been suggested that patients with histories of seizures or patients who have electroencephalograph abnormalities are more prone to lithium toxicity, and lithium should be used with particular caution in this group.

Lithium toxicity may be fatal. When this occurs, the terminal event is often associated with the pulmonary complications which result from the accumulation of very viscous, difficult to remove secretions in the respiratory tract.[22,23] Death may also occur on the basis of cardiac arrhythmias.

The primary concerns in treatment of lithium toxicity are supportive measures for the patient's vital processes and measures to rid the patient of the offending drug.

Gastrointestinal absorption of large amounts of lithium is generally decreased in patients with impaired consciousness. Therefore, gastric lavage through a wide bore tube followed by saline cathartics may usefully dispose of quantities of lithium before it enters the general circulation even if drug ingestion has not immediately preceded treatment for toxicity. Charcoal, however, does not absorb lithium effectively.

The kidney is the important organ for eliminating lithium which has been absorbed. Unfortunately, toxicity may lead to a decrease in the renal clearance of lithium—an event which, as previously mentioned, can rapidly become part of a vicious cycle at the outset of the lithium toxicity. If the serum sodium level is low, a saline infusion can substantially increase the excretion of lithium, but such an infusion is generally of little value when serum sodium concentrations are normal. Dialysis, however, can be of definite benefit in the emergency elimination of lithium, and both peritoneal dialysis and hemodialysis have been used to advantage in this situation—at times in conjunction with each other. Dialysis is maintained until plasma lithium concentrations fall below therapeutic levels, because remobilization of the ion from bone and other "spaces" can result later in a rebound rise in lithium levels after the dialysis is discontinued. Consequently, lithium levels should be followed every four to six hours during treatment of lithium toxicity. Other plasma electrolytes should also be followed as should the electrocardiogram and chest x-ray. Kidney excretion of lithium is favored by a reclining as opposed to an upright position. For reasons stated above, careful attention is to be paid to the bronchial toilet during lithium toxicity, and assisted respiration may become indicated.

General clinical monitoring of the patient is quite important in addition to laboratory monitoring. Intracellular concentrations of lithium, responsible for severe toxic manifestations, may be increasing even as plasma levels fall and are slower to return to normal levels than the peripherally measurable plasma drug concentration.

General Side Effects of Lithium

Lithium has side effects that may affect the nervous system even within the normal therapeutic range of plasma concentrations. The most common of these are a fine hand tremor and muscular weakness. The incidence of hand tremor decreases with maintenance time on lithium, but at one time or another as many as half of patients treated with lithium may complain of at least some degree of hand tremor.[24] Men have been reported to complain of this hand tremor more frequently than women.[24] In essence, this is a benign side effect, not associated with any parkinsonian-type features, but can potentially be a realistic problem to anyone whose work or avocation is dependent on fine hand coordination. When this is the case, the beta-adrenergic blocking agent propranolol may be used to counteract the tremor. The usual dose is 10–20 mg orally three times a day. Muscular weakness is commonly experienced in the first week of lithium treatment, but this effect is almost always short-lived and no special treatment for this complaint is indicated.

An organic brain syndrome in the absence of signs of toxicity has also been reported with lithium.[25] This syndrome is often accompanied by visual hallucinations and perplexity. It has been noted to clear within several days after the discontinuation of the lithium.

The issue which has occasioned the most concern in terms of the possible long-term adverse lithium effects is the question of potential kidney damage.[21,26–28]

Physiologically, lithium has little if any effect on glomerular function. The decrease in glomerular filtration rates over the course of increasing durations of lithium treatment parallels the decrease that would be expected on the basis of increasing age alone.

Renal tubular function, however, is a different story. To a greater or lesser extent, varying among individuals, the presence of the lithium ion results in an impairment of water reabsorption in the renal tubules. When this effect is sufficient to become clinically apparent, as is the case with as many as 50% of patients initially and 25% of patients later in the course of treatment, the presentation is that of diabetes insipidus with polyuria and secondary polydipsia. The urine is of low specific gravity and low osmolality, and the ability to concentrate the urine is impaired. Urine volumes of 5 or 6 L a day are not unusual, and much higher volumes than this have been reported. Nephrogenic diabetes insipidus involves no pituitary gland dysfunction. Rather, the kidney is unresponsive to vasopressin. (This has led to rational, although not necessarily successful, attempts to utilize this property of lithium at the level of the renal tubules to counteract symptomatology in the syndrome of inappropriate ADH.) Under ordinary circumstances, nephrogenic diabetes insipidus is not dangerous; it is important principally because of the annoyance of polyuria (and nocturia) and polydipsia to the patient. However, during negative water balance, such as in the case of extreme heat, fever, heavy sweating, or major surgery, dehydration becomes a risk. Dehydration, of course, is a serious problem in patients who are receiving lithium treatment because it brings with it the danger of lithium toxicity. Patients with lithium-induced diabetes insipidus should be instructed to take steps to be certain that they have access to sufficient supplies of water, such as, for example, by taking a canteen of water with them on long automobile trips.

Most of the time, nephrogenic diabetes insipidus responds favorably to a reduction of lithium dosage. Occasionally, however, it does not and the expression of this syndrome may rarely even persist for some time after the discontinuation of lithium treatment. For patients who need to be treated with lithium and for whom reduction of serum level is either ineffective in controlling the renal symptoms or inadvisable psychiatrically, a thiazide diuretic may be employed. In many cases, thiazide diuretics suppress nephrogenic diabetes insipidus. The safest way to initiate diuretic treatment in a patient receiving lithium is first to discontinue the lithium, then adjust the diuretic to the desired dosage, and finally restart the lithium with lower dose. Typically, half the previous lithium dose is needed. Frequent serum lithium determinations should be made as the lithium is reinstituted to assure that toxicity is avoided.

In 1977 a report with frightening implications was published concerning histological changes in the kidneys of patients who had been treated with lithium.[29] In autopsy or biopsy specimens abnormally high rates were observed of tubular atrophy, interstitial fibrosis, and sclerotic glomeruli. Eight of the 14 patients involved had impairment of renal concentrating ability, and the histological changes appeared to correlate with diminution of renal function. It was noted, however, that these patients had had episodes of lithium toxicity during the course of their treatment. The findings of histological changes in patients who have had lithium treatment have been replicated, but the apparent significance of these changes varies with the control group employed.[26–30] More nephropathy has been found in lithium patients than in healthy controls (kidney donors), but changes similar to those in the lithium patients were found in patients with long-term affective disorders who had not received lithium treatment, raising the question of whether the kidney lesions are a feature of the affective disorder itself, an indirect or nonspecific consequence of the affective disorder, or the result of some other treatment factor. Furthermore, although some glomeruli may be sclerotic in lithium-treated patients, generally normal filtration rates seem to be maintained, and the reserve and compensatory renal capacity seems to be adequate. Caution, to be sure, is still appropriate, and the complete story may not as yet have been written, but the evidence at present is that the lithium probably does not cause significant nephropathy. There have been no reported cases of terminal azotemia clearly related to lithium's effects on the kidney, whereas there have certainly been suicides associated with the discontinuation of lithium treatment.

The major cardiac side effect of lithium is in patients with the sick-sinus syndrome. In these patients, lithium can interrupt the rhythmic functioning of the sinus mode, leaving the heart without its normal pacemaker—an event associated with obvious dangers.[30,31] If such a patient were nevertheless in definite psychiatric need of lithium, this could be an indication for placement of an artificial cardiac pacemaker that would then protect the patient from the risk of asystole or dangerous cardiac rhythms that might otherwise result from the sick-sinus syndrome. Myocarditis is a serious, but very rare, complication of lithium treatment.[32,33] Innocuous T-wave flattening or inversion frequently occurs on the electrocardiogram of lithium-treated patients. With sensitive enough monitoring, T-way changes would probably be detected in a majority of patients receiving lithium. The similarity of these changes to those produced by hypokalemia is thought to reflect the replacement by lithium of potassium within the myocardium—an intracellular electrolyte shift which is not reflected peripherally in the plasma.

A final effect of lithium on the heart may occur in utero. A disproportionate number of cardiovascular abnormalities, particularly the otherwise very rare Ebstein anomaly, have been noted in babies born to women undergoing lithium therapy during pregnancy—especially during the first trimester.[34] Since the first trimester may be well advanced before a woman realizes that she is pregnant, females of child-bearing potential should be cautioned about this risk and advised about birth control if they are sexually active. Lithium should be discontinued before attempts at conception.

Caution is also necessary at the time of parturition for women taking lithium. Typically, renal clearance of lithium increases by 50% to 100% during pregnancy, but this reverts to baseline rates immediately after delivery. Thus, patients maintained on the same dose of lithium postpartum as had been required to maintain therapeutic levels during pregnancy are at significant risk for becoming lithium toxic. The most conservative course is to discontinue lithium at the time of delivery and then cautiously reinstitute treatment at lower dosages after a day or two, monitoring serum levels closely. In this circumstance it is to be remembered as well that lithium passes into the mother's milk. It is therefore inadvisable for lithium-treated mothers to nurse.

Lithium is concentrated in the thyroid gland, and lithium is known to lead to decreases in circulating levels of thyroid hormones which are generally benign.[21] Initially triiodothyronine response to thyroid-stimulating hormone is diminished, although this apparently returns to normal after approximately six weeks. Euthyroid goiter has been reported in approximately 4% of lithium-treated patients,[35,36] but about 8% may become clinically hypothyroid in the course of lithium therapy.[36] A benign reversible exophthalmos may also be associated. Thus, it is appropriate to monitor patients on lithium for hypothyroidism, being cautious not to confuse it with depression, and to administer supplemental thyroid medication where indicated. There is evidence that patients with preexisting thyroid abnormalities may be particularly prone to the effects of lithium on the thyroid,[37] but this need not be a contraindication to lithium treatment as long as thyroid functioning is monitored and appropriate supplements are given to maintain suitable circulating thyroid hormone levels. The most sensitive laboratory test to detect hypothyroidism is a thyroid-stimulating hormone level, which should be obtained twice yearly.

Acneiform and maculopapular skin lesions as well as folliculitis have occasionally been observed with lithium treatment. These are not allergic and are significant only in terms of their cosmetic implications, which are generally rather minor. They disappear with discontinuation of lithium treatment and often do not recur when it is reinstituted.

Particularly at the time when lithium therapy is initiated, a number of patients experience a variety of generally mild gastrointestinal symptoms. These include abdominal discomfort, nausea, vomiting, bloating, anorexia, and/or diarrhea.[21] These symptoms seem to occur more frequently and more severely when the serum lithium concentration is increasing rapidly. Thus, patients experiencing this form of distress may benefit from a temporary discontinuation of the lithium or reduction in dose followed by a more gradual buildup to the desired therapeutic serum level.

Patients receiving lithium often are prone to gain weight, an issue which can be a sticking point for certain individuals. This can be a fluid-space or edematous weight gain based on electrolyte shifts accompanying the lithium treatment, but true increases in tissue mass can also occur. This may in part be due to an insulin-like effect of lithium on body metabolism and gluconeogenesis. Another common mechanism is, no doubt, the ingestion of calorie-rich beverages by patients with marked, or even subtle, polydipsia. In either of these cases, calorie restriction is the preferred and effective method of weight control.

A small minority of patients may experience potency disturbances when undergoing lithium treatment.[22] In such cases a reduction in lithium dose may be tried, but drug discontinuation would need to be judged from a risk/benefit perspective.

A relative leukocytosis with lymphocytopenia has been observed in a majority of patients undergoing lithium treatment. This effect is highly statistically significant, and the overabundance of neutrophils that is involved frequently carries patients far above the normal range of white blood cell counts. The neutrophils, however, are apparently normal functionally, and no adverse consequences of these lithium-related leukocyte count abnormalities are known.

Acknowledgment

This work was supported, in part, through grant number 1-R01-MH34309 from the National Institute of Mental Health.

REFERENCES

1. Kessler KA: Tricyclic antidepressants: Mode of action and clinical use, in Lipton MA, DiMascio A, Killam KF (eds): *Psychopharmacology: A Generation of Progress.* New York, Raven Press, 1978, pp 1289–1302.
2. Klein DF, Gittleman R, Quitkin F, et al: *Diagnosis and Drug Treatment of Psychiatric Disorders: Adults and Children.* ed 2. Baltimore, The Williams & Wilkins Co, 1980, pp 449–492.
3. van der Kolk BA, Shader RI, Greenblatt DJ: Autonomic effects of psychotropic drugs, in Lipton MA, DiMascio A, Killam KF (eds): *Psychopharmacology: A Generation of Progress.* New York, Raven Press, 1978, pp 1009–1020.
4. Richelson E: Tricyclic antidepressants and neurotransmitter receptors. *Psychiatr Ann* 1979;9:186–195.
5. Snyder SH, Yamamura HI: Antidepressants and the muscarinic acetylcholine receptor. *Arch Gen Psychiatry* 1977;34:236–239.
6. Siris SG, Glassman AH, Stetner F: The value of plasma concentrations in assessing the effects of tricyclic antidepressants, in Schoolar JC, Claghorn J (eds): *The Kinetics of Psychiatric Drugs.* New York, Brunner/Mazel, 1979.
7. Glassman AH, Bigger JT: Cardiovascular effects of therapeutic doses of tricyclic antidepressants. *Arch Gen Psychiatry* 1981;38:815–820.
8. U'Prichard DC, Greenberg DA, Sheehan PP, et al: Tricyclic antidepressants: Therapeutic properties and affinity for alpha-noradrenergic receptor binding sites in the brain. *Science* 1978;199:197–198.
9. Glassman AH, Perel JM, Shostak M, et al: Clinical implications of imipramine plasma levels for depressive illness. *Arch Gen Psychiatry* 1977;34:197–204.
10. Freyschuss U, Sjoqvist F, Tuck D, et al: Circulatory effects in man of nortriptyline, a tricyclic antidepressant. *Pharmacol Clin* 1970;2:68–71.

11. Vohra J, Burrows GD, Sloman G: Assessment of cardiovascular side effects of therapeutic doses of tricyclic antidepressant drugs. *Aust NZ J Med* 1975;5:7–11.
12. Roose SP, Glassman AH, Siris SG, et al: Comparison of imipramine- and nortriptyline-induced orthostatic hypotension: A meaningful difference. *J Clin Pharmacol* 1981;1:316–319.
13. Ostow M: Orthostatic hypotension and psychic energizers: A clinical note. *Psychosomatics* 1966;7:224–225.
14. Burrows GD, Vohra J, Dumovic P, et al: TCA drugs and cardiac conduction. *Prog Neuropsychopharmacol* 1977;1:329.
15. Bunney WE Jr: Psychopharmacology of the switch process in affective disorders, in Lipton MA, DiMascio A, Killam KF (eds): *Psychopharmacology: A Generation of Progress.* New York, Raven Press, 1978, pp 1249–1259.
16. Prien RF, Klett CJ, Caffey EM Jr: Lithium carbonate and imipramine in prevention of affective episodes. *Arch Gen Psychiatry* 1973;29:420–425.
17. Siris SG, Chertoff HR, Perel JM: Rapid cycling affective disorder during imipramine treatment: A case report. *Am J Psychiatry* 1979;136:341–342.
18. Wehr TA, Goodwin FK: Rapid cycling in manic-depressives induced by tricyclic antidepressants. *Arch Gen Psychiatry* 1979;36:555–559.
19. Robinson DS, Nies A, Ravaris CL, et al: Clinical psychopharmacology of phenelzine: MAO activity and clinical response, in Lipton MA, DiMascio A, Killam KF (eds): *Psychopharmacology: A Generation of Progress.* New York, Raven Press, 1978, pp 961–973.
20. Gelenberg AJ: MAO inhibitors in sickness and in health. *Biol Ther Psychiatry* 1982;5:25–28.
21. Reisberg B, Gershon S: Side effects associated with lithium therapy. *Arch Gen Psychiatry* 1979;36:879–887.
22. Hollister LE: *Clinical Pharmacology of Psychotherapeutic Drugs.* New York, Churchill-Livingstone, 1978, pp 214–226.
23. Schou M: Lithium in psychiatry, a review, in Efron DH, Cole JO, Levine J, et al (eds): *Psychopharmacology: A Review of Progress 1957–1967,* PHS publication no. 1866. Washington, DC, Government Printing Office, 1968, p 701.
24. Vestergaard P, Amdisen A, Schou M: Clinically significant side effects of lithium treatment: A survey of 237 patients in long term treatment. *Acta Psychiatr Scand* 1980;62:193–200.
25. Rifkin A, Quitkin F, Klein DF: Organic brain syndrome during lithium carbonate treatment. *Compr Psychiatry* 1973;14:251–254.
26. Jenner FA: Lithium and the question of kidney damage. *Arch Gen Psychiatry* 1979;36:888–890.
27. Schou M, Vestergaard P: Lithium and the kidney scare. *Psychosomatics* 1981;22:92–94.
28. Lippman S: Is lithium bad for the kidneys? *J Clin Psychiatry* 1982;43:220–224.
29. Hestbeck J, Hansen HE, Amdisen A, et al: Chronic renal lesions following long-term treatment with lithium. *Kidney Int* 1977;12:205–213.
30. Roose SP, Nurnberger JI, Dunner DL, et al: Cardiac sinus node dysfunction during lithium treatment. *Am J Psychiatry* 1979;136:804–806.
31. Wilson J, Kraus E, Bailas M, et al: Reversible sinus node abnormalities due to lithium carbonate therapy. *N Engl J Med* 1976;294:1223–1224.
32. Tseng H: Interstitial myocarditis probably related to lithium carbonate intoxication. *Arch Pathol* 1971;92:444–448.

33. Swedberg K, Winblad B: Heart failure as a complication of lithium treatment. *Acta Med Scand* 1974;196:279–280.
34. Weinstein MR, Goldfield MD: Cardiovascular malformations with lithium use during pregnancy. *Am J Psychiatry* 1975;132:529–531.
35. Schou M, Amdisen A, Eskajaer-Jensen S, et al: Occurrence of goiter during lithium treatment. *Br Med J* 1968;3:710–713.
36. Shopsin B: Effects of lithium on thyroid function: A review. *Dis Nerv Syst* 1970;31:237–244.
37. Burman KD, Dimond RC, Earll JM, et al: Sensitivity to lithium in treated Graves' disease. *J Clin Endocrinol Metab* 1976;43:606–613.

CHAPTER 7

BIOLOGICAL THEORIES IN SCHIZOPHRENIA

KATHERINE M. NOLL
JOHN M. DAVIS

Disorders in which an individual, apparently normal during the early part of life, at some time before old age and without apparent physical cause loses the ability to reason, have long been a concern of psychiatry. These disorders are called dementias, to distinguish them from amentia (in which the ability to reason never developed). A major organizing characteristic used in theories concerning it has been the age at which symptoms first become evident. A variety of dementias with onset early in life and culminating in psychosis were recognized before the time of Kraepelin. The best described of these was hebephrenia, or "adolescent mind" (so called because the onset of symptoms occurred approximately at puberty). Kraepelin believed that the endogenous psychoses with early onset were related, and adopted the term *dementia praecox* to describe them. He believed that in all cases there was at least some degree of mental deterioration over time even when floridly psychotic symptoms were in remission. Under this rubric he included hebephrenic, catatonic, and paranoid forms.[1] Bleuler agreed that the disorders in which reasoning ability was lost were related, but argued that deterioration was not always a foregone conclusion, particularly in the cases showing catatonic or paranoid symptoms. He believed that the distinguishing and uniting feature was the alteration of the individual's normal personality such that various cognitive and emotional functions seemed separated from each other. To emphasize these points he used the term "schizophrenia" or "divided mind." This included the three types described by Kraepelin, but he also added a fourth type in which floridly psychotic symptoms were rare, which he called "simple" schizophrenia. Together he referred to these as the "group of schizophrenias."[2]

Bleuler stated, however, that a diagnosis of manic-depressive illness should be made only by ruling out schizophrenia. Bleuler described carefully the symptoms characterizing these patients. However, it was the disordering of thought patterns that came to be identified with the term schizophrenia. Schneider's list of "first rank symptoms" served to widen the definition of schizophrenia, whereas a diagnosis of manic-depressive illness was reserved for patients with "pure" affective traits and no evidence of any thought disorder. The extreme form this point of view reached can be characterized by Lewis and Piotrowski's assertion[3] that "even a trace of schizophrenia is schizophrenia." By the 1950s, in the United States in particular the diagnostic label of schizophrenia had come to be used to identify virtually any psychosis of unknown origin.[4]

Whether the functional psychoses were related was relatively unimportant up to the 1950s, as the diagnosis had little impact on treatment. (It seems ironic that Ugo Cerletti's first patient successfully treated with convulsive electric shock was probably manic rather than schizophrenic.) The antipsychotic drugs that appeared in the 1950s seemed to relieve at least the floridly psychotic symptoms of most patients diagnosed as schizophrenic, and this seemed to lend credence to belief in the commonality of these disorders. The facts that some patients responded to electroconvulsive therapy and others did not, and that some recovered more rapidly under treatment with antipsychotic drugs than others, did not seem to have much impact on the concept of schizophrenia as a relatively unitary disorder. Even the evident difference between the chronic and progressive as opposed to episodic and nondeteriorating course of the illness was not seen as a major distinction—perhaps because the course of the illness could not be predicted from the presenting symptoms. However, as relatively successful somatic treatments began to accumulate, research into biological aspects of "schizophrenia" burgeoned rapidly through the 1960s and 1970s. It became increasingly evident that major factors in the etiology of these patients' symptoms were being obscured by the actual heterogeneity of the disorders being subsumed under this classification.[5-10] The traditional subcategories based on the most prominent symptoms failed to provide adequate homogeneity to facilitate precision in research on biological factors in schizophrenia. In contrast to the views of Bleuler and his followers, several reviewers recently concluded that a diagnosis of chronic schizophrenia is unwarranted on the basis of the cross-section of presenting symptoms,[11,12] but that the *presence* of affective symptoms predicts a long-term course more like that of an affective disorder or a reactive psychosis.[4,13,14]

This discovery of the heterogeneity of disorders with onset in or soon after adolescence, psychosis with disordered thought, and in many cases progressive deterioration of intellect and normal personality has necessitated introducing a discussion of biological theories of schizophrenia with a discussion of differential diagnosis. For "schizophrenia" to be a useful concept, it should be distinguished from other disorders with similar symptoms. Furthermore, genuine understanding of the etiology of schizophrenic symptoms in any given patient (with the ultimate goal being treatment and even prevention of the disorders) requires an adequate number of subclassifications to permit ultimate understanding of the true origins of the symptoms. At present it is not possible to make this breakdown with complete accuracy since there is apparent discrepancy in the research results and biological theories of schizophrenia. This may arise from many different etiologies having the same or very similar symptoms as a final common pathway. The efforts of Kraepelin and Bleuler to integrate the psychoses of youth may ultimately have hindered understanding their causes.

CLASSIFICATION AND DIFFERENTIAL DIAGNOSIS

Himmelhoch[15] has provided an excellent discussion of the philosophical issues involved in deciding what to include and what not to include in the diagnostic classification of schizophrenia. Paraphrasing Molière, he notes that "there are schizophrenias and schizophrenias," and a large number of neurologic, infectious, metabolic, and autoimmune diseases mimic the symptoms of schizophrenia. Although many of these can, through very careful examination, be distinguished from "true" schizophrenia, sometimes the symptoms are mimicked perfectly. How much overinclusion takes place depends to some extent on the symptom criteria used to make the diagnosis. Bleuler's criteria have led to the overinclusion of affective disorders, and only some of these may be eliminated by requiring the presence of Schneider's first-rank symptoms. The distinction between "good prognosis" and "poor prognosis" also relates to the issue of distinguishing between schizophrenia and the affective disorders. This prognostic classification attends more to the individual's history than to his or her current symptoms. Himmelhoch notes the "plethora of biochemical hypotheses," which he suspects may represent a variety of subgroups of schizophrenia. However, he argues that there is a group of patients, particularly from the "poor prognosis group," who "demonstrate a certain monolithic obstinacy that is not so easily broken down into qualitatively separate entities." He maintains that these patients do represent a homogeneous group which has been the core of genetic studies in schizophrenia. He notes the fact that all of the current genetic hypotheses of schizophrenia are essentially "diathesis-stress" models; they explain both the variety of symptom patterns and the lack of complete concordance in monozygotic twins by the interaction of environmental and experiential factors with the underlying predisposition to produce the schizophrenic outcome.

While partial penetrance in a genetic trait makes delineation of the mode of transmission difficult, heterogeneity cannot be ruled out as the reason no one theory of genetic transmission has adequately described all of the pedigrees studied. Despite Himmelhoch's assertion that sometimes schizophrenia *is* schizophrenia, those disorders that are identifiable with a particular pathologic cause (particularly when this has led to symptom remission through treatment other than antipsychotic medication) no longer tend to be considered as true schizophrenias. It seems possible that as more and more patients' symptoms are found to be attributable to an identifiable cause, the number of patients in the group of "true" schizophrenics may be whittled to nothing. Perhaps the question is *which* of the causes of schizophreniform symptoms is to be considered "true" schizophrenia, or whether the concept of schizophrenia may evaporate once all of the etiologies have been described and all patients can be assigned to one of them. Alternatively, it may still be useful to return to the concept of "the group of schizophrenias," in recognition of the similarity of symptoms despite the differences in source. As treatment implications seem to be a major factor in classification, it is likely that those who remain diagnosed as schizophrenic will be those for whom there remains no real "cure."

Pending resolution of this issue, we can now only distinguish among those groups of patients with schizophreniform symptoms who appear, on biological grounds at least, to be different in some significant way. The biological aspects that have been consistently identified can be noted, and the theories to account for some or all of them can be discussed. However, it should also be noted that most current research on schizophrenia is done with heterogeneous groups of patients; therefore, significant factors which are characteristic of only a small percentage of the whole patient group will tend to disappear in studies of large groups of patients or will fail to be replicated when small groups of patients are studied. Thus negative findings do not necessarily invalidate a particular hypothesis of the etiology of schizophrenia. However, they may indicate the need for more studies to identify those patients for whom the hypothesis may be correct.

The most important distinction appears to be that which Kraepelin and Bleuler attempted to make: the distinction between schizophrenia and affective psychoses. As the two most important functions of diagnosis are to predict the course of the illness and to indicate the most effective treatment, it is appropriate that efforts to make this distinction should concentrate on these issues. Although it has long been recognized that affective psychoses appear to have a better outcome than schizophrenia, the 30- to 40-year follow-up study in progress at the University of Iowa supports this observation with data on a large number of patients and control subjects.[16] Diagnosis was made by reviewing chart materials and applying current diagnostic criteria. Researchers used operational criteria of the following outcome variables: marital status, residential status, occupational status, and presence of psychiatric symptoms at follow-up. They found that although both patient groups showed some long-term impairment compared with surgical controls, outcome was substantially better for affective patients on all four measures. There was no difference in outcome between patients whose index hospitalization had been for mania and those hospitalized for depression.

The use of the term "schizophrenic" is most likely to be questioned for patients with schizoaffective symptoms and those seen as "acute" or "good prognosis" schizophrenics. Taylor and Abrams have been questioning the inclusion of these patients in the schizophrenic classification for some time. They note that few met the more rigorous research criteria for schizophrenia, whereas many later met those for mania,[17] and most showed complete remission of symptoms with treatment and were more likely to have relatives with affective disorders or alcoholism.[18] They also note that the presence of symptoms traditionally believed to indicate schizophrenia, such as formal thought disorder, first-rank symptoms, auditory hallucinations, persecutory delusions, and catatonia, do not have predictive value in the presence of symptoms meeting the Feighner et al criteria[19] for mania.[20-22]

A set of symptoms that was found to have predictive value was premorbid inferiority feelings.[23] These patients' families showed an excess of neither schizophrenia nor affective disorders. Symptom onset was more likely to have been associated with stress, and these patients showed less thought disorder and lower rate of relapse than schizophrenic patients without premorbid inferiority feelings.

With increased use of lithium to treat affective psychoses, treatment considerations made the schizophrenia-affective psychosis distinction even more important. Hirschowitz et al[24] studied a sample of patients admitted with schizophrenic or schizoaffective symptoms. Eighty percent of those with a good prognosis (by the criteria of McCabe et al[25]) showed substantial remission of symptoms, including "schizophrenic" symptoms, in a two-week trial on lithium alone. Edelstein et al[26] found that a reduction in thought disturbance in response to infused physostigmine (a muscarinic cholinergic agonist found to reduce manic symptoms in manic patients) predicted a clinical response to lithium. Antidepressant and antipsychotic responses to lithium could also be predicted by *worsening* of thought disorder in response to amphetamine.[27] Lithium is generally considered to be more effective than antipsychotic drugs in bringing about remission of symptoms in manic patients. It also has fewer severe side effects, and there is little risk of tardive dyskinesia. These facts make identification of lithium-responsive "schizophrenic" patients important. In addition, patients with good prognosis also seem more likely to show significant improvement without drugs over a 30-day period and to improve when *removed* from antipsychotic medication.[28] The authors of this study recommend maintenance on antipsychotic medication for these patients, but at substantially lower doses than those used to maintain remission in other schiziphrenic patients.

A new approach to making the schizophrenic-affective disorder distinction is discriminant function analysis,[29,30] which uses available symptom and life-history data. Although this approach seems to be quite successful in discriminating schizophrenic from affective patients in a large group of mixed psychotic patients, application of the function to patients with schizo-affective symptoms failed to show a clearly bimodal distribution.[29,31] However, in both cases the number of patients falling on the affective side of the discrimination was larger than the number falling on the schizophrenic side.

This introduces the question of the distinction of schizo-affective disorder from schizophrenia and affective psychoses. The viscissitudes of this diagnostic category may be illustrated by the changes in its status during the development of DSM-III. The Washington University group who developed the research diagnostic criteria (RDC) discovered that the majority of patients diagnosed as schizo-affective had a long-term course that was episodic and showed full remission between episodes. Furthermore, this patient group had a higher percentage of affectively ill than schizophrenic relatives. These factors led them to conclude that it was a variant on the bipolar affective disorders. Thus in the first draft of DSM-III, schizo-affective disorder was neither classified as a form of schizophrenia nor given a separate status. This led to a considerable outcry by a number of researchers who felt that its status as an affective disorder had not been adequately demonstrated; and it was pointed out that a significant number, between 10% and 40% of these patients, had a more schizophrenic-like course and outcome. The final compromise was to include it in DSM-III as a separate diagnostic entity, with no direct relation to either the schizophrenias or the affective disorders.

This disagreement continues. The majority of authors seem to agree that these patients should not necessarily be returned to the schizophrenic category, but agreement ends there. Several studies failed to find any difference between patients diagnosed as schizo-affective by RDC or DSM-III criteria and manic or bipolar patients[11,20,32]; several studies (including those previously mentioned by Fowler et al[31] and Brockington et al[29]) found significant heterogeneity in this group and concluded that it could not be subsumed under either of the two major functional psychoses[10,33,34] in terms of symptoms, outcome, or genetic distribution in pedigrees. However, one apparent prognostic improvement is suggested by Himmelhoch et al.[35] These researchers noted that the presence of "interepisodic thought disorder" predicted a chronic and deteriorating course, no matter how prominent these patients' affective symptoms might be during the acute stage of the illness. McGlashan and Carpenter[36] also have argued that affective symptoms are not inconsistent with a diagnosis of schizophrenia, although they ultimately argue for maintaining a separate category for these patients. As a final note on this controversy, Carpenter et al,[37] reporting on data from the International pilot study of schizophrenia, noted that to their surprise, acute schizophrenia and schizo-affective subtypes were not distinguishable at two and five-year outcome from other schizophrenic subtypes (although this might be accounted for by the exclusion from the study of patients with well-established chronicity).

Another diagnostic group traditionally included with the schizophrenias is characterized by intense negative affect, impulsive behavior, unstable interpersonal relationships, bizarre responses on projective tests, and brief decompensations into psychosis under stress (which frequently remit rapidly without treatment). This group, though not included in DSM-I or DSM-II, was traditionally referred to as "borderline schizophrenia" on the basis of the thought disorder evident on projective testing and during psychotic episodes. However, as more attention has been given to this concept, its relationship to schizophrenia has been questioned. The adjective "borderline" has been used with a variety of other terms such as "syndrome," "personality," "organization," and "character"; sometimes the term is used alone. In an effort to determine whether this was a valid diagnostic entity, Spitzer et al[38] polled members of the American Psychiatric Association. They determined that the term was being applied to two fairly distinct symptom patterns, which were incorporated into DSM-III as borderline personality disorder and schizotypal personality disorder. The exact relationship of these two entities to schizophrenia or the affective disorders remains ambiguous.[39,40] Follow-up studies of these patients have shown that they do not become chronic schizophrenics, but it is not as easy to distinguish them from patients with affective disorders.[41] Stone[39] has suggested that these patients may have genetic loadings for both affective disorder and schizophrenia, but that these are modest enough not to produce the full profile of symptoms. He also suggests that these patients may have a fairly high genetic loading for schizophrenia, but have had optimal environmental conditions that protected them from developing classic schizophrenia. More work needs to be done to define the relationship between this diagnostically demonstrable disorder and schizophrenia and affective disorders.[42]

A final group of disorders that has been questioned regarding its relationship to classic schizophrenia is that of the paranoid psychoses. Both Kraepelin and Bleuler included these in their descriptions of schizophrenia (dementia praecox), although Bleuler noted that some of these patients did not have a chronic and deteriorating course. The fact that systematic delusions of persecution can occur in individuals with little other evidence of psychosis led to the distinction of paranoia and paranoid states from schizophrenia in earlier diagnostic manuals. However, paranoid schizophrenia was still diagnosed in individuals showing delusions of persecution in generalized psychotic decompensation. Two recent lines of evidence suggest that it may not be appropriate to include this with other types of schizophrenia. Potkin et al[43] found significantly lower platelet monoamine oxidase activity in chronic paranoid schizophrenics than in chronic nonparanoid schizophrenics. Kendler and Hays[44] and Kendler and Davis[45] found that relatives of paranoid schizophrenic patients showed no increased risk of schizophrenia over that of the general population, whereas there was increased risk for schizophrenia in the relatives of nonparanoid schizophrenics. The finding of increased risk in schizophrenics' relatives is not unanimous, at least using DSM-III criteria (see Pope et al[46]). The inclusion of paranoid schizophrenic patients in studies of biological factors in schizophrenia may also mitigate the validity of the findings for all "schizophrenic" patients.

GENETIC DIATHESIS OF SCHIZOPHRENIA

Since the appearance of Franz Kallman's germinal paper on the genetics of schizophrenia in 1938,[47] many efforts have been made to identify and sort out any genetic contribution to schizophrenia. A number of factors have made the pattern of transmission in terms of Mendelian genetics difficult if not ultimately impossible to elucidate. One of these factors is the already-discussed probability of heterogeneity. Another perhaps even more pervasive problem is the variability of presentation. The lack of perfect concordance for schizophrenia in identical twins indicates that the penetrance of the genetic factor is not complete. Although inclusion in genetic studies of individuals with schizoid or schizotypal personality characteristics ("schizophrenia spectrum disorders" is often used as an all-inclusive term) appears to increase the evidence for genetic diathesis. However, there are still some influential theorists who argue that genetic factors have not been conclusively demonstrated to play a role in the etiology of schizophrenia.[48]

In a major review of studies of genetic factors in schizophrenia, Kessler[49] indicated that three major lines of research have pointed to a genetic involvement in the etiology of schizophrenia: family studies, twin studies, and adoption studies. In family studies, the incidence of schizophrenia or schizophrenia-like disorders among the relatives of schizophrenic patients (the Iowa studies have used the word "proband" to identify the index patient) is compared with the incidence of these disorders among relatives of nonschizophrenic control individuals. To indicate a genetic factor, incidence should be higher among first-degree relatives of the schizophrenic proband than among distantly related individuals, and overall incidence should be higher among probands' relatives than in unrelated individuals. Confounding this is the fact that individuals with a high degree of shared genes generally also have a high degree of shared environment. So although family studies such as Rosenthal's[50] have invariably shown increased risk for schizophrenia spectrum disorders in schizophrenics' relatives, this still does not rule out environmental factors as adequate causes of the symptoms.

Twin studies have provided a less easily assailed line of evidence. Whereas monozygotic twins have identical genetic inheritance, dizygotic twins have no more genetic similarity than any other pair of siblings, although they should have as nearly identical environments as do monozygotic twins. Therefore, if the incidence of schizophrenia is significantly higher in monozygotic than in dizygotic twins, this is a strong indicator of a genetic role in etiology. Nearly a dozen major twin studies have been reported worldwide, and all show higher rates of concordance in monozygotic twins than in dizygotic twins.[49] Indeed, in a study of monozygotic twins raised separately, Slater and Cowie[51] found a 65% concordance for schizophrenia in the twins of identified schizophrenic probands.

The studies with the most relevance to this may be the adoption studies. Not only do they allow a more complete separation of genetic and environmental influences, but they also can be done prospectively as well as retrospectively, so that the evaluation of environmental factors is not as likely to be contaminated by outcome. The most elegant and exhaustive of these has been the Danish study (detailed discussion of which may be found in Rosenthal et al's *The Transmission of Schizophrenia*[52]), made possible by the completeness of Danish adoption records. Using the "crossfostering" strategy,[53] these researchers studied not only adopted-away children of schizophrenic parents and adopted-away children of normal parents raised by normal adoptive parents, but also children born to normal parents and adopted by schizophrenic parents. This study showed expected elevated rates of a number of psychopathological conditions in the biological offspring of schizophrenic parents as compared with control adoptees. However, it *failed* to show an increase in psychopathology compared with controls of the children adopted by schizophrenic parents. Thus, the study not only supported the hypothesis of genetic factors in etiology, but also provided evidence *against* a significant role for environmental factors. A further analysis from this study has indicated the separation, both biologically and environmentally, of major depressive disorder from the schizophrenia spectrum.[54]

A number of efforts have been made, on the basis of pedigrees of schizophrenic patients, to identify the exact mode of transmission for the predisposition to the spectrum of disorders. Matthysse and Kidd[55] assessed two of the more common models, the single major locus (one-gene) model and the multifactorial model. These both allow for variability in expression of the underlying genetic pattern and essentially represent the extremes of the single-gene as opposed to the multiple-gene hypothesis. Using the data from several family studies, they found that the data were not consistent with either of these models. Using a different data set and separating paranoid from nonparanoid subtypes, Baron[56] also failed to find support for either single-locus or multifactorial-polygenic patterns of inheritance. He suggested a number of methodological faults that may continue to make assessment of inheritance data difficult, such as the failure to take into account factors from nongenetic contributions, the assessment of the "spectrum" disorders, heterogeneity, the possible role of assortive mating, and assessment of risk in relation to age of onset.

Another aspect of the genetics of schizophrenia has involved the human leukocyte antigens (HLA). HLA antigens have been found to be associated with a number of disorders in humans, particularly those that involve an autoimmune component (one of the theories of schizophrenia, which will be discussed further). A special characteristic of the disorders associated with HLA antigens is that they are familial, but show a non-Mendelian pattern of inheritance with considerable variability in presentation.[57] This has led to a search for an association between HLA antigens and schizophrenia. However, no consistent pattern of association has emerged, even when considerable effort has been made to break patient groups down into subtypes and pool data from several subject populations. McGuffin et al[58] found an increased incidence of HLA-BW5 and a decreased incidence of HLA-AW29 and BW17 in a large, mixed group of schizophrenic patients and an increase in HLA-A1 and a decrease in HLA-A2 and HLA-BW17 in a subgroup with Schneiderian symptoms. Crowe et al[59] found an excess of HLA-AW26 among hebephrenic patients compared with a large group of population controls, but no consistent differences on any of the other antigens studied. They failed to replicate any of the previously reported associations. Gattaz and Beckmann[60] found an increase in HLA-B27 in a patient group, but after correction for the number of antigens tested, this held only for chronic schizophrenics and patients with poor prognosis. Pooling two studies, Gattaz et al[61] found that HLA-B27 was significantly increased in the patient group; noting the high association of this marker with certain arthropathies and the fact that these arthropathies are not found in persons with schizophrenia, they suggested that HLA-B27 might serve as a marker for vulnerability to schizophrenia or other abnormalities. They further indicated that this antigen might be useful in differentiating various subtypes of the illness. McGuffin et al[57] failed to find this association, although they did find an increase in HLA-A9 in paranoid patients and an increase in HLA-A1 in hebephrenic patients. In light of the confusion, it seems reasonable to conclude with them that "possession of a particular HLA antigen is neither a necessary prerequisite nor a sufficient cause" for various subtypes of schizophrenia.

Thus no clear pattern of transmission appears likely to be identified in the near future. Kessler[49] concludes that this problem is rarely handled adequately in genetic counseling. He suggests that individuals involved in genetic counseling of schizophrenic patients and their relatives need to proceed extremely carefully and to recognize the possible short-term and long-term consequences of such counseling on the individual and his or her family.

BIOLOGICAL ABNORMALITIES IN SCHIZOPHRENIA

To indicate that some aspect of schizophrenia is genetically transmitted is, de facto, to assert a biochemical component. Since the earliest discussions of the schizophrenic syndrome, various efforts have been made to identify physiological and biochemical factors associated with it. It was hoped that the "real cause" of schizophrenia might be identified by reasoning out the sources of pathological findings. Thus, much work has been done to identify ways in which the physiology and biochemistry of schizophrenic patients differs from that of "normal" individuals and nonschizophrenic patients. The findings thus far have failed to indicate a single etiological source of the widespread pathology of schizophrenia. As various aspects of bodily function in schizophrenic patients have been studied, it has become evident that little of their physiological functioning is normal. To what extent this indicates overall failure of physical function in schizophrenia and to what extent it is an artifact of pooling groups of patients with differing disorders is unclear.

Birth Season and Perinatal Complications

Schizophrenic patients appear to have suffered, in the course of their premorbid lives, more "insults" of both a physiological and psychological type than have their nonschizophrenic siblings. This succession of insults seems to have begun at birth or even before.[62] A frequent criticism of this finding is that it represents retrospective data and that the individual's history is colored by their subsequent illness. In light of this, as a part of the Danish study, prospective data were gathered on the births of offspring to severely schizophrenic mothers. These offspring have now been followed into adulthood, and the correlation between the occurrence of birth complications and later psychiatric illness has been assessed.[63] The study divided the offspring into three groups: those with clear-cut schizophrenia; those with schizophrenic symptoms, but not the full syndrome (comparable to DSM-III schizotypal personality disorder and referred to by the authors as "borderline schizophrenia"); and those with no evidence of mental disorder. The schizophrenic offspring had the highest incidence of reported complications during pregnancy or birth;

those with borderline schizophrenic symptoms had the least; and the group with no mental disorder was intermediate. This finding suggests that the schizophrenic and borderline schizophrenic offspring had the schizophrenic diathesis, but that its expression was modulated by the amount of stress experienced during the mother's pregnancy and at the child's birth. The other offspring, having no genetic diathesis, were essentially unaffected by the presence or absence of birth complications, at least insofar as these affected their subsequent mental health.

A related finding, for which the relationship to the disorder is less evident, is that of the seasonal variation of births of schizophrenic patients. Although it is clear that individuals who later become schizophrenic are born at all times of the year, a large number of studies from a great variety of geographical locations have found an excess of schizophrenics to have been born during the winter months.[64–68] Three findings indicate that there is a relationship to the cold season: the relationship holds for data from New South Wales in the southern hemisphere where the seasons are reversed;[64] the relationship is more clear cut the more severe the climate;[65,67] and more schizophrenics were born in the years with the coldest winters.[66] However, the exact relationship between birth during a cold winter and schizophrenia remains unclear. A number of intriguing hypotheses have been proposed, including the "genetic gain" hypothesis. This hypothesis states that individuals with the schizophrenic diathesis are actually more robust than others in infancy and therefore more likely to survive a severe winter. Another hypothesis is that mothers who convey the schizophrenic diathesis are more likely to conceive during the spring and early summer months; and a third, that birth during the winter is more associated with viral infections or other stresses which may lead to precipitation of the disorder in predisposed individuals. Shur[68] assessed a large group of schizophrenic patients for degree of genetic risk. High risk was indicated by the presence of schizophrenia in a first- or second-degree relative, and low risk was suggested by the absence of affected relatives. He found that fewer patients with high genetic risk were born during the winter than those with low genetic risk, which he interpreted as support for the hypothesis of winter illness and stress as a precipitating factor. The relationship between this finding and the immunological theories of schizophrenia will be discussed later.

Visual and Vestibular Dysfunction

A number of studies have found abnormalities in muscular coordinative systems of schizophrenic patients. One of the earliest findings was that of abnormal smooth-pursuit eye-tracking patterns.[69] Abnormal eye-tracking patterns had previously been observed in individuals with vestibular disturbances of a variety of etiologies. Velocity arrests (a halt in eye movement during visual pursuit of a swinging pendulum) were present in virtually all of a group of schizophrenic patients, whereas this pattern was rare in normal subjects.[69] Replication of this study by Shagass et al[70] verified this finding, but they also observed this pattern in patients with other diagnoses with a history of psychosis. Iacono and Lykken,[71] studying monozygotic twins, found a high degree of concordance for eye-tracking patterns. This suggests genetic control and indicates that this abnormality may be a genetic marker for susceptibility to psychotic decompensation. Not all visual functions are affected, however. Levin et al[72] found that saccadic eye movements in schizophrenic patients are normal. Both smooth and saccadic eye movements are controlled at the brainstem level[73] and are related to vestibular function. Irrigation of the ear canal with fluid at a temperature above or below normal body temperature produces a vestibular response in the form of ocular nystagmus, through deflection of the cupula of the semicircular canals by convection currents. Myers et al[74] found that severely ill, chronic, drug-free schizophrenic patients showed a substantially reduced vestibular response compared with nonpatients using this technique. Levy et al[75] failed to replicate this finding, although they did find patients to have more dysrhythmic responses. Fish and Dixon[76] found vestibular hyporeactivity in infants born to schizophrenic mothers; this hyporeactivity was associated with other evidence of developmental disorders in these high-risk children and with evidence of psychopathology at age 10. The authors related these findings to disturbance of brain-stem arousal mechanisms, an explanation consistent with that postulated by Levy et al[75] to explain their finding of dysrhythmic responses.

Muscle Abnormalities

One possible explanation for abnormal visual movements in schizophrenic patients relates to abnormalities in muscle tissue in these patients. Meltzer[77] has reported significantly elevated levels of serum creatine phosphokinase in patients experiencing acute psychotic episodes, a finding verified by a number of other laboratories. Although some researchers have argued that this is associated with increased activity, Meltzer has argued that the finding holds even when activity level is controlled. Schubert et al,[78] using strict RDC criteria (which require at least six months' duration of symptoms, thus eliminating most acute psychotic episodes and favoring chronic schizophrenia), verified Meltzer's finding and suggested that the creatine phosphokinase is released from muscle tissue as a result of increased membrane permeability, possibly related to sympathetic nervous system dominance. Meltzer's studies have indicated a number of abnormalities in the muscle tissue of schizophrenic patients.[79] In addition to abnormal bands in schizophrenics' muscle tissue, Ross-Stanton and Meltzer[80] have observed excessive branching of subterminal motor nerves and multiple innervation of skeletal muscle fibers in psychotic patients. Branching was particularly marked in paranoid schizophrenic patients.

Autonomic Abnormalities

A frequent observation in schizophrenic patients is that arousal is disturbed. Zahn[81] reviewed efforts to correlate autonomic nervous system characteristics with genetic predisposition to schizophrenia. He found reports suggesting that although children at high risk for schizophrenia show evidence of high levels of autonomic arousal, schizophrenic patients show a diminished autonomic response to stress. There is considerable evidence for heritability of some autonomic response patterns as measured by electrodermal activity. There is also reason to believe that some aspects of this measure are influenced by learning and by psychological state.

EEG and Evoked Potentials

Although visual and vestibular responses are coordinated at the brainstem level, studies of cortical function in schizophrenic patients also show abnormalities. Reviewing electroencephalogram (EEG) studies of schizophrenic patients, Shagass[82,83] observed that there have been many reports of abnormal EEG wave forms, not only in terms of the pattern of the waves but also temporal lobe spiking. This suggests that schizophrenia may in some ways resemble an epileptiform disorder. Abrams and Taylor[84] also found abnormal left temporal lobe EEGs in schizophrenics. In addition, there are a number of reports of spiking in subcortical structures in these patients. However, Shagass[83] notes that this characterized those schizophrenic patients described as "reactive"; patients with chronic or "process" schizophrenia show less EEG abnormality. The main finding for chronic patients was reduced frequency, suggesting cortical underarousal rather than overarousal. Stevens et al[85] found that spiking in temporal lobe structures was particularly common in patients who were hallucinating or showing other typically schizophrenic behaviors. In a study comparing chronic, nonparanoid schizophrenics with alcoholic and normal individuals, Coger et al[86] found similarities in abnormal brain wave patterns in alcoholics and schizophrenics, but noted that in the schizophrenics these abnormalities were observed primarily in the left temporal region.

Another area of recent interest is the study of evoked potentials, which are the patterns of cortical response generated by specific sensory stimuli. Particular interest has been placed on the relationship between variations in magnitude of the sensory stimuli and variations in magnitude of response. If the magnitude of response increases more than the magnitude of the stimulus, the individual is said to be a sensory "augmenter"; if the magnitude of response increases less than the magnitude of the stimulus, the individual is a sensory "reducer." Although most studies have shown marked sensory reducing in schizophrenic patients,[82,87] these patients have also shown greater variability of response.[82] Shagass et al[88] reported a particularly unusual characteristic of the somatosensory evoked potential (as contrasted with visual or auditory evoked potentials) in chronic schizophrenic patients. The early part of the cortical response (before 100 ms poststimulus) showed more stability than that seen in other patients or controls, whereas the response after 100 ms poststimulus showed more variability than that seen in other patients or controls. This is hypothesized to reflect a defect of sensory gating or filtering mechanisms at a subcortical level. One possible site for the abnormality might be the brainstem reticular activating system. However, it should be noted that little evidence has been found for significant histological changes in postmortem examination of schizophrenic brain tissue.[89] The abnormality was observed only at the primary projection area for somatosensory input to the cortical region of the brain. Other abnormalities of cortical function in schizophrenic patients will be discussed.

Neurological Abnormalities

Although many researchers have argued that schizophrenic patients show behavioral evidence of what appear to be neurological abnormalities, it has proved difficult to demonstrate differences from normal brain function and structure. Pathological findings observed in the past often turned out to be attributable to factors other than the schizophrenic disorder itself. More recently, new techniques for studying brain structure and activity have clarified this issue and provided more concrete evidence for morphological differences between schizophrenic and normal brains. Before the advent of computer-assisted tomography (CAT scans), the study of brain morphology in living patients required pneumoencephalography, a painful and risky procedure often very difficult to justify on grounds of the patient's diagnosis or treatment. However, Reitan reported in 1976[90] that the accumulation of evidence over the years indicated, particularly in the case of chronic and deteriorating schizophrenics, that there is dilation of the lateral ventricles of the brain that appears to be correlated with duration of illness. The question remained whether this was related to the schizophrenia itself or to some other factor, such as duration of use of antipsychotic medication, institutional neglect, dietary deficiency, or experience of treatments believed to be accompanied by some amount of brain damage such as electroconvulsive therapy. In 1976, in one of the first studies to utilize the CAT scan, Johnstone et al[91] noted that those schizophrenic patients with the greatest evidence of cerebral atrophy also showed the greatest cognitive impairment. In response to criticisms that their findings might be due to treatment-related factors, Crow and Johnstone[92] noted that these findings were the most striking in patients who had *not* received any of the aforementioned treatments. With the spread of the use of the relatively safe and noninvasive CAT scan, other studies rapidly replicated these findings. Weinberger et al[93] observed significant ventricular enlargement in chronic schizophrenic patients which was especially marked in those *not* treated with shock therapy. Schizo-affective and nonschizophrenic patients did not show this abnormality. In further studies, these researchers[94,95] also found that ventricular enlargement was associated with poor premorbid social adjustment and with poor response to treatment. They felt that this might identify a genetically separate group of patients, since the HLA profiles of this group were different from those of patients without ventricular enlargement. In a further study,[96] they found that although ventricular size is highly correlated in siblings in nonschizophrenic families, it is not correlated in families with a chronic schizophrenic patient. In those families, the schizophrenic patient had larger ventricles than any of his or her siblings. However, the discordant siblings also had ventricles that were larger than those of the controls, again suggesting some genetic factor related to the schizophrenic diathesis. This finding was replicated by Reveley et al,[97] who found that although ventricle size is much more highly correlated in normal monozygotic twins than in normal dizygotic twins, this high correlation was not observed in seven pairs of monozygotic twins discordant for schizophrenia (although, again, they observed that the nonschizophrenic twin tended to have larger ventricles than the controls). They hypothesized that the ventricular difference (and the difference in diagnosis) might be related to some other factor, such as perinatal complications, which in the presence of a genetic diathesis pushed the symptomatic twin toward later decompensation.

Golden et al,[98] using the Luria-Nebraska neuropsychological battery, found statistically significant correlations between ventricle-brain ratio and abnormal performance on a number of scales of this test. A further study by these researchers[99] compared brain tissue density measured by CAT scan for a group of patients meeting DSM-III criteria for chronic schizophrenia and a matched group of normal subjects. They found that the schizophrenic patients showed reduced tissue density in the anterior left hemisphere compared with the controls.

Andreason et al,[100] studying a group of young, nonhospitalized patients meeting DSM-III criteria for schizophrenia, also found ventricular enlargement in this group, although not in as marked a degree as that observed in other studies with older and longer-hospitalized patients. They also found[101] that patients with ventricular enlargement showed a preponderance of the "negative" symptoms of schizophrenia (such as poverty of speech, affective flattening, anhedonia, and "avolition"). Patients with normal ventricles were characterized by the more "positive" symptoms of schizophrenia (hallucinations, delusions, bizarre behavior, formal thought disorder). They felt, in agreement with Weinberger's group, that ventricular size, particularly in combination with symptom pattern, may provide a meaningful classification distinction.

Findings from CAT scan data with respect to ventricular enlargement have led to a search for other morphological changes in brain tissue associated with schizophrenia. A study reported by Weinberger et al[102] and replicated by Coffman et al[103] of atrophy of the cerebellar vermis in schizophrenic patients led to investigations of this finding by other researchers. Nasrallah et al[104] investigated CAT scans from schizophrenic, manic, and control patients and found more evidence of cerebellar atrophy in the manic patients than in the schizophrenic patients. Luchins et al[105] did postmortem studies on the cerebellar vermis in schizophrenic and control subjects. Noting observations by others that normal human cerebral asymmetry is absent or reversed in chronic schizophrenic patients, they found that those who showed evidence of vermian atrophy failed to show reversal of asymmetry. Lippmann et al[106] found dimensions of the cerebellar vermis to be smaller than normal in both schizophrenic and bipolar patients, but this effect was especially pronounced in bipolar patients with a history of alcohol abuse. Heath et al[107] found CAT scan evidence of cerebellar vermal atrophy in 50% of a group of patients with "functional psychosis" (50 schizophrenic and 64 nonschizophrenic) and in 38% of a group of patients with seizures. These researchers postulated that atrophy of the cerebellar vermis reduces the cerebellum's inhibitory influence on the activity of forebrain structures involved in the control of both emotions and seizure activity. Heath et al have also reported success in treating otherwise treatment-nonresponsive psychotic patients by implantation of a "cerebellar pacemaker."[108] How this finding actually relates to "true" schizophrenia, however, remains to be clarified.

Another abnormality of schizophrenic brain structure reported in the research literature is that of increased width of the sylvian fissure, the interhemispheric fissure, and the three broadest cortical sulci.[109] These measures, like enlargement of cerebral ventricles, suggest progressive tissue loss from the cerebral cortex in these patients. However, in the group of patients studied in this way, there was no correlation between the presence of these cortical abnormalities and ventricular enlargement. The authors suggest that more than one process may be involved in cortical tissue loss in schizophrenic patients.

A frequently reported finding, alluded to earlier, has been the abnormality of cerebral lateralization in schizophrenic patients. Differences in cortical hemispheric function have been recognized since Broca's report of the localization of speech function in the left hemisphere in the 1800s, but the extent of hemispheric differentiation did not become clear until publication of Sperry's work with commisurotomized patients in the 1950s. Since then, a number of measures of hemispheric dominance and lateralization have been devised and used. One of these is initial lateral eye movements, shown to be associated with activation of the contralateral frontal lobes during tasks involving cognitive processing. Schizophrenic thought disorder and speech patterns have appeared to be related to abnormal function of the left hemisphere, a hypothesis reinforced by the similarity of schizophrenic symptoms to those of left temporal lobe epilepsy. However, Schweitzer et al[110] noted that schizophrenic patients appear to initiate thought in their left hemispheres significantly more often than controls. They observed that this seems inappropriate, given the evidence of left hemisphere dysfunction in schizophrenic patients. However, this finding was supported by Gur,[111] who observed that schizophrenics, like right-hemisphere-damaged patients who presumably must rely on their left hemisphere, when asked to detect differences between pairs of altered pictures presented simultaneously or successively, respond more rapidly in the successive presentation. This supports the hypothesis that schizophrenics tend to overactivate their dysfunctional hemisphere.

Normal right-handed individuals usually show cerebral asymmetry on CAT scans, with wider right frontal and left occipital lobes. However, Luchins et al[112] found that right-handed schizophrenic patients showed an increased frequency of both frontal and occipital reversals compared with controls. This finding was restricted to patients *without* evidence of cerebral atrophy, indicating that the contributions of these factors to schizophrenic pathology can be separated and may represent different etiologies. These authors subsequently replicated this finding.[113] Among black patients, reversed asymmetry was associated with increased frequency of HLA-A2 antigen.[114] Additionally, Chaugule and Master[115] noted that schizophrenic patients, when compared with affective psychotics, neurotics, and normal controls, were significantly more likely to be nondextral (not completely right-handed), a finding in agreement with that of Luchins et al[116] studying MZ schizophrenic twins. Andreason et al[117] also found an excess of left-handedness in schizophrenic patients, and these patients also had high ventricular/brain ratios. In some cases, failure to be completely dextral is found in individuals who are left-hemisphere dominant for speech, suggesting a possible injury to the left motor cortex, often thought to have occurred at or before birth. Another hypothesis concerns abnormal interhemispheric conduction in schizophrenics, a finding reported by Gulman et al.[118] Reviews of the data on hemispheric asymmetry and its meaning have been written by Newlin et al[119] and Merrin.[120]

The recent development of positron-emission tomography (the PET scan) has permitted the study of cerebral glucose utilization similar to the use of the CAT scan to study brain tissue. As cerebral glucose utilization is believed to reflect the activity of various parts of the brain, this advance permits the observation of the actual functional activity of various brain regions. In 1974, Ingvar and Franzen,[121] using xenon radiography, had observed reduced blood flow to the frontal lobes of older chronic schizophrenic patients during mental activation. In addition, they noted relatively high occipitotemporal blood flow in these same patients. In a later review of this research, Ingvar[122] postulated that this hypofrontal activity in deteriorated schizophrenic patients might be related to malfunction of dopaminergic projections to this region via the medial forebrain bundle. This finding was dramatically verified with the development of the PET scan,[123] although these researchers did not find definite indications of the source of the reduction in frontal lobe activation in schizophrenic patients. This particular research seems to have excited the general public's interest in schizophrenia; the popular and general scientific press has been filled with reports of these findings and their implications in recent months.

Neurotransmitter Abnormalities

Dopamine Historically, the implication of the catecholamine neurotransmitter dopamine in the schizophrenic process came from several sources. The first drug observed to have antipsychotic properties, reserpine, acts by depleting neuronal stores of the monoamine neurotransmitters (serotonin and the catecholamines dopamine and norepinephrine) and preventing storage and release of new transmitter. In addition, the epidemics of amphetamine abuse in the 1950s and 1960s produced a large number of cases of psychosis essentially indistinguishable from paranoid schizophrenia.[124,125] These amphetamine psychoses were found to respond to treatment with antipsychotic drugs, which also blocked the stereotypic behavior syndrome produced in rats by amphetamines.[125] The appearance of stereotypic behavior in rats was also prevented by alpha-methyl-para-tyrosine, a drug that inhibits the enzyme tyrosine hydroxylase and therefore depletes the catecholamines; inhibition of dopamine-beta-hydroxylase, the enzyme which converts dopamine to norepinephrine, did not prevent the appearance of the stereotyped behavior. In addition, the appearance of Parkinson's disease-like extrapyramidal symptoms in patients taking large doses of antipsychotic drugs also pointed to the importance of dopamine, as Parkinson's disease was known to be associated with the destruction of dopaminergic neurons of the basal ganglia. The addition of a tyrosine hydroxylase inhibitor to the medication of some schizophrenic patients was found to potentiate the antipsychotic action of neuroleptic drugs,[126] although the combination of these two treatments is rarely used. By 1974, the "dopamine hypothesis of schizophrenia" was in considerable vogue, although there were still some problems with it.[127,128] The area of the brain most likely to be involved appeared to be the mesolimbic dopamine system;[129] Parkinson's disease and schizophrenia were not mutually exclusive,[125] apparently ruling out the nigrostriatal dopamine tract as the primary site of the abnormality.

One of the first problems with the hypothesis that schizophrenia results from excessive release of dopamine came from studies of the accumulation of its metabolites in the cerebrospinal fluid of schizophrenic patients. Bowers[130] found that schizophrenic patients had *lower* levels of probenecid-accumulated homovanillic acid (the major metabolite of dopamine) than patients with affective disorders, and that patients with poor prognosis had lower levels than patients with good prognosis. In addition, treatment with antipsychotic drugs led to increases in cerebrospinal fluid homovanillic acid in both schizophrenic groups. Post et al[131] failed to replicate this finding, but their study employed exclusively acute schizophrenic patients. Nevertheless, Bird[132] found elevated levels of dopamine post mortem in the nucleus accumbens (a primary projection site of the mesolimbic dopamine tract) of schizophrenic patients as compared with controls, and this was true of those not treated with antipsychotic drugs as well as of those with a history of drug treatment.

Another problematic finding for a simple hyperdopaminergic theory was that of the effects of dopamine agonist drug treatments. A number of studies have reported worsening of psychotic symptoms in schizophrenic patients given levodopa, the immediate precursor of dopamine.[133,134] However, it is the positive symptoms of schizophrenia that appear to be exacerbated by this treatment. In patients maintained on neuroleptic drugs, the addition of moderate doses of levodopa has been reported to result in improvement of the negative symptoms (apathy, withdrawal, poverty of speech, etc) of schizophrenia.[135,136] In addition, this treatment was noted to be helpful in some young schizophrenic children not also maintained on neuroleptics.[137] The relationship between the positive and negative symptoms of schizophrenia and their relation to dopamine is discussed by MacKay[138] and Crow.[139]

One frequently studied dopamine receptor stimulant is apomorphine. Its use is limited to some extent by the violent emesis produced by large doses. However, in doses low enough to avoid severe vomiting, actual improvement of schizophrenic symptoms has been reported,[140,141] although these findings were for chronic, neuroleptic-resistant patients in one study[140] and for schizo-affective, manic-type patients in another.[141] This effect was hypothesized to be a possible consequence of stimulation of *presynaptic* rather than postsynaptic dopamine receptors; the significance of this distinction is that presynaptic receptors (sometimes called autoreceptors) are believed to be involved in a mechanism for regulation of transmitter release by feedback inhibition—that is, stimulation of presynaptic receptors may lead to a decrease in transmitter release from the presynaptic neuron.[142]

Because of the paradoxical effects of dopamine agonists and reports that dopamine receptor binding predicted the antipsychotic potency of neuroleptic drugs,[143] considerable attention has been devoted recently to the study of dopamine receptors. A number of studies have been done to characterize the dopamine autoreceptor and identify binding properties and effects of various drugs on it,[144–146] although some researchers remain unconvinced of the autoreceptor's existence.[147] Meltzer[148] has reviewed these studies and their implications for psychiatry.

Kebabian et al[149] reported that in certain brain areas, dopamine stimulates increased production of cyclic adenosine monophosphate (cAMP), a substance believed to act as a "second messenger" in a number of intracellular activities. This led to the investigation of antipsychotic drug effects on dopamine-stimulated cAMP production. The butyrophenone neuroleptics such as haloperidol, which were clinically the most potent of the antipsychotic drugs, showed very little inhibition of dopamine-induced cAMP formation in vitro, leading Snyder[150] to postulate initially two different states of the dopamine postsynaptic receptor. However, additional research suggested that (as with nicotinic and muscarinic acetylcholine receptors) there is more than one type of dopamine receptor in the brain[151,152] and that one of them (Snyder's DA-1 type) is linked to the production of cAMP while the other (DA-2) is not. The antipsychotic effects of neuroleptic drugs apparently take place at the DA-2 receptor and not at the DA-1 receptor.[153] Henn et al[154] have suggested that the important cAMP-related dopamine synapses occur on glial rather than neuronal cells and are thus involved in cell metabolism and regulation rather than direct neuronal interactions. Snyder[153] postulates that the butyrophenones bind the DA-2 receptor selectively; this would account for their higher potency. He also suggests that if tardive dyskinesia is mediated through DA-1 receptors, the DA-2-selective receptor blocking agents should produce less risk of this unpleasant side effect of neuroleptic drugs. An important additional finding is that these DA-2 receptors appear to be located largely in the cortical projection areas of the corticostriate dopamine tract. This finding seems significant in light of the earlier-discussed findings of the PET scan studies of cortical glucose utilization in schizophrenic patients. Cross et al[155] found an increase in DA-2 receptors in post mortem brain samples from schizophrenic patients, whether or not they had been treated with neuroleptics. This is in accord with other findings of increased dopamine receptors[156,157] and dopamine postsynaptic supersensitivity[158] in schizophrenic patients. These data and their implications are reviewed by Langer et al.[159]

Some other studies complicating the picture of the relationship between dopamine and symptoms of schizophrenia are those showing an inverse relationship between extrapyramidal symptoms and clinical response to chlorpromazine[160] and studies showing little relationship between symptom-worsening in response to dextroamphetamine and treatment response to pimozide, a highly specific dopamine receptor blocker.[161,162] Thus, there is considerable confusion concerning the actual role played by dopamine, its receptors, and autoreceptors in the positive and negative symptoms of schizophrenia. Reviews of the evidence generally end by pointing up the inconclusiveness that still remains about the role of dopamine in this disorder (eg, Carlsson[163] and van Praag[164]). It seems appropriate to conclude with Alpert and Friedhoff[165] that "Dopamine appears important but cannot be viewed as a simple pathogen."

Norepinephrine Although most research on the role of catecholamines in schizophrenia has concentrated on dopamine, there is some evidence implicating norepinephrine in schizophrenic pathogenic processes. Early in the 1970s several reports appeared of significant improvement in psychotic symptoms in some patients with large doses of propranolol.[166,167] As propranolol acts by blockading beta-adrenergic norepinephrine receptors, this implied a role for norepinephrine in generating schizophrenic symptoms. However, the therapeutic effects of propranolol appeared to be restricted to a particular group of patients, those with acute or schizoaffective rather than chronic course.[167–169] In reviewing this work, Gruzelier and Yorkston[170] observed that patients showing a therapeutic response to propranolol were overresponsive to sensory stimuli before treatment. They hypothesized that for these patients in particular, anxiety may be an important factor in the psychotic process. That propranolol's therapeutic effect is not mediated, even indirectly, via dopamine blockade was shown by two studies[171,172] in which there was no increase in prolactin in the cerebrospinal fluid of either responsive or nonresponsive patients. As an increase in prolactin is a reliable indicator of dopamine blockade and occurred in these patients when neuroleptics were added to their medication regime;[172] therefore, an incidental dopamine blockade cannot account for the therapeutic effects of propranolol in these cases. Freedman[173] suggests that neuroleptic drugs do block the sensitization of brain stem, cortex, and cerebellum to sensory input which is induced by overactivity of noradrenergic projections to these areas. This overactivity may characterize the brain function of acutely schizophrenic patients and result in the clinical experience of sensory flooding reported by these patients. Above-normal concentrations of norepinephrine have been found in the cerebrospinal fluid of schizophrenic patients, particularly those with paranoid symptoms.[174,175] This elevation was reduced by treatment with pimozide[175] and coincided with reduction in psychotic symptoms. In postmortem studies of brain tissue from chronic paranoid schizophrenic patients, elevated levels of norepinephrine were found in certain limbic forebrain areas,[176,177] particularly the nucleus accumbens. Norepinephrine release in the brain is regulated by presynaptic $alpha_2$ receptors. Sternberg et al[178] found that clonidine, an $alpha_2$ receptor stimulant, reduced plasma 3-methoxy, 4-hydroxyphenylethyleneglycol, the primary metabolite of norepinephrine, levels in normal persons, but not in schizophrenic patients. This indicates a subsensitivity of presynaptic receptors in these patients and therefore impaired regulation of norepinephrine release. However, clonidine has not been shown to have antipsychotic properties.[179] Thus, as with dopamine, the exact role played by norepinephrine in the generation of psychotic symptoms remains obscure.

Serotonin One of the earliest factors implicating serotonin in schizophrenia was the finding that the hallucinogenic compound LSD binds to serotonergic receptors and appears to exert its hallucinogenic action there. However, schizophrenic patients given LSD reported that its effects, while interesting, were different from the hallucinations concomitant with their psychosis.[180] Nevertheless, evidence that serotonergic neurotransmission is in some way abnormal in schizophrenia continues to crop up. The similarity of schizophrenia to coeliac disease (which will be discussed further) has suggested a possible role of serotonin in the generation of these symptoms, as serotonin is increased in coeliac patients and has been implicated in causing the symptoms of this disorder.[181] Bender[182,183] has observed a significant increase in serum tryptophan (the dietary amino acid that can cross the blood-brain barrier and is the precursor of brain serotonin) and brain tryptophan uptake in patients withdrawn from chlorpromazine. This increase was correlated with exacerbation of schizophrenic symptoms (although these patients had significantly reduced levels of plasma tryptophan compared with controls while taking chlorpromazine). Although antipsychotic drugs have been shown to bind serotonin receptors[184,185] and to inhibit serotonin-stimulated production of cAMP,[184] the hypothesis that overproduction of serotonin or hypersensitivity of serotonin receptors[183] is pathogenic in schizophrenia does not appear to fit with other evidence. For example, newly hospitalized schizophrenic patients were found to have lower plasma tryptophan levels than controls before treatment,[186] and their tryptophan levels increased with treatment. Further, increase in plasma tryptophan was correlated with clinical improvement in patients who improved, whereas tryptophan levels did not increase in patients who did not respond to treatment.[187] Wyatt et al[188] found that treatment with L-5-hydroxytryptophan (another serotonin precursor) improved symptoms in six of seven chronic undifferentiated schizophrenic patients who had been resistant to phenothiazines and in one of four chronic paranoid schizophrenic patients. Chouinard et al[189] treated 32 chronic schizophrenic patients with tryptophan and benserazide, an inhibitor of liver tryptophan pyrrolase, an enzyme which converts plasma tryptophan to niacin. These researchers found that although this combination was not as effective in symptom reduction as chlorpromazine (and four patients were removed from the study because of acute worsening of symptoms), in general the tryptophan treatment did decrease psychotic symptoms and particularly decreased depressive mood and guilt feelings, a finding consistent with tryptophan's known antidepressant activity. Sardesai et al[190] studied a protein found in the serum alpha-2-globulin fraction in schizophrenic patients and known to increase intracellular tryptophan in these patients; they found that this protein increased the action of liver tryptophan oxygenase (pyrrolase) in rats. However, as schizophrenics not only do not have an excess of niacin but, in fact, often are deficient in this compound, tryptophan metabolism by this pathway is apparently blocked further on. The result of this protein, however, would be to deprive the brain of tryptophan and thereby reduce brain serotonin. Another suggestion that serotonin deficiency may be implicated in schizophrenic symptoms is that long-term amphetamine treatment decreases serotonin;[191] it also produces a psychosis indistinguishable from paranoid schizophrenia as mentioned earlier.[180] Freedman et al[192] found that both chronic undifferentiated and chronic paranoid schizophrenic patients had elevated platelet serotonin levels accompanied by low platelet monoamine oxidase activity, but the paranoid patients had low levels of plasma tryptophan as well. However, a report of severely reduced postsynaptic serotonin receptors (illustrated by binding of tritiated LSD) in postmortem samples of frontal cortex from schizophrenic patients[193] was thought by Whittaker et al[194] to have resulted from long-term chlorpromazine treatment, as this effect can be demonstrated in rats and is not found in patients drug free for the year preceding their death.

Thus, it appears that the evidence concerning the role of serotonin in schizophrenia is, if anything, more confusing than that of the catecholamines. In addition to ambiguity concerning whether schizophrenic symptoms are related to elevated or deficient brain serotonin, there is the possibility of psychosis produced by abnormally methylated derivatives of this neurotransmitter, which will be discussed later.

Gamma-amino butyric acid (GABA) The discovery of the role of GABA agonist effects in the anxiolytic properties of the benzodiazepine antianxiety drugs has led to considerable interest in this neurotransmitter and its action in various psychopathological conditions. Its postsynaptic action appears to be primarily inhibitory, and it is found to interact with a number of other neurotransmitters. As GABA is one of the products of the respiratory cycle, its presence does not always indicate a role as a neurotransmitter, but the presence of the enzymes which mediate its formation and breakdown (glutamic acid decarboxylase and GABA transaminase) are thought to be indicative of a significant cellular role for this compound. As mentioned earlier, there is reason to implicate anxiety in the generation of schizophrenic symptoms in some patients. The report of Bird et al[195] of not only increased dopamine but also reduced glutamic acid decarboxylase in postmortem tissue samples from schizophrenic brains created considerable interest in the possibility of a role for abnormal GABA-ergic transmission in schizophrenia.[196-198] The reduction in glutamic acid decarboxylase was particularly striking in the nucleus accumbens, where dopamine concentrations were noted to be elevated.[199] This suggests the possibility that there may normally be inhibitory GABA-ergic synapses on dopaminergic neurons in the nucleus accumbens[200] and that these are reduced in schizophrenia. This possibility is discussed by Perry et al,[201] who found significantly reduced levels of GABA itself, compared with control subjects, in the nucleus accumbens in post mortem samples of brain tissue from both schizophrenic patients and patients with Huntington's chorea (a disorder also often accompanied by psychotic symptoms). That this effect was not a result of neuroleptic use is suggested by the finding of Marco et al[202] that several antipsychotic agents produced increases rather than decreases in GABA turnover in the nucleus accumbens of rat brain. However, Gold et al[203] found decreased levels of GABA in the CSF of depressed patients but not psychotic patients when compared with neurologic controls. Even though withdrawal from the GABA agonist drug baclofen has been reported to result in hallucinations,[204] trials of baclofen[205,206] and other GABA-ergic agonists such as muscimol,[207] gamma-hydroxybutyrate,[208] and even diazepam[209] failed to produce evidence of significant antipsychotic effects in schizophrenic patients. Thus GABA joins the list of neurotransmitters apparently disordered in at least some schizophrenic patients, but this abnormality does not in itself appear sufficient to account for the disorder.

MAO Activity

Monoamine oxidase (MAO) is an enzyme which occurs in virtually all tissues of the body in several isozymes (all will be referred to as MAO). It is the major means by which many of the neurotransmitters are broken down; not only does it have serotonin and the catecholamines as substrates, but it is also important in the catabolism of a number of other neurotransmitters and neuromodulators such as octopamine, tyramine, phenylethylamine, and tryptamine. Its importance in psychological functions is suggested by the fact that one major category of antidepressant drugs is believed to have its clinical effect through inhibiting the activity of the MAOs and thereby prolonging the functional life of the monoamine neurotransmitters. Thus, the observation of Murphy and Wyatt in 1972[210] that some schizophrenic patients had diminished platelet MAO activity led to considerable research on this subject. Wyatt et al[211] reported the following year that low platelet MAO activity occurred in both monozygotic twins discordant for schizophrenia and might therefore constitute a genetic marker for vulnerability to schizophrenia (although apparently not a direct cause in itself). However, these same researchers failed to find reduced platelet MAO activity in a group of acute schizophrenic patients.[212] Subsequent reports varied, with some finding the effect in chronic patients[213–216] and some failing to find it;[217,218] one group[219] failed to find differences between schizophrenic and control patients in their own sample in MAO activity in platelets, erythrocytes, or skin cell fibroblasts, but did find reduced MAO activity in platelet samples from chronic schizophrenic patients provided by colleagues at the National Institute of Mental Health. Meltzer and Arora[220] found reduced MAO activity in muscle tissue from both schizophrenic and other psychotic patients. Reveley et al[221] failed to find differences in MAO activity in postmortem caudate and frontal cortex tissue samples from schizophrenic and schizophrenic-like patients and normal controls. Schildkraut et al[222] found that reduced MAO activity in platelets occurred in a subgroup of chronic schizophrenic patients with auditory hallucinations and delusions, a finding verified by Meltzer et al[223] and replicated by Schildkraut et al.[224] In reviewing reports published before 1979, Wyatt et al[225] noted that while most studies had reported diminished MAO activity in chronic schizophrenic patients, the data on its activity in acute schizophrenic patients remained inconclusive, and an etiological relationship between low platelet MAO activity and schizophrenia had not been demonstrated. In fact, low platelet MAO activity has been observed to be significantly related to a variety of psychopathology and behavior pathology, particularly if paired with some other marker such as evoked potential augmenting[226] or high erythrocyte/plasma lithium ratio in vitro.[227] An excellent discussion of the research on MAO activity and schizophrenia, and the issues involved in evaluating this work, is provided by Meltzer.[228]

Phenylethylamine

One effect of a significant reduction in MAO would be an increase in a number of compounds which normally are broken down by this enzyme. One substance of interest in this line is phenylethylamine, a relative of the catecholamines found in the nervous system (although not demonstrated to act as a neurotransmitter itself). It is particularly interesting because its chemical structure is very similar to that of the amphetamines.[229] It has many properties in common with amphetamines, including similar behavioral effects [229–232] and the ability to produce release of catecholamines from nerve terminals.[232] MAO-inhibiting drugs potentiate the behavioral effects of phenylethylamine in animals.[231] Thus, it would seem likely that increased levels of phenylethylamine in the nervous system might have effects similar to those of amphetamines in humans. As mentioned previously, amphetamine produces a paranoid schizophrenia-like psychosis in humans for which threshold dose levels vary considerably among individuals.[233,234] Nervous system levels of this compound can be estimated from the amount excreted in urine. Although depressed patients excrete less of it than normal individuals, manic patients (whose behavior in many ways mimics the early effects of amphetamine) excrete more than normal, and schizophrenic patients excrete more than manic patients. In the study by Fischer et al,[229] there was no overlap between the normal group and the schizophrenic group, an important point particularly in a search for possible etiological factors. This finding has been replicated and in fact has been found to be particularly true of chronic paranoid schizophrenic patients,[235] the precise group that would be predicted to result from chronic amphetamine overdose. The finding has been replicated with urine samples from Indian patients and controls, from whom the samples were analyzed blind to the diagnostic category.[236] As promising as this may be in terms of a possible genuine etiological hypothesis, there are many factors that must be considered before any causal relationship is proved. These are discussed by Jeste et al.[236] Although it seems unlikely that paranoid schizophrenia would result from a simple excess of this amphetamine-like compound in the nervous system (the Indian study did show overlap between patient and control values), Gold and Bowers[234] have noted the fact that some individuals show extreme sensitivity to low doses of amphetamines and have speculated that this low-dose, amphetamine-precipitated psychosis indicates a neurobiological vulnerability to schizophrenia. One way that this might occur could be via receptors, perhaps receptors also stimulated by dopamine;[230] this would explain the antipsychotic effect of dopamine receptor-blocking neuroleptic drugs even in the absence of excessive amounts of dopamine itself in the central nervous system. If this should prove to be an adequate explanation of paranoid schizophrenia, it still would probably not account for all schizophrenias but only those resembling amphetamine-induced psychosis.

Dopamine Beta-Hydroxylase

Another factor which could affect the catecholamine system in schizophrenia would be alterations of dopamine-beta-hydroxylase, the enzyme which catalyzes the conversion of dopamine to norepinephrine in noradrenergic neurons. Failure of this enzyme to be normally active would result in an accumulation of dopamine over a period of time, as it would not be further metabolized. Fusaric acid, an agent that inhibits dopamine-beta-hydroxylase, has been demonstrated to increase psychosis in manic patients.[237] Disulfiram (Antabuse), another inhibitor of dopamine-beta-hydroxylase, has also been shown to increase psychosis in schizophrenic patients[238] and to induce schizophrenia-like symptoms in a person with a history of a schizophreniform psychosis but asymptomatic immediately before taking the drug.[239] Dopamine-beta-hydroxylase requires ascorbic acid (vitamin C) as a cofactor, and schizophrenic patients have been noted to have low blood levels of vitamin C.[240] In addition, several researchers have noted a significantly increased need for vitamin C in schizophrenic patients as compared with normal individuals.[241,242] A deficit in dopamine-beta-hydroxylase has also been reported in postmortem brain samples from schizophrenic patients.[243]

Mineral Abnormalities

Another factor necessary for normal activity of dopamine-beta-hydroxylase is copper. Schizophrenic patients have long been observed to have excessive amounts of copper in their serum[244,245] and to show bluish-brown pigmentation of the skin containing copper. This can be treated by the copper-chelating agent D-penicillamine.[246] However, Baron et al[245] found serum copper content in both schizophrenic and normal persons to be unrelated to serum dopamine-beta-hydroxylase activity. Patients treated with D-penicillamine, especially in combination with neuroleptic drugs, were reported to show considerable symptom improvement,[244,246] and chlorpromazine in itself reduces brain copper levels in experimental animals.[247] The exact relation of this treatment to symptom improvement is still not understood.

Endocrine Abnormalities

Another area in which schizophrenic patients show abnormalities is in endocrine function; however, the study of abnormal endocrine function in schizophrenia appears to have been somewhat neglected in recent years even though techniques for endocrine assessment have improved.[248] The hormone which has been most studied in schizophrenic patients is prolactin, not so much for its effects on the nervous system as because it is itself to some extent regulated by dopamine, which inhibits its release; a rise in serum prolactin is a reliable indicator of the dopamine-blocking properties of neuroleptic drugs.[249] Although there is some evidence of reduced prolactin levels in drug-free chronic schizophrenic patients with normal ventricular size,[250] suggesting elevated dopamine levels in the central nervous system, this effect has not been found in acutely disturbed, newly admitted patients.[251] In fact, as a rise in serum prolactin is usually a concomitant of stress, this could be expected in acutely disturbed schizophrenic patients and might mask other factors affecting prolactin levels.

The thyroid system has also been observed to function abnormally in schizophrenic patients. Thyroid disease has been noted to occur more frequently in the mothers of schizophrenic patients than in a carefully matched control sample,[252] and protirelin (thyrotropin-releasing hormone) has been reported to reduce psychotic symptoms when administered intravenously[253] and to improve some of the negative symptoms of schizophrenia when administered orally.[254] Patients were shown to have lower levels of triiodothyronine than control subjects; although patients had normal levels of thyroxine, they had fewer binding sites for this hormone than did controls.[253]

It has frequently been observed that chronic schizophrenic patients, particularly male patients, often show a considerable deficit in normal sexual interest and behavior; this deficit has been observable from soon after puberty in many cases. Studying gonadotrophin secretion in chronic schizophrenic male patients, Ferrier et al[255] found that although prolactin and testosterone levels were normal in these patients, luteinizing hormone and follicle-stimulating hormone were significantly reduced in patients compared with normal subjects. These abnormalities are consistent not only with a diminution in sexual interest, but also with the reduction in fertility often noted in schizophrenic patients. The extent of the abnormality was related to the length of illness and age at onset, as well as severity of positive symptoms, such that the more severe the illness the more reduced were the two hormone levels. These levels were not related to medication status. Whether these same abnormalities are also seen in female chronic schizophrenic patients remains to be reported.

Prostaglandin Abnormalities

The prostaglandins, first identified in the 1930s, are unsaturated fatty acids with a 20-carbon chain and a cyclopentane ring synthesized from cell membrane lipids and dietary fatty acids.[256,257] The name of these compounds derives from the fact that they were first identified in semen, but further studies have shown them to be present in virtually all tissues of the body. They play a great variety of roles in the body and appear to be particularly important in inflammatory processes, fever, and pain sensitivity. Many commonly used analgesic and antipyretic agents such as aspirin and acetaminophen have as an important aspect of their action the inhibition of prostaglandin synthesis.[256] Prostaglandins are classified in three main series depending on the number of double bonds in their side chains; the PGE and PGF series are particularly important, as these are found in brain tissue.[257] The Hedqvist hypothesis[258] states that E-type prostaglandins inhibit the sympathetic nervous system through a feedback control mechanism.

The implication of these compounds, the PGE series in particular, in schizophrenia originated with the report of Abdulla and Hamadah[259] that adenosine diphosphate stimulates the release of PGE_1 in the platelets of normal persons and patients with affective illnesses, but not in the platelets of schizophrenic patients. This suggested that schizophrenic patients might be deficient in PGE_1; Rotrosen et al[260] noted a significant reduction in PGE_1-stimulated cAMP accumulation in platelets from schizophrenic patients, an apparent verification of this hypothesis, although this reduction was unaffected by antipsychotic drugs. The hypothesis that schizophrenia is a prostaglandin E_1 deficiency disease has been most thoroughly espoused by Horrobin et al.[261–263] They note as evidence for this hypothesis that all effective antipsychotic drugs (except clozapine[264]) stimulate secretion of prolactin, which is a potent stimulator of prostaglandin synthesis; that schizophrenic patients are resistant to pain and inflammation, but are virtually free from rheumatoid arthritis (associated with PG excess); and that high doses of antiprostaglandin drugs often produce schizophrenia-like psychotic symptoms (see also Turner[265] and Tollefson and Garvey[266]). Litvin[267] noted high renin concentrations in the blood of three untreated paranoid schizophrenic patients, which would also be consistent with prostaglandin deficiency. However, Feldberg[268] asserted that schizophrenia may be associated with PGE series excess. He observed that injection of PGE_1 into the cerebral ventricles of cats produces a catalepsy similar to catatonic behavior in humans (although note Taylor and Abrams' assertion quoted earlier that catatonia is more characteristic of affective psychoses than of schizophrenia). He also notes that febrile episodes are often accompanied by psychosis and that some schizophrenic patients have febrile episodes concurrent with exacerbations of their psychotic symptoms. A report by Mathe et al[269] of increased levels of PGE in the cerebrospinal fluid of schizophrenic patients appeared to support this theory rather than Horrobin's. However, treatment of acute schizophrenic patients with prostaglandin E suppressant drugs by Falloon et al[270] failed to produce any remission of symptoms (although patients were noted to have elevated body temperature). Horrobin et al[263] argue that both hypotheses (PGE_1 deficiency and PGE excess) could be true in that they might represent different groups of schizophrenic patients. In addition, they note that PGE_1 has a bell-shaped dose-response curve, with high concentrations having similar effects to low concentrations. Other evidence exists concerning the relationship of prostaglandins and brain function relevant to schizophrenia.

Serotonin promotes PGE release in the brain (and as discussed earlier, serotonin appears to be deficient in at least some schizophrenic patients[271]). E-series prostaglandins are potent anticonvulsants, probably through potentiation of the GABA-ergic system both by promoting GABA release and by stimulating GABA receptors.[256]

Vincent et al[272] observed that the normal effects of PGE_1 are inhibited in rats deficient in essential fatty acids, particularly linoleic acid. This observation is consistent with the hypothesis of Rudin[273] that some schizophreniform, manic-depressive-like, and phobic neurotic disorders result from a type of "substrate pellagra" secondary to essential fatty acid deficiency. In this study, 12 treatment-resistant patients with pellagraform symptoms were treated with linseed oil (which is very high in linoleic and linolenic acids), and 8 showed moderate to marked improvement of symptoms; relapse followed withdrawal of linseed oil supplements.

Rudin notes that this work is consistent with the prostaglandin theories of schizophrenia, but argues that the essential fatty acid deficiency is the basic factor underlying the disorder.

Opiates and Endorphins

When it was discovered that the 61-90 section of the polypeptide chain beta-lipotropin had many of the properties of opiate compounds, it was named beta-endorphin (a contraction of "endogenous morphine"), and the search was begun for its actions in the human nervous system.[274,275] The fact that opiates affect many of the brain functions that are disordered in mental illness (such as mood, sleep, pain sensitivity, etc) suggested the investigation of a possible role for the endorphins in mental illness.[276] The report by Jaquet and Marks[277] that microinjection of beta-endorphin into the brains of rats produced a cataleptic state reminiscent of schizophrenic catatonia further spurred this research. A number of slightly differing opiate peptides have been isolated from beta-lipotropin, and these have been investigated in a variety of ways.[276]

Three main hypotheses have been researched: (1) that schizophrenia involves endorphin excess, which can be studied by assaying endorphin levels in patients compared with normal persons, by giving narcotic antagonists (opiate receptor blocking agents) to schizophrenic patients, or by dialyzing schizophrenic patients; (2) that schizophrenia involves a deficit of endorphins, which can be investigated by administering opiate peptides to patients; and (3) that endorphins in schizophrenics are abnormal or unbalanced, which can be investigated by altering endorphin equilibrium or analyzing dialyzates from these patients. Excellent discussions of these research strategies are provided by Volavka et al,[278] Davis et al,[279] Buchsbaum et al,[280] van Praag and Verhoeven,[281] and van Ree and de Wied.[282]

Endorphin excess Terenius et al[283] developed several techniques for the analysis of opiate peptides from human serum and cerebrospinal fluid. A number of reports of cerebrospinal fluid sample analysis showed differences between patients and normal controls,[284-287] with acute schizophrenic patients showing an excess of cerebrospinal fluid opioids and chronic schizophrenic patients apparently deficient when compared with controls. However, not all studies found this; Naber et al[288] found that although schizophrenic men had higher levels of immunoreactive opioids (though not beta-endorphin) than normal men, they did not differ significantly from other patients. Brambilla et al[289] assayed plasma levels of beta-endorphin, beta-lipotropin, and adrenocorticotropic hormone and found that alterations in levels of these compounds did not distinguish schizophrenics from other patients. Some of the more interesting data on this subject have come from studies in which schizophrenic patients were treated with renal dialysis. The initial report of Wagemaker and Cade in 1977[290] that they had successfully used dialysis to bring about remission of schizophrenic symptoms in a number of young patients with Schneiderian first-rank symptoms was greeted with considerable enthusiasm, and a number of studies were initiated to test this treatment. Several papers appeared speculating as to the mechanism by which this treatment might have an effect (for example, Cohen et al[291]), and one of the suspected mechanisms was the presence of opioid compounds. However, reports rapidly appeared of schizophrenic patients showing no benefit from dialysis.[292-296] Reports of improvement were primarily in affective rather than schizophrenic symptoms.[297,298] One report did discuss some reduction in hallucinations or the frightening quality of hallucinations,[299] but the effect was in no way as spectacular as that reported by Wagemaker and Cade.

Another strategy for testing the hypothesis of excess endorphins in schizophrenic patients is to give opiate antagonists to patients and observe them for a potential reduction in symptoms. The two most commonly used of these are naloxone (which is administered to newborn infants to aid in recovery from the effects of anesthesias administered to the mother during labor) and naltrexone. An initial report of a therapeutic effect of naloxone in schizophrenia by Gunne et al[300] led to a number of attempts to replicate that finding, but the results were generally negative,[301-303] although these early studies used relatively low doses of naloxone intravenously. Later studies using higher doses showed more significant reductions in symptoms, particularly hallucinations.[304-306] Pickar et al[306] summarized these studies, and the increase in successful outcomes with higher doses is evident. These authors reported that in their own study, conducted with a large number of patients from World Health Organization collaborating research centers, patients who were also receiving neuroleptic medication were more likely to show significant general symptom reduction with naloxone. Studies with naltrexone, a longer-lasting oral antagonist, have so far been negative.[307–309]

Endorphin deficiency In the past, opiate drugs have generally not been used in the treatment of schizophrenia, primarily because of their high addiction potential, but also because they have not been reported to have significant therapeutic value. However, the synthesis of beta-endorphin in the laboratory was followed by research to determine whether it might have a therapeutic effect in schizophrenia. The initial study by Kline et al[310] produced mixed results in a single-blind design; repeated doses of the compound were not effective. Berger et al[311] found that schizophrenic patients injected intravenously with a bolus of beta-endorphin from an albumin-coated syringe showed an increase in serum prolactin (suggesting inhibition of dopamine neurotransmission); although in some of the patients there was a statistically significant reduction in symptoms of schizophrenia after beta-endorphin as measured by the Brief Psychiatric Rating Scale, the reduction was not clinically apparent to either the patients or the nursing staff. Although Gerner et al[312] found an improvement in depressed patients after beta-endorphin infusion, schizophrenic patients showed a nonsignificant worsening with the drug; however, Pickar et al[313] did not observe beneficial effects of intravenous beta-endorphin in either schizophrenic or depressed patients.

The most successful results of endorphin treatment of schizophrenic patients have been reported by researchers at the State University of Utrecht in the Netherlands. These researchers studied the activity of fragments of the beta-lipotropin chain in animals and found that the nonopiate-like peptide des-tyrosine-gamma endorphin (DT-gamma-E), the 62-77 fragment of the polypeptide chain, had neuroleptic-like activity. It did not have the usual sedative and locomotor effects of haloperidol. In the belief that this might constitute an "endogenous neuroleptic," they treated a group of otherwise neuroleptic-resistant schizophrenic patients with the compound.[314] They subsequently replicated their results in double-blind studies.[315] Positive results were also reported by Emrich et al[316] using the same compound. Further research with DT-gamma-E[317–319] has indicated that although it provides a dramatic therapeutic effect in some patients, particularly hebephrenic and paranoid patients, it is essentially ineffective in schizo-affective patients and those with "residual" schizophrenic symptoms.[318] These researchers noted that the effect of DT-gamma-E on various aspects of neural and endocrine function suggest that it has a major impact on the dopamine system in the brain, but that the effect is different from that of neuroleptics. Research on the effects of this compound on catecholamine systems in rat brain suggest that it functions to some extent as a dopamine antagonist in some areas.[320] Other researchers have reported it to produce dramatic increases in melatonin in rat pineal gland.[321] The Utrecht researchers suggest that the defect underlying the schizophrenic symptoms of those patients showing a dramatic therapeutic response to this treatment is faulty cleavage of the gamma-endorphin fragment from the original polypeptide chain.[282,318] This error has its effect particularly in the nucleus accumbens,[282] an area of the brain which has frequently been implicated in schizophrenic symptoms and treatment effects (see earlier sections).

Abnormal endorphins Although the Utrecht researchers' work suggests that endorphins may result from faulty cleavage from the original polypeptide chain, Palmour et al[322] reported finding leucine^5-beta-endorphin in the dialysates of schizophrenic patients, suggesting another hypothesis. As methionine is usually found in this locus of the endorphin chain, this altered form of the fragment could be genetically determined and might constitute a predisposition to psychosis. However, two further studies, one using 2[323] and one using 98 schizophrenic patients,[324] failed to find any evidence of this abnormal endorphin in schizophrenic patients.

Digestive production of opioid peptides from exogenous sources is also a possibility relating schizophrenia with endogenous opiates. Zioudrou et al[325] reported the production of opioid peptides in pepsin hydrolysates of wheat gluten and alpha-casein (a milk protein). It was demonstrated these are produced in vivo and are not degraded in the gut. These opiates could be absorbed into the gut, cross the blood-brain barrier, and act as opiates in the brain. The significance of this finding is in its implications relative to theories of abnormal reaction to gluten and milk in the etiology of schizophrenia.

Abnormal Reaction to Gluten

Mental and behavioral disturbances have long been associated with coeliac disease, a disorder involving sensitivity of the small intestine to a component of the wheat gluten protein. However, it was not until Dohan's comprehensive study of the relationship between the availability of wheat flour and the incidence of schizophrenia appeared[326] that an association was made between wheat gluten and schizophrenia. Dohan argued that in coeliac disease, there is a hereditary abnormality which is made symptomatic by the consumption of wheat and certain other cereals; this amounts to a diathesis-stress origin of the disorder's symptoms. On the hypothesis that it is this same sensitivity to wheat gluten which produces the symptoms of schizophrenia, he analyzed not only the incidence of schizophrenia in various countries as it correlated with the consumption of wheat, but also changes in the incidence of schizophrenia correlated with shortages of wheat during World War II. His predictions were borne out to a remarkable degree, in that the incidence of schizophrenia correlated highly with wheat consumption in various countries and had covaried with wheat availability during the war. Dohan and his colleagues[327] further tested the hypothesis of a correlation between coeliac symptoms and schizophrenia by placing a group of schizophrenic patients on a gluten-free, milk-free diet such as that used to treat coeliac disease. Even though these patients did not show evidence of malabsorption from the small intestine, they showed substantial symptomatic improvement on the diet. This work was replicated by Singh and Kay[328] with neuroleptic-treated schizophrenic patients with a variety of symptom patterns. These patients, as a group, showed marked improvement while on the milk- and gluten-free diet, and their symptoms worsened when they were given a "gluten challenge." As the study was done double blind, their results seemed reasonably compelling, although the study was challenged by some authors on other methodological grounds.[329,330] In a later discussion of this research, Singh[331] noted that anticholinergic and neuroleptic drugs appear to have opposite effects on the drug-responsive aspects of schizophrenia, whereas gluten appears to affect those symptoms which are not responsive to neuroleptic drugs. Further attempts to study the effects of gluten-free diets and gluten challenge on schizophrenic patients have had mixed results. Rice et al[332] essentially replicated the study of Singh and Kay;[333] of the 16 patients who completed their study, two improved significantly on the gluten-free diet and one of these showed significant worsening during the gluten challenge. They concluded that the gluten hypothesis of schizophrenia might apply to some, but not all, schizophrenic patients. Potkin et al[334] studied eight young schizophrenic patients, none of whom showed either improvement on the cereal- and milk-free diet or worsening with gluten challenge; nor did any show an inflammatory response (as measured by serum alpha$_1$-glycoprotein) to the gluten challenge. Some research has suggested that the effect of the gluten-free diet, when successful, may be to increase blood levels of neuroleptic, the absorption of which may be inhibited by gluten.[335] However, Osborne et al[336] studied five neuroleptic-resistant patients with a constant dose of butaperazine. These patients failed to show a therapeutic response to the diet and showed no change in plasma butaperazine levels when placed on or removed from the diet. Storms et al[337] studied 26 schizophrenic patients, who were given a cereal- and milk-free diet; half were then given cookies containing gluten, and half were given cookies containing only gluten-free peanut flour. Contrary to expectations, the gluten-challenged patients appeared to show improvement (primarily in mood), whereas the gluten-free patients did not. Hekkens[338] found gluten (gliadin, the protein in wheat gluten to which coeliac patients are reactive) antibodies in 2 of 20 schizophrenic patients in quantities resembling that found in coeliac patients, and Manowitz[339] reported that the profile of plasma amino acids in fasting schizophrenic patients resembles that of coeliac patients more than that of normal controls. However, Kinnell et al[340] found that few of 98 schizophrenic patients and 90 of their unaffected relatives had serum antibodies to oats, wheat, gluten, chicken, calf, or milk protein. McGuffin et al[341] also failed to find more antibodies to gluten in schizophrenic patients than in controls or patients with affective disorders.

In light of these varying reports, it is interesting that Russian psychiatry has used fasting in the treatment of mental illness since 1946.[342] Patients are usually maintained abstinent from food for 20 to 30 days. Impressive symptom remissions are noted in a large number of patients, especially those who are relatively young, have some insight into their illness, and who have not been chronically ill over long periods of time. Because of differences in Russian diagnostic categories, it is difficult to determine which type of patients benefit most.

In reviewing work done before 1978, Dohan[343] discussed four hypotheses concerning the possible pathogenic mechanisms which might underlie schizophrenic symptoms triggered by food proteins. One is that the peptic-pancreatic digestion of certain food proteins produces polypeptides that are psychotoxic; the second, subsidiary to the first, is that in schizophrenia-predisposed individuals, normal barriers to these peptides entering the brain are defective, and thus the psychotoxic properties are able to be manifested. The third and fourth hypotheses concern the genetic relationship between schizophrenia and coeliac disease: that the defect in the gut barrier to these peptides is genetic and is common to both disorders, and that other, dissimilar genes determine which disorder will be manifest.

Viral and Immunological Abnormalities in Schizophrenia

It has been known for a long time that some kinds of viral infection, particularly meningal or encephalitic infections, are frequently manifested with symptoms of psychosis.[344] In addition, slow virus infections can result in diseases of the brain such as Kuru or Creutzfeld-Jacob disease,[345] in which psychosis is a major part of the symptomatology. This has led to speculation that the symptoms of schizophrenia may result from either viral infection, especially of a slow-acting type, or from destruction of brain tissue through an autoimmune process possibly triggered by a viral infection (such as is thought to be the etiological factor in multiple sclerosis). One of the agents suspected has been herpes simplex virus, as a brain infection by this virus has been shown to be associated with significant alterations in neurotransmitters and their release.[344] These researchers also investigated cytomegalovirus, varicella zoster virus, and measles virus, primarily by means of antibody levels in serum from patients and controls. They found, however, that patients with affective psychoses and dementias had higher levels of antibodies to the viruses than did schizophrenic patients. Torrey et al[346] also failed to find elevated antibodies to measles, herpes simplex virus I, cytomegalovirus, and rubella virus in serum or cerebrospinal fluid of schizophrenic patients, although 6 of 17 multiple-admission schizophrenic patients had elevated levels of immunoglobulin G (IgG) or measles antibody. A more recent report, however, indicated that 20 of 178 schizophrenic patients had elevated levels of IgM against cytomegalovirus in their serum (as did 3 of 17 patients with bipolar affective disorders[347]).

Russian researchers (discussed by Durell and Archer[348]) have reported finding unusual immunoglobulins in the brains of schizophrenic patients. Heath and Krupp[349] found a protein fraction in schizophrenic serum they named "taraxein" which produced schizophreniform behavior in monkeys; however, this finding has not been duplicated. These reports have spurred further efforts to determine whether some cases of apparent schizophrenia could result from viral or autoimmune processes. These may result from unusual viruses, but it is also possible that they could result from common viruses which persist after primary infection in these patients and ultimately produce pathology by cell destruction or by autoimmune pathology after antigenic alteration of host cells.[350]

Pulkkinen[351] studied concentrations of IgA, IgG, and IgM in the serum of 76 schizophrenic patients. He found the highest concentrations of IgM in the patients who were behaviorally withdrawn at the time of admission and the lowest in those with paranoid symptoms. Further, elevations (relative to other patients) of IgA and IgM at admission predicted a shorter hospitalization. Low IgM in paranoid patients was hypothesized to be related to stress (presumably higher in these than other patients), which may result in hypofunction of their immune system. It has recently been demonstrated that stress does result in hypofunction of the immune system and that this effect is mediated via the endogenous opiates.[352] This would seem to have impact on both the endorphin and viral theories of schizophrenia. Tyrrell et al[353] reported finding a virus-like agent with cytopathic properties in the cerebrospinal fluid of 13 of 38 schizophrenic patients; a similar agent was found in 8 of 11 patients with serious or chronic nervous system disease, but in only 1 of 25 patients with surgical or general medical conditions. These authors and their colleagues[354] reported that the patients with this agent had higher IgA levels than those without it, but that there was no systematic difference in their symptoms. In a discussion of research on immunoglobulins in schizophrenia, Bock[355] noted that these proteins are not normally synthesized inside the blood-brain barrier, but that they are synthesized there under various pathological conditions involving the immune apparatus. Thus CSF studies are particularly relevant in a study of schizophrenia. Her research also found anu replicated deficits in serum IgM in schizophrenic patients (though none were catatonic or paranoid). These results, then, are apparently not in agreement with those of Pulkkinen.[351]

In a review of several studies on humoral and cellular immunity in schizophrenia done in their laboratory, Vartanian et al[356] reported several interesting findings: the schizophrenic patients they studied had a very high antibody titre against a brain $alpha_2$ glycoprotein found in *glial* cells—much higher than titres found in normal controls or in patients with other neurological autoimmune disorders like multiple sclerosis or amyotrophic lateral sclerosis. The schizophrenic patients had more elevated levels of B lymphocytes and fewer than normal T lymphocytes. Serum from 81% of 50 schizophrenic patients prevented DNA synthesis in lymphocytes from normal individuals; and there was high activity against thymus gland leukocytes in schizophrenics, manic-depressive psychotics, and patients with thyrotoxic goiter, but not in normal controls, or patients with senile dementia, appendicitis, and other diseases. Stevens[357] has reported that postmortem examination of tissue from schizophrenic brains has shown substantial fibrillary gliosis, which would be consistent with Vartanian et al's[356] report of antiglial antibodies. Stevens noted that glial cells are rarely examined in postmortem studies of schizophrenic brain tissue, yet alterations of the glia could have a tremendous impact on neural functioning. Pandey, Gupta, and Chaturvedi[358] replicated the finding of antibrain antibodies in nearly half of 54 schizophrenic patients; these were present in none of 27 controls. They did not discuss whether the antibodies were against proteins of neural or glial origin. The antibodies were more likely to be found in patients with a positive family history of schizophrenia and in patients with several prior episodes of schizophrenia. These authors reasoned that their evidence is consistent with a process produced by a slow virus infection.

Goldstein et al[359] note that long-term use of chlorpromazine has been linked to the presence of atypical lymphocytes in the blood of schizophrenic patients and to the development of systemic lupus erythematosus, an autoimmune disorder, in psychotic patients. This suggests that some or even many of the findings of immunological abnormalities in schizophrenia could be secondary to neuroleptic use rather than to the disorder itself. This is particularly important in light of Rudin's[360] argument that systemic lupus erythematosus may provide a model for schizophrenia. Systemic lupus erythematosus is associated with schizophreniform psychoses and has central nervous system pathology revealed by immunofluorescent immune complex deposits in the choroid plexus. The choroid plexus is the site of the generation of cerebrospinal fluid from blood plasma and therefore is an important component of the blood-brain barrier. A disorder of the choroid plexus could produce some of the effects noted earlier such as abnormal transport of gut-produced polypeptides into the brain. Rudin has also argued[361] that viral coat peptides and cereal grain glutens could produce this autoimmunity-generated "leak" between the blood and the brain. According to this theory, the same disorder could be caused by at least two of the mechanisms already shown to be associated with schizophrenia—allergy to cereal glutens or infection by viruses. The issue of cause and effect seems significant here and remains to be more carefully examined. If neuroleptic use were the cause, worsening over time might be expected in any patients receiving long-term neuroleptic therapy, and there should have been a distinct change in the general character of schizophrenia after the advent of neuroleptics. Both of these effects remain to be demonstrated.

Abnormal Methylation of Neurotransmitters or Related Substances

The "transmethylation hypothesis" of schizophrenia was first proposed by Osgood and Smythies[362] after they noted that the transfer of a methyl group to each of the hydroxyl groups of norepinephrine would transform this compound into one very similar to mescaline. Monomethylation is one of the usual means by which catecholamines are inactivated in the nervous system. However, these initial breakdown products might easily serve as substrates for some abnormal enzyme action by which they became dimethylated or trimethylated hallucinogenic compounds. The theory was later extended to include serotonin and tryptamine, which could be transformed into bufotenine or dimethyltryptamine (DMT).[363] This hypothesis rests on the idea that the hallucinations of schizophrenia are the same as those caused by the hallucinogenic compounds produced by the abnormal methylation. Subsequent experience has indicated that this is not the case. Although patients report that amphetamine makes their psychoses worse, they find the effects of hallucinogenic drugs different from the hallucinations concomitant with their psychoses.[180] The first and perhaps strongest piece of evidence in support of the transmethylation hypothesis was the report by Pollin et al[364] that methionine (a methyl donor) administered with a monoamine oxidase inhibitor caused an increase in schizophrenic symptoms in patients who were in partial remission. A number of other laboratories confirmed this finding, but the hypothesis that these effects resulted from abnormal methylation of neurotransmitters or their metabolites was not demonstrated. Another approach to testing the hypothesis was the effort to find and identify abnormally methylated hallucinogenic compounds in the serum and urine of schizophrenic patients. What appeared to be an abnormal catecholamine breakdown product, dimethyl phenylethylamine (DMPEA), was the first such compound to be reported. Given the observation noted above, phenylethylamine itself might be considered to be more pathogenic than DMPEA. This compound, when assayed in the urine of schizophrenics, was observed in the final stage of analysis as the famous "pink spot." It was first reported by Friedhoff and Van Winkle[365,366] and confirmed by Bourdillon et al.[367] However, considerable controversy arose over these findings, and some of the findings were argued to be attributable to artifacts of the assay procedure or to aspects of the patients' diet or inaccuracies in diagnosis.[368,369] Later, bufotenine was reported in the urine of acute schizophrenics and chronic patients off medication who were experiencing an exacerbation of their symptoms.[370–372] Saavedra and Axelrod[373] reported finding an enzyme in brain tissue that would convert tryptamine into hallucinogenic methylated compounds. This enzyme's activity was inhibited in normal brain tissue. Bidder et al[374] reported finding DMT in blood and urine of psychiatric patients, but not in that of control individuals. Rosengarten and Friedhoff[363] published a detailed and carefully organized review of the research that had been done on the transmethylation hypothesis before 1976. While evidence supported the possibility of psychosis produced by endogenously generated hallucinogens, they concluded that the data were still inconclusive as to whether this actually occurred and resulted in schizophrenic symptoms.

Relatively little research relevant to the transmethylation hypothesis of schizophrenia has appeared since this review[363] was published. Oon et al[375] reported finding *N*-methyltryptamine and DMT in nanogram amounts in the urine of 19 normal human subjects. Acidification of the subjects' urine produced a transient increase in DMT excretion, but giving the subjects methionine did not affect DMT excretion. Gillin et al[376] also reviewed the "psychedelic" model of schizophrenia. They noted that DMT concentrations were not found to differ between schizophrenics and controls and that the effects of artificially administered DMT did not really resemble the symptoms of schizophrenia. Another finding against the hypothesis was that of Baldessarini et al[377] that neither methionine nor *S*-adenosyl-methionine (the metabolite believed to be actually responsible for endogenous methylation) produced an increase in methylated catecholamines in rat tissues and actually decreased the concentrations of DMT. Maj et al[378] also reported failing to find increased plasma *S*-adenosyl-methionine in schizophrenic patients and argued that although the psychotogenic effects of administration of methyl donors to schizophrenic patients had been demonstrated too reliably to be questioned, they believed that the production of psychotomimetic substances by methylation of transmitters or their metabolites would be unlikely to be the mechanism by which this effect is mediated. Thus, the transmethylation hypothesis, although still provocative, has so far failed to provide an adequate demonstration that this is, in fact, the agent responsible for even a subtype of schizophrenia.

BIOLOGICAL THEORIES OF SCHIZOPHRENIA

Thus far, we have reviewed nosological issues concerning schizophrenia, evidence for genetic transmission of schizophrenia or the predisposition to develop it under the right environmental circumstances, and evidence of biological abnormalities associated with the disorder. Some of these biological abnormalities have generated various hypotheses and theories concerning the etiology of schizophrenia itself or at least of some of its symptoms. For various reasons, although some of these hypotheses are compelling in many ways, none has yet provided an adequate explanation for all or even most cases of schizophrenia. We will first review the hypotheses with the strongest arguments, then mention some of the more unusual theories of schizophrenia, and finally close with a discussion of some recent theories that integrate various ideas in novel and often comprehensive ways.

Theories Previously Discussed

Dopamine theory The theory of schizophrenia with the strongest evidence behind it is the theory that the symptoms of schizophrenia result from abnormal stimulation of dopamine receptors. Several dopamine receptors have been hypothesized, and not all are involved in schizophrenia, nor do all brain regions receive dopaminergic projections. The evidence favoring this theory is based on the fact that all drugs that have proved to reduce symptoms of schizophrenia act on the dopamine system, either directly or indirectly, to reduce stimulation of postsynaptic dopamine receptors. The problems with this theory are: (1) that the same drugs, apparently by the same mechanism, reduce psychotic symptoms in disorders other than schizophrenia (few theorists still believe that all psychosis is schizophrenic); (2) that not all symptoms of schizophrenia can be demonstrated to result from abnormal dopaminergic neurotransmission; (3) that chronically schizophrenic patients show evidence of reduced, rather than excessive, dopamine turnover in the central nervous system; and (4) that schizophrenic patients whose overt psychosis is brought into remission by the use of dopamine receptor-blocking drugs continue to have other persistent symptoms of both a biological and a psychological-behavioral nature.

Other neurotransmitters Theories involving the other known neurotransmitters tend to follow the format that the symptoms of schizophrenia result either from a deficit of the neurotransmitter (GABA and possibly serotonin) or an excess of it (norepinephrine and possibly serotonin). However, treatments affecting these neurotransmitters are considerably less successful in reducing the symptoms of schizophrenia than are the dopamine-blocking neuroleptics. One hypothesis related both to the dopamine theory and to norepinephrine is that proposed by Stein and Wise.[379] They argue that in schizophrenics the brain produces a neurotoxin from dopamine called 6-hydroxydopamine; it is taken up into catecholamine neurons (or acts on catecholamine receptors) in such a way that its immediate effects produce the positive symptoms of psychosis, and the slow destruction of the catecholamine neurons ultimately produces the negative symptoms of schizophrenia. Thus, the treatments for schizophrenia that block catecholamine receptors (as do both the neuroleptics and propranolol) would not only reduce the immediate effects of the neurotoxin, but also reduce the long-term damage to the catecholamine systems caused by it. This hypothesis has gotten little attention recently, and it has been argued that there is no evidence of 6-hydroxydopamine in the brains of schizophrenics. However, the biochemist R.N. Adams (personal communication, K.N.) has noted that 6-hydroxydopamine is so unstable that its breakdown requires seconds or less; none would be expected to be found in postmortem brain samples even if it had been present. In addition, Adams has also demonstrated that in the absence of vitamin C in the brain, the inhibition of dopamine-beta-hydroxylase could result in the build-up of large amounts of dopamine. Under these conditions dopamine can autooxidize into dopamine-orthoquinone, which is very unstable and rapidly degenerates into 6-hydroxydopamine. In this context it seems useful to note the reports of various authors, discussed earlier, of excessively high need for vitamin C by schizophrenics.

Low MAO activity Low MAO activity could alter concentrations of a large number of body substances with considerable impact on the central nervous system; in fact, one of the two treatments that consistently worsen schizophrenic symptoms involves use of an MAO inhibitor with *S*-adenosyl-methionine. However, low MAO activity is found in a large number of persons, the vast majority of whom show little or no evidence of disordered thought or behavior. In addition, MAO-inhibiting drugs fail to produce psychosis in most people (although there have been reports of manic-like reactions in some depressed patients treated with MAO inhibitors).

Phenylethylamine Amphetamines are the only exogenous agents demonstrated to produce a psychosis in normal subjects; indistinguishable from a type of schizophrenia the evidence suggests that all normal individuals will develop a paranoid schizophrenia-like illness when given chronic high doses of amphetamine, with the only variability having to do with how much amphetamine or what length of dosage is required to produce this effect. Schizophrenic patients have been shown to excrete high amounts of phenylethylamine, an endogenous congener of the catecholamines with many amphetamine-like properties. Chronic paranoid schizophrenics in particular have been shown to excrete phenylethylamine in large quantity. Thus, the theory states that schizophrenics produce excess amounts of phenylethylamine and/or produce normal amounts but fail to break it down, perhaps because of low MAO activity.

Baldessarini and Fischer,[380] in a paper arguing that mental disorders may be caused by the actions of false transmitters on postsynaptic receptors, noted that beta-hydroxylation of phenylethylamine allows it to be taken up into and released from both norepinephrine and dopamine neurons. Studies of the effects of phenylethylamine and its beta-hydroxylated derivatives on the dopamine receptors Snyder believes are involved in the antischizophrenic effects of neuroleptics would be instructive.

PGE excess or deficiency The main problem with the PGE excess theory of schizophrenia is that antiprostaglandin drugs have not been shown to have any beneficial effects for schizophrenic patients. However, Horrobin has elaborated on a theory of schizophrenia related to a deficit of PGE_1.[381] As it encompasses a number of the theories of schizophrenia, it will be discussed in the section on integrative theories of schizophrenia. In this context, it may be shown to account for much of the evidence about abnormalities in schizophrenia.

Endorphin excess, deficiency, or abnormality With the exception of benefit to some schizophrenic patients from treatment with naloxone (primarily the reduction of hallucinations), the endorphin excess hypothesis does not account for many cases of schizophrenia. The cataplexy produced in animals by large doses of endogenous opiates seems a less than adequate model of schizophrenia; indeed, catatonia may not be specific to schizophrenia. Although the dialysis studies have suggested that some patients may benefit significantly from this treatment, it has not been demonstrated that an opioid compound is actually removed through dialysis. The best evidence of an important role of abnormal endogenous opiates in schizophrenia seems to be the repeated success of the Utrecht researchers in treating some subtypes of schizophrenic patients with des-tyrosine-gamma-endorphin. The patients responding to this treatment seem to be those most resistant to neuroleptics; rather than mimicking neuroleptic action, the compound appears to ameliorate some of the negative symptoms of schizophrenia as well as positive symptoms. These researchers' hypothesis of some types of schizophrenia being produced by abnormal cleavage of the gamma-endorphin fraction from the original polypeptide chain[282] seems to be an abnormality readily explained by common mechanisms of genetic mutation. An analysis of patterns of genetic transmission in families of individuals responding to this treatment would seem to be in order.

Gluten theory Schizophrenia clearly is not identical to coeliac disease, although Buscaino[382] has reported that over 90% of schizophrenic patients he autopsied showed evidence of colitis or other enteric disease (manic-depressive patients did not show these changes). However, reports of some success in treating schizophrenic patients with a milk- and gluten-free diet have not been entirely invalidated. The effect seems to be restricted to a relatively small number of schizophrenic patients. If the gluten theory has validity, it is as a subset of the immunological theories.

Viral and immunological theories These fall into two major groups: one proposing that because of deficiencies in normal immunological processes (necessary to explain the familial nature of schizophrenia) schizophrenics harbor a virus, which over a long period of time damages the brain and produces the symptoms of schizophrenia; and one reasoning that a reaction either to a virus or to some other protein induces an autoimmune reaction in the potential schizophrenic which itself results in the nervous system damage characteristic of some kinds of schizophrenia. Rudin argues that autoimmune damage to the choroid plexus as a source of the symptoms of schizophrenia can be consistent with, or a cause of, the "substrate pellagra" he believes is at the root of some cases of schizophrenia.[273]

Transmethylation hypothesis The hypothesis that schizophrenia is caused by "psychedelic" substances produced by abnormal methylation of neurotransmitters or their metabolites is weakened by the fact that the effects of psychedelic drugs are unlike actual schizophrenia. Also, it has yet to be demonstrated conclusively that schizophrenic patients produce these abnormally methylated compounds in a part of the nervous system where they would result in psychosis. Although it is not yet totally discredited, even the early supporters of the transmethylation hypothesis now voice doubts about its adequacy as the explanation of schizophrenia.

Unusual Theories of Schizophrenia

Digestive toxins Baruk[383] has described a number of cases of patients with infections of coliform bacilli that produced psychotic symptoms, particularly those resembling catatonia. He has argued that these bacilli produce a neurotropic toxin in the gut that may then result in schizophrenic-like symptoms. He also identified a type of psychosis that he believed to be of biliary origin and noted that he and his colleagues were trying to identify the substance responsible and to identify patients suffering from a schizophrenia with these origins. As noted earlier, Buscaino[382] observed evidence of enteric pathology in over 90% of 88 schizophrenic patients he autopsied. However, neither antibiotics nor gall bladder removal has been associated with remission of symptoms of schizophrenia, and it seems unlikely that this will account for a significant proportion of patients.

Abnormal interhemispheric connections On the basis of the finding of Rosenthal and Bigelow[384] that schizophrenic patients had a corpus callosum perpendicularly wider than normal, Randall[385] reasoned that there are extra myelinated fibers in these patients, fibers connecting brain areas that would not ordinarily be connected. This could result in "aberrant and extraneous neural input" to the affected areas of the brain and therefore would "produce bizarre output in the modality of its specialized function." For example, the schizophrenic's experience of "thoughts heard aloud" could result from these thoughts being transmitted from the side of the brain initiating them to a contralateral cognitive area, resulting in the patient's perception that the words were coming from outside. The action of neuroleptics, then, would be to suppress conduction in these interhemispheric connections.[386] This theory seems neuropsychologically naive.

Melatonin deficiency Noting that a deficiency of melatonin will lead to a reduction in PGE_1 Riscalla[387] reasoned that since melatonin production is inhibited by visual system response to light, pineal melatonin production is increased in people who are blind. Thus, blindness should protect individuals from schizophrenia if schizophrenia is caused by a deficiency of PGE_1. She surveyed the patient population of a large state mental hospital and found that of 32 blind patients, none who were schizophrenic had been totally blind on admission; two schizophrenic patients who were partially blind appeared to have become so after becoming schizophrenic. She argued that this demonstrated a rarity of coexistence of schizophrenia and blindness. This hypothesis should of course be considered a subset of the prostaglandin theory, although it appears to be a melatonin deficiency theory. In line with this, Smith[388] observed that of a group of 30 schizophrenic patients, only 3 exhibited normal levels and diurnal rhythms in serum melatonin. The rest either had low melatonin levels with shallow diurnal rhythm or high levels of melatonin with little discernible diurnal rhythm. These findings do not seem to be completely congruent with a melatonin deficiency theory of schizophrenia, although they may verify an abnormality of melatonin regulation as an important factor in schizophrenia.

Integrative Theories

In reviewing the literature on biological theories of schizophrenia, two papers[261,389] stood out as appearing to account for more than the usual number of findings. Unless the concept of schizophrenia is really to be broken down into a multitude of relatively unrelated disorders with widely differing etiologies, the wide variety of findings in schizophrenic patients must be shown to be related to each other in some meaningful ways. Further, if the disorder, or perhaps small number of disorders, comes from a genetic factor which in some way predisposes its bearers from an early age to the deterioration shown by these patients, it seems more parsimonious to assume that a small number of genetic factors are involved and that a final elucidation of schizophrenia will show some relatively simple genetically mediated sources. Thus, it is somewhat exciting to encounter papers which integrate a variety of reported findings in such a way that much of what has been reported about schizophrenic patients seems to evolve logically from a relatively parsimonious source. The first of these papers was published in a widely circulated journal and has been available for several years; the second is from a somewhat more obscure source and was not quoted in any of the other papers discussed in this review.

PGE_1 deficiency Horrobin[261] published a review in *The Lancet* in which he proposed that most of the major findings in schizophrenia could be accounted for as results of a deficiency of one of the prostaglandins, specifically, PGE_1. He argued that this theory reconciled the dopamine, prostaglandin, opioid, pineal deficiency, zinc deficiency, wheat sensitivity, and autoimmune hypotheses of schizophrenia. He reasoned that although it is possible for several ultimate causes to be operating, all schizophrenic outcomes are mediated through PGE_1 deficiency at one point. Thus, the relation to the opiate or endorphin hypothesis is that any of the three possibilities—excess, deficiency, or abnormal kinds of endogenous opiates—would lead to a deficiency of PGE_1. As dopamine and PGE_1 appear to have antagonistic actions in the central nervous system this deficiency would result in, among other things, dopamine supersensitivity (which would then be to some extent a secondary aspect of schizophrenia). Melatonin deficiency also results in reduced PGE_1, and melatonin levels are somewhat reduced in most people toward the end of the winter, which is the period of the highest number of births of individuals who later become schizophrenic. Zinc deficiency could also be a cause of PGE_1 deficiency, as could deficiency of essential fatty acids (as Rudin has argued) or an abnormality in metabolizing fatty acids into prostaglandins. Furthermore, he noted that several other factors can block conversion of linoleic acid to prostaglandins, and these have been associated with mental and behavioral abnormalities. He reasoned that dopamine blockade would treat only part of the symptoms of schizophrenia, since dopamine supersensitivity is a result rather than a cause of PGE_1 deficiency. He predicted that drugs that increase PGE_1 synthesis will be more effective treatments for schizophrenia than neuroleptics and will have fewer unwanted side effects. He noted several reports of success with this approach, and that it seems to be particularly effective when several PGE_1 stimulants are combined.

Hyperformaldehydism This theory, described by Barker et al,[389] proposes that the genetically determined lesion in schizophrenia is a defect in the disposition of one-carbon compounds in the nervous system leading to hyperformaldehydism. They note that formaldehyde in the human body is derived primarily from methyl groups provided by dietary intake of methionine and choline and from the de novo synthesis of methionine. Formaldehyde is normally oxidized to formate (formic acid) by any of several aldehyde dehydrogenases that are highly variable in their activities in different subcellular fractions. There is apparently a specific formaldehyde dehydrogenase in mammalian tissues which is both nicotinamide adenine dinucleotide and glutathione dependent. Formate is oxidized mainly by a folate-dependent pathway. Thus increased demethylation of methyl donors could lead to increases in formaldehyde, but only if there were a lesion in the system mediating breakdown of formaldehyde to formate or of formate to carbon dioxide. They propose that the most likely candidate is the specific formaldehyde dehydrogenase of mammalian tissue. As this is folate-dependent, a deficiency of tetrahydrofolate would lead to a buildup of formaldehyde and formate, and in fact severe folate deficiency has been associated with neurological and psychotic symptoms. The authors propose that in schizophrenia, it might be more reasonable to consider an "effective folate deficiency," where folate is present but is "trapped" in one or another form. They note that excess formaldehyde or formate could themselves "trap" folate by condensing with it to form derivatives that could not activate the formaldehyde dehydrogenase. This could then become a self-perpetuating abnormality. They report that the administration of methionine to folate-deficient nonschizophrenic persons leads to the production of psychotic symptoms.

They then observe that reactions of catecholamines and indoleamines with aldehydes produce cyclized products of the tetrahydroisoquinoline and tetrahydro-beta-carboline classes. Dopamine is particularly reactive in this way, and its reaction with formaldehyde is much greater than that observed with acetaldehyde (the reaction proposed by some to account for alcohol addiction). The next most reactive transmitter is norepinephrine, so this theory would propose that the dopaminergic and noradrenergic systems would be expected to be the most affected. In severe forms, other transmitter systems would also be affected. This would indeed produce an abnormality at the dopamine receptor, and any treatment increasing dopamine levels would be expected to worsen symptoms.

In addition, this theory accounts for the symptom-worsening effects of methyl donor treatments, without resulting in the presence of psychedelic-like drugs. The authors note that the tetrahydroisoquinolines and tetrahydro-beta-carbolines have been shown to affect biogenic amine transport systems, synaptic membranes, and synaptic vesicles. They also have uptake and storage like neurotransmitters, are released from nerve terminals with neurotransmitters, stimulate the release of naturally occurring biogenic amines, and have agonist and antagonist effects on both presynaptic and postsynaptic receptors. However, they are not substrates for MAO, but in fact inhibit this enzyme. The authors report increased formaldehyde levels in the urine of schizophrenics. They end their paper by proposing a number of hypotheses that could be tested relevant to their theory.

Much work remains to be done in the study of schizophrenia, its causes, and ways to treat it more certainly, safely, and effectively than is now possible; the most to be hoped for is the discovery of effective means of preventing this devastating disorder. Although these answers are not yet in sight, this overview should suggest that scientific efforts continue to make inroads into the darkness surrounding schizophrenia. Some answers may be found within our lifetimes.

REFERENCES

1. Altschule MD: *The Development of Traditional Psychopathology.* New York, John Wiley and Sons, Inc, 1976.
2. Bleuler E: *Dementia praecox oder Gruppe der Schizophrenien.* Leipzig and Wien, F. Deuticke, 1911 (English translation, 1950).
3. Lewis NDC, Piotrowski ZA: Clinical diagnosis of manic-depressive psychosis, in Hoch P, Zubin J (eds): *Depression.* New York, Grune and Stratton, 1954.
4. Pope HG Jr, Lipinski JF Jr: Diagnosis in schizophrenia and manic-depressive illness. *Arch Gen Psychiatry* 1978;35:811–828.
5. Baxter CF, Melnechuk T: New initiatives in schizophrenia research, in Baxter CF, Melnechuk T (eds): *Perspectives in Schizophrenia Research.* New York, Raven Press, 1980.
6. Bowers MB Jr: Biochemical processes in schizophrenia: An update, in Keith SJ, Mosher LR (eds): *Special Report: Schizophrenia 1980.* Washington, DC, U.S. Government Printing Office, 1980.
7. Buchsbaum MS, Haier RJ: Biological homogeneity, symptom heterogeneity, and the diagnosis of schizophrenia. *Schizophr Bull* 1978;4:473–475.
8. Haier RJ: The diagnosis of schizophrenia: A review of recent developments, in Keith SJ, Mosher LR (eds): *Special Report: Schizophrenia 1980.* Washington, DC, U.S. Government Printing Office, 1980.
9. Meltzer HY: Biology of schizophrenia subtypes: A review and proposal for method of study. *Schizophr Bull* 1979;5:460–479.
10. Mendlewicz J, Linkowski P, Wilmotte J: Relationship between schizoaffective illness and affective disorders or schizophrenia. *J Affective Disord* 1980; 2:289–302.
11. Pope HG Jr, Lipinski JF, Cohen BM, et al: "Schizoaffective disorder": An invalid diagnosis? A comparison of schizoaffective disorder, schizophrenia, and affective disorder. *Am J Psychiatry* 1980;137:921–927.
12. Kendell RE, Brockington IF: The identification of disease entities and the relationship between schizophrenic and affective psychoses. *Br J Psychiatry* 1980;137:324–331.
13. Kazanetz EP: Differentiating exogenous psychiatric illness from schizophrenia. *Arch Gen Psychiatry* 1979;36:740–745.
14. Roff JD: Long-term outcome for a set of schizophrenic subtypes, in Wirt RD, Winokur G, Roff M (eds): *Life History Research in Psychopathology,* vol IV. Minneapolis, University of Minnesota Press, 1975, pp 211–236.
15. Himmelhoch JM: What is schizophrenia?, in Bergsma D, Goldstein AL (eds):

Birth Defects: Original Article Series, vol XIV, no. 5. New York, A.R. Liss, 1978, pp 19–39.
16. Tsuang MT, Woolson RF, Fleming JA: Long-term outcome of major psychoses. I. Schizophrenia and affective disorders compared with psychiatrically symptom-free surgical conditions. *Arch Gen Psychiatry* 1979; 36:1295–1301.
17. Taylor MA, Gaztanaga P, Abrams R: Manic depressive illness and acute schizophrenia: A clinical, family history, and treatment-response study. *Am J Psychiatry* 1974;131:678–682.
18. Taylor MA, Abrams R: Manic-depressive illness and good prognosis schizophrenia. *Am J Psychiatry* 1975;132:741–742.
19. Feighner JP, Robins E, Guze SB, et al: Diagnostic criteria for use in psychiatric research. *Arch Gen Psychiatry* 1972;26:57–63.
20. Abrams R, Taylor MA: Catatonia: A prospective clinical study. *Arch Gen Psychiatry* 1976;33:579–581.
21. Abrams R, Taylor MA: Importance of schizophrenic symptoms in the diagnosis of mania. *Am J Psychiatry* 1981;138:658–661.
22. Taylor MA, Abrams R: Catatonia: Prevalence and importance in the manic phase of manic-depressive illness. *Arch Gen Psychiatry* 1977;34:1223–1225.
23. Kendler KS, Hays P: Schizophrenia with premorbid inferiority feelings: a distinct subgroup? *Arch Gen Psychiatry* 1982;39:643–647.
24. Hirschowitz J, Casper R, Garver DL, et al: Lithium response in good prognosis schizophrenia. *Am J Psychiatry* 1980;137:916–920.
25. McCabe MS, Fowler RC, Cadoret RJ, et al: Familial differences in schizophrenia with good and poor prognosis. *Psychol Med* 1971;1:326–332.
26. Edelstein P, Schultz JR, Hirschowitz J, et al: Physostigmine and lithium response in the schizophrenias. *Am J Psychiatry* 1981;138:1078–1081.
27. van Kammen DP, Docherty JP, Marder SR, et al: Acute amphetamine response predicts antidepressant and antipsychotic responses to lithium carbonate in schizophrenic patients. *Psychiatry Res* 1981;4:313–325.
28. Marder SR, van Kammen DP, Docherty JP, et al: Predicting drug-free improvement in schizophrenic psychosis. *Arch Gen Psychiatry* 1979;36:1080–1085.
29. Brockington IF, Kendell RE, Wainwright S, et al: The distinction between the affective psychoses and schizophrenia. *Br J Psychiatry* 1979;135:243–248.
30. Fowler RC, Liskow BI, Tanna VL, et al: Schizophrenia-primary affective disorder discrimination. I. Development of a data-based diagnostic index. *Arch Gen Psychiatry* 1980;37:811–814.
31. Fowler RC, Mezzich J, Liskow BI, et al: Schizophrenia-primary affective disorder discrimination. II. Where unclassified psychosis stands. *Arch Gen Psychiatry* 1980;37:815–817.
32. Rosenthal NE, Rosenthal LN, Stallone F, et al: Toward the validation of RDC schizoaffective disorder. *Arch Gen Psychiatry* 1980;37:804–810.
33. Baron M, Gruen R, Asnis L, et al: Schizoaffective illness, schizophrenia and affective disorders: Morbidity risk and genetic transmission. *Acta Psychiatr Scand* 1982;65:253–262.
34. Brockington IF, Perris C, Kendell RE, et al: The course and outcome of cycloid psychosis. *Psychol Med* 1982;12:97–105.
35. Himmelhoch JM, Fuchs CZ, May SJ, et al: When a schizoaffective diagnosis has meaning. *J Nerv Ment Dis* 1981;169:227–282.
36. McGlashan TH, Carpenter WT Jr: Affective symptoms and the diagnosis of schizophrenia. *Schizophr Bull* 1979;5:547–553.
37. Carpenter WT Jr, Strauss JS, Bartko JJ: Beyond diagnosis: The phenomenology

of schizophrenia. *Am J Psychiatry* 1981;138:948–953.
38. Spitzer RL, Endicott J, Gibbon M: Crossing the border into borderline personality and borderline schizophrenia. *Arch Gen Psychiatry* 1979;36:17–24.
39. Stone MH: Assessing vulnerability to schizophrenia or manic-depression in borderline states. *Schizophr Bull* 1979;5:105–110.
40. Gunderson JG: The relatedness of borderline and schizophrenic disorders. *Schizophr Bull* 1979;5:17–22.
41. Liebowitz MR: Is borderline a distinct entity? *Schizophr Bull* 1979;5:23–37.
42. Soloff PH: A comparison of borderline with depressed and schizophrenic patients on a new diagnostic interview. *Compr Psychiatry* 1981;22:291–300.
43. Potkin SG, Cannon HE, Murphy DL, et al: Are paranoid schizophrenics biologically different from other schizophrenics? *N Engl J Med* 1978;298: 61–66.
44. Kendler KS, Hays P: Paranoid psychosis (delusional disorder) and schizophrenia: a family history study. *Arch Gen Psychiatry* 1981;38: 547–551.
45. Kendler KS, Davis KL: The genetics and biochemistry of paranoid schizophrenia and other paranoid psychoses. *Schizophr Bull* 1981;7:689–709.
46. Pope HG Jr, Jonas JM, Cohen BM, et al: Failure to find evidence of schizophrenia in first-degree relatives of schizophrenic probands. *Am J Psychiatry* 1982;139:826–828.
47. Kallmann F: *The Genetics of Schizophrenia.* New York, Augustin, 1938.
48. Lidz T, Blatt S, Cook B: Critique of the Danish-American studies of the adopted-away offspring of schizophrenic parents. *Am J Psychiatry* 1981;138: 1063–1068.
49. Kessler S: The genetics of schizophrenia: A review, in Keith SJ, Mosher LR (eds): *Special Report: Schizophrenia 1980.* Washington, DC, U.S. Government Printing Office, 1980.
50. Rosenthal D: *Genetic Theory and Abnormal Behavior.* New York, McGraw-Hill Book Co, 1970.
51. Slater E, Cowie V: *The Genetics of Mental Disorders.* London, Oxford University Press, 1971.
52. Rosenthal D, Wender PH, Kety SS, et al: Schizophrenics' offspring reared in adoptive homes, in Rosenthal D, Kety SS (eds): *The Transmission of Schizophrenia.* Oxford, Pergamon Press Ltd, 1968.
53. Wender PH, Rosenthal D, Kety SS, et al: Crossfostering: A research strategy for clarifying the role of genetic and experimental factors in the etiology of schizophrenia. *Arch Gen Psychiatry* 1974;30:121–128.
54. Kendler KS, Gruenberg AM, Strauss JS: An independent analysis of the Copenhagen sample of the Danish adoption study of schizophrenia. IV. The relationship between major depressive disorder and schizophrenia. *Arch Gen Psychiatry* 1982;39:639–642.
55. Matthysse SW, Kidd KK: Estimating the genetic contribution to schizophrenia. *Am J Psychiatry* 1976;133:185–191.
56. Baron M: Genetic models of schizophrenia. *Acta Psychiatr Scand* 1982;65: 263–275.
57. McGuffin P, Farmer AE, Yonace AH: HLA antigens and subtypes of schizophrenia. *Psychiatry Res* 1981;5:115–122.
58. McGuffin P, Farmer AE, Rajah SM: Histocompatibility antigens and schizophrenia. *Br J Psychiatry* 1978;132:149–151.
59. Crowe RR, Thompson JS, Flink R, et al: HLA antigens and schizophrenia. *Arch Gen Psychiatry* 1979;36:231–233.

60. Gattaz WF, Beckmann H: HLA antigens and schizophrenia. *Lancet* 1980;1: 98–99.
61. Gattaz WF, Beckmann H, Mendlewicz J: HLA antigens and schizophrenia: a pool of two studies. *Psychiatry Res* 1981;5:123–128.
62. McNeil TF, Kaij L: Obstetric factors in the development of schizophrenia: Complications in the birth of preschizophrenics and in reproduction by schizophrenic parents, in Wynne LC, Cromwell RL, Mathysse S (eds): *The Nature of Schizophrenia.* New York, John Wiley & Sons, Inc, 1978.
63. Parnas J, Schulsinger F, Teasdale TW, et al: Perinatal complications and clinical outcome within the schizophrenia spectrum. *Br J Psychiatry* 1982; 140:416–420.
64. Birth season and schizophrenia. *Br Med J* 1978;1:527–528.
65. Torrey EF, Torrey BB: A shifting seasonality of schizophrenic births. *Br J Psychiatry* 1979;134:183–186.
66. Hare E, Moran P: A relation between seasonal temperature and the birth rate of schizophrenic patients. *Acta Psychiatr Scand* 1981;63:396–405.
67. Watson CG, Kucala T, Angulski G, et al: Season of birth and schizophrenia: A response to the Lewis and Griffin critique. *J Abnorm Psychol* 1982;91:120–125.
68. Shur E: Season of birth in high and low genetic risk schizophrenics. *Br J Psychiatry* 1982;140:410–415.
69. Holzman PS, Proctor LR, Hughes DW: Eye-tracking patterns in schizophrenia. *Science* 1973;181:179–181.
70. Shagass C, Amadeo M, Overton DA: Eye-tracking performance in psychiatric patients. *Biol Psychiatry* 1974;9:245–260.
71. Iacono WG, Lykken DT: Eye-tracking and psychopathology: New procedures applied to a sample of normal monozygotic twins. *Arch Gen Psychiatry* 1979;36:1361–1369.
72. Levin S, Holzman PS, Rothenberg SJ, et al: Saccadic eye movements in psychotic patients. *Psychiatry Res* 1981;5:47–58.
73. Raphan T, Cohen B: Brainstem mechanisms for rapid and slow eye movements. *Annu Rev Physiol* 1978;40:527–552.
74. Myers S, Caldwell D, Purcell G: Vestibular dysfunction in schizophrenia. *Biol Psychiatry* 1973;7:255–261.
75. Levy DL, Holzman PS, Proctor LR: Vestibular responses in schizophrenia. *Arch Gen Psychiatry* 1978;35:972–981.
76. Fish B, Dixon WJ: Vestibular hyporeactivity in infants at risk for schizophrenia: Association with critical developmental disorders. *Arch Gen Psychiatry* 1978;35:963–971.
77. Meltzer HY: Neuromuscular abnormalities in the major mental illnesses. I. Serum enzyme studies, in Freeman DS (ed): *Biology of the Major Psychoses: A Comparative Analysis.* New York, Raven Press, 1975.
78. Schubert DSP, Brocco K, Miller FT, et al: Serum creatine phosphokinase levels in patients meeting the St. Louis research diagnostic criteria for schizophrenia. *Am J Psychiatry* 1982;139:491–493.
79. Meltzer HY: Neuromuscular dysfunction in schizophrenia. *Schizophr Bull* 1976;2:106–135.
80. Ross-Stanton J, Meltzer HY: Motor neuron branching patterns in psychotic patients. *Arch Gen Psychiatry* 1981;38:1097–1103.
81. Zahn TP: Autonomic nervous system characteristics possibly related to a genetic predisposition to schizophrenia. *Schizophr Bull* 1977;3:49–60.
82. Shagass C: EEG and evoked potentials in the psychoses, in Freedman DX

(ed): *Biology of the Major Psychoses,* vol 54. New York, Raven Press, 1975, pp 101–127.
83. Shagass C: An electrophysiological view of schizophrenia. *Biol Psychiatry* 1976;11:3–30.
84. Abrams R, Taylor MA: Differential EEG patterns in affective disorder and schizophrenia. *Arch Gen Psychiatry* 1979;36:1355–1358.
85. Stevens JR, Bigelow L, Denney D, et al: Telemetered EEG-EOG during psychotic behaviors of schizophrenia. *Arch Gen Psychiatry* 1979;36:251–262.
86. Coger RW, Dymond AM, Serafetinides EA: Electroencephalographic similarities between chronic alcoholics and chronic, nonparanoid schizophrenics. *Arch Gen Psychiatry* 1979;36:91–94.
87. Buchsbaum M: Average evoked response agumenting/reducing in schizophrenia and affective disorders, in Freedman DX (ed): *Biology of the Major Psychoses,* vol 54. New York, Raven Press, 1975, pp 129–142.
88. Shagass C, Roemer RA, Straumanis JJ, et al: Temporal variability of somatosensory, visual, and auditory evoked potentials in schizophrenia. *Arch Gen Psychiatry* 1979;36:1341–1351.
89. Hankoff LD, Peress NS: Neuropathology of the brain stem in psychiatric disorders. *Biol Psychiatry* 1981;16:945–952.
90. Reitan RM: Neurological and physiological bases of psychopathology. *Annu Rev Psychol* 1976;27:189–216.
91. Johnstone EC, Crow TJ, Frith CD, et al: Cerebral ventricular size and cognitive impairment in chronic schizophrenia. *Lancet* 1976;2:924–926.
92. Crow TJ, Johnstone ED: Cerebral atrophy and cognitive impairment in chronic schizophrenia. *Lancet* 1977;1:357.
93. Weinberger DR, Torrey EF, Neophytides AN, et al: Lateral cerebral ventricular enlargement in chronic schizophrenia. *Arch Gen Psychiatry* 1979;36: 735–739.
94. Weinberger DR, Bigelow LB, Kleinman JE, et al: Cerebral ventricular enlargement in chronic schizophrenia. *Arch Gen Psychiatry* 1980;37:11–13.
95. Weinberger DR, Cannon-Spoor E, Potkin SG, et al: Poor premorbid adjustment and CT scan abnormalities in chronic schizophrenia. *Am J Psychiatry* 1980;137:1410–1413.
96. Weinberger DR, DeLisi LE, Neophytides AN, et al: Familial aspects of CT scan abnormalities in chronic schizophrenic patients. *Psychiatry Res* 1981;4: 65–71.
97. Reveley AM, Reveley MA, Clifford CA, et al: Cerebral ventricular size in twins discordant for schizophrenia. *Lancet* 1982;1:540–541.
98. Golden CJ, Moses JA Jr, Zelazowski R, et al: Cerebral ventricular size and neuropsychological impairment in young chronic schizophrenics. *Arch Gen Psychiatry* 1980;37:619–623.
99. Golden CJ, Graber B, Coffman J, et al: Structural brain deficits in schizophrenia. *Arch Gen Psychiatry* 1981;38:1014–1017.
100. Andreasen NC, Smith MR, Jacoby CG, et al: Ventricular enlargement in schizophrenia: Definition and prevalence. *Am J Psychiatry* 1982;139: 292–296.
101. Andreasen NC, Olsen SA, Dennert JW, et al: Ventricular enlargement in schizophrenia: Relationship to positive and negative symptoms. *Am J Psychiatry* 1982;139:297–302.
102. Weinberger DR, Torrey EF, Wyatt RJ: Cerebellar atrophy in chronic schizophrenia. *Lancet* 1979;2:718–719.
103. Coffman JA, Mefferd J, Golden CJ, et al: Cerebellar atrophy in chronic schizophrenia. *Lancet* 1981;1:666.

104. Nasrallah HA, Jacoby CG, McCalley-Whitters M: Cerebellar atrophy in schizophrenia and mania. *Lancet* 1981;1:1102.
105. Luchins DJ, Morihisa JM, Weinberger DR, et al: Cerebral asymmetry and cerebellar atrophy in schizophrenia: A controlled postmortem study. *Am J Psychiatry* 1981;138:1501–1503.
106. Lippmann S, Manshadi M, Baldwin H, et al: Cerebellar vermis dimensions on computerized tomographic scans of schizophrenic and bipolar patients. *Am J Psychiatry* 1982;139:667–668.
107. Heath RG, Franklin DE, Walker CF, et al: Cerebellar vermal atrophy in psychiatric patients. *Biol Psychiatry* 1982;17:561–583.
108. Heath RG, Llewellyn RC, Rouchell AM: The cerebellar pacemaker for intractable behavioral disorders and epilepsy: Follow-up report. *Biol Psychiatry* 1980;15:243–256.
109. Weinberger DR, Wyatt RJ: Structural brain abnormalities in chronic schizophrenia: Computed tomography findings, in Baxter C, Melnechuk T (eds): *Perspectives in Schizophrenia Research.* New York, Raven Press, 1980.
110. Schweitzer L, Becker E, Welsh H: Abnormalities of cerebral lateralization in schizophrenia patients. *Arch Gen Psychiatry* 1978;35:982–985.
111. Gur RE: Cognitive concomitants of hemispheric dysfunction in schizophrenia. *Arch Gen Psychiatry* 1979;36:269–274.
112. Luchins DJ, Weinberger DR, Wyatt RJ: Schizophrenia: Evidence of a subgroup with reversed cerebral asymmetry. *Arch Gen Psychiatry* 1979;36: 1309–1311.
113. Luchins DJ, Weinberger DR, Wyatt RJ: Schizophrenia and cerebral asymmetry detected by computed tomography. *Am J Psychiatry* 1982;139: 753–757.
114. Luchins DJ, Weinberger DR, Torrey EF, et al: HLA-A2 antigen in schizophrenic patients with reversed cerebral asymmetry. *Br J Psychiatry* 1981; 138;240–243.
115. Chaugule VB, Master RS: Impaired cerebral dominance and schizophrenia. *Br J Psychiatry* 1981;139:23–24.
116. Luchins D, Pollin W, Wyatt RJ: Laterality in monozygotic schizophrenic twins: An alternative hypothesis. *Biol Psychiatry* 1980;15:87–93.
117. Andreasen NC, Dennert JW, Olsen SA, et al: Hemispheric asymmetries and schizophrenia. *Am J Psychiatry* 1982;139:427–430.
118. Gulmann NC, Wildschiodtz G, Orbaek K: Alteration of interhemisphere conduction through corpus callosum in chronic schizophrenia. *Biol Psychiatry* 1982;17:585–594.
119. Newlin DB, Carpenter B, Golden CJ: Hemispheric asymmetries in schizophrenia. *Biol Psychiatry* 1981;16:561–582.
120. Merrin EL: Clinical characterization of schizophrenic patients and cerebral asymmetry: Review and hypothesis. *Compr Psychiatry* 1982;23:55–67.
121. Ingvar DH, Franzen G: Abnormalities of cerebral blood flow distribution in patients with chronic schizophrenia. *Acta Psychiatr Scand* 1974;50:425–462.
122. Ingvar DH: Abnormal distribution of cerebral activity in chronic schizophrenia: A neurophysiological interpretation, in Baxter C, Melnechuk T (eds): *Perspectives in Schizophrenia Research.* New York, Raven Press, 1980.
123. Buchsbaum MS, Ingvar DH, Kessler R, et al: Cerebral glucography with positron tomography. *Arch Gen Psychiatry* 1982;39:251–259.
124. Snyder SH: Amphetamine psychosis: A "model" schizophrenia mediated by catecholamines. *Am J Psychiatry* 1973;130:61–67.
125. Crow TJ: An evaluation of the dopamine hypothesis of schizophrenia, in

Hemmings G, Hemmings WA, (eds): *Biological Basis of Schizophrenia.* Baltimore, North Park Press, 1978.

126. Carlsson A, Persson T, Roos BE, et al: Potentiation of phenothiazines by alpha-methyltyrosine in treatment of chronic schizophrenia. *J Neural Transm* 1972;33:83–90.
127. Matthysse S: Dopamine and the pharmacology of schizophrenia: The state of the evidence. *Psychiatry Res* 1974;11:107–113.
128. Luchins D: The dopamine hypothesis of schizophrenia: A critical analysis. *Neuropsychobiology* 1975;1:365–378.
129. Stevens JR, Livermore A Jr: Kindling of the mesolimbic dopamine system: Animal model of psychosis. *Neurology* 1978;28:36–46.
130. Bowers MB Jr: Central dopamine turnover in schizophrenic syndromes. *Arch Gen Psychiatry* 1974;31:50–54.
131. Post RM, Fink E, Carpenter WT Jr, et al: Cerebrospinal fluid amine metabolites in acute schizophrenia. *Arch Gen Psychiatry* 1975;32:1063–1069.
132. Bird ED, Neurochemical findings in the postmortem schizophrenic brain, in Hemmings G, Hemmings WA (eds): *Biological Basis of Schizophrenia.* Baltimore, North Park Press, 1978.
133. Celesia G, Barr A: Psychosis and other psychiatric manifestations of levodopa therapy. *Arch Neurol* 1970;23:1993–2000.
134. Goodwin F: Psychiatric side effects of levodopa in man. *JAMA* 1971;218: 1915–1920.
135. Gerlach J, Luhdorf K: The effect of l-dopa on young patients with simple schizophrenia, treated with neuroleptic drugs: A double-blind crossover trial with madopar and placebo. *Psychopharmacologia* 1975;44:105–110.
136. Buchanan FH, Parton RV, Warren JW, et al: Double blind trial of l-dopa in chronic schizophrenia. *Aust NZ J Psychiatry* 1975;9:269–271.
137. Campbell M, Small AM, Collins PJ, et al: Levodopa and levoamphetamine: A crossover study in young schizophrenic children. *Curr Ther Res* 1976; 19:70–86.
138. Mackay AVP: Positive and negative schizophrenic symptoms and the role of dopamine. *Br J Psychiatry* 1980;137:379–383.
139. Crow TJ: Positive and negative schizophrenic symptoms and the role of dopamine. *Br J Psychiatry* 1980;137:383–386.
140. Tamminga CA, Schaffer MH, Smith RC, et al: Schizophrenic symptoms improve with apomorphine. *Science* 1978;200:567–568.
141. Corsini GU, Pitzalis GF, Bernardi F, et al: The use of dopamine agonists in the treatment of schizophrenia. *Neuropharmacology* 1981;20:1309–1313.
142. Groves PM, Wilson CJ, Young SJ, et al: Self-inhibition by dopaminergic neurons: An alternative to the "neuronal feedback loop" hypothesis for the mode of action of certain psychotropic drugs. *Science* 1975;190:522–529.
143. Creese I, Burt DR, Snyder SH: Dopamine receptor binding predicts clinical and pharmacological potencies of antischizophrenic drugs. *Science* 1976; 192:481–483.
144. Walters JR, Roth RH: Dopaminergic neurons: An in vivo system for measuring drug interactions with presynaptic receptors. *Arch Pharm* 1976;296:5–14.
145. Westfall TC, Besson M, Giorguieff M, et al: The role of presynaptic receptors in the release and synthesis of ^{3}H-dopamine by slices of rat striatum. *Arch Pharm* 1976;292:279–287.
146. Serra G, Argiolas A, Gessa GL: Opposite changes in dopamine autoreceptors sensitivity induced by chronic antidepressants and neuroleptics, in Gessa GL, Corsini GU (eds): *Apomorphine and Other Dopaminomimetics:*

Basis Pharmacology, vol 1. New York, Raven Press, 1981, pp 133–142.
147. Cerrito F, Maura G, Raiteri M: Do presynaptic dopamine autoreceptors exist?, in Gessa GL, Corsini GU (eds): *Apomorphine and Other Dopaminomimetics: Basic Pharmacology*, vol 1. New York, Raven Press, 1981, pp 123–132.
148. Meltzer HY: Relevance of dopamine autoreceptors for psychiatry: Preclinical and clinical studies. *Schizophr Bull* 1980;6:456–475.
149. Kebabian JW, Petzold GI, Greengard P: Dopamine-sensitive adenylate cyclase in caudate nucleus of rat brain and its similarity to the "dopamine receptor." *Proc Natl Acad Sci USA* 1972;69:2145–2149.
150. Snyder SH: The dopamine hypothesis of schizophrenia: Focus on the dopamine receptor. *Am J Psychiatry* 1976;133:197–202.
151. Tye NC, Horsman L, Wright FC, et al: Two dopamine receptors: supportive evidence with the rat rotational model. *Eur J Pharmacol* 1977;45:87–90.
152. Schwarcz R, Fuxe K, Agnati LF, et al: Effects of bromocriptine on ^{3}H-spiroperidol binding sites in rat striatum. Evidence for actions of dopamine receptors not linked to adenylate cyclase. *Life Sci* 1978;23:465–470.
153. Snyder SH: Dopamine receptors, neuroleptics, and schizophrenia. *Am J Psychiatry* 1981;138:460–464.
154. Henn FA, Anderson DJ, Sellstrom A: Possible relationship between glial cells, dopamine and the effects of antipsychotic drugs. *Nature* 1977;266: 637–638.
155. Cross AJ, Crow TJ, Owen F: ^{3}H-fluphenthixol binding in post-mortem brains of schizophrenics: Evidence for a selective increase in dopamine D2 receptors. *Psychopharmacology* 1981;74:122–124.
156. Lee T, Seeman P: Elevation of brain neuroleptic/dopamine receptors in schizophrenia. *Am J Psychiatry* 1980;137:191–197.
157. Seeman P, Lee T, Bird ED, et al: Elevation of brain neuroleptic/dopamine receptors in schizophrenia, in Baxter C, Melnechuk T (eds): *Perspectives in Schizophrenia Research*. New York, Raven Press, 1980.
158. Pandey GN, Garver DL, Tamminga C, et al: Postsynaptic supersensitivity in schizophrenia. *Am J Psychiatry* 1977;134:518–522.
159. Langer DH, Brown GL, Docherty JP: Dopamine receptor supersensitivity and schizophrenia: A review. *Schizophr Bull* 1981;7:208–224.
160. Alpert M, Diamond F, Weisenfreund J, et al: The neuroleptic hypothesis: Study of the covariation of extrapyramidal and therapeutic drug effects. *Br J Psychiatry* 1978;133:169–175.
161. van Kammen DP, Docherty JP, Marder SR, et al: Antipsychotic effects of pimozide in schizophrenia: Treatment response prediction with acute dextroamphetamine response. *Arch Gen Psychiatry* 1982;39:261–266.
162. van Kammen DP, Docherty JP, Marder SR, et al: Long-term pimozide pretreatment differentially affects behavioral responses to dextroamphetamine in schizophrenia. *Arch Gen Psychiatry* 1982;39:275–281.
163. Carlsson A: Does dopamine have a role in schizophrenia? *Biol Psychiatry* 1978;13:3–21.
164. van Praag HM, Dopamine and the development of disorders of human behaviour, in Horn AS, Korf J, Westerink BHC (eds): *The Neurobiology of Dopamine*. New York, Academic Press, Inc, 1979.
165. Alpert M, Friedhoff AJ: An un-dopamine hypothesis of schizophrenia. *Schizophr Bull* 1980;6:387–390.
166. Atsmon A, Blum I, Wijsenbeek H, et al: The short-term effects of adrenergic-blocking agents in a small group of psychotic patients. *Psychiatr Neurol Neurochir* 1971;74:251–258.

167. Atsmon A, Blum I, Steiner M, et al: Further studies with propranolol in psychotic patients: Relation to initial psychiatric state, urinary catecholamines and 3-methoxy-4-hydroxyphenylglycol excretion. *Psychopharmacologia* 1972;27:249–254.
168. Gardos G, Cole JO, Volicer L, et al: A dose-response study of propranolol in chronic schizophrenics. *Curr Ther Res* 1973;15:314–323.
169. Rackensperger W, Gaupp R, Mattke DJ, et al: Behandlung von akuten schizophrenen psychosen mit beta-receptoren-blockern. *Arch Psychiatr Nervenkr* 1974;219:29–36.
170. Gruzelier JH, Yorkston NJ: Propranolol and schizophrenia: Objective evidence of efficacy, in Hemmings G, Hemmings WA (eds): *Biological Basis of Schizophrenia.* Baltimore, University Park Press, 1978.
171. Belmaker RH, Ebstein RP, Dasberg H, et al: The effect of propranolol treatment in schizophrenia on CSF amine metabolites and prolactin. *Psychopharmacology* 1979;63:293–296.
172. Hanssen T, Heyden T, Sundberg I, et al: Propranolol in schizophrenia: Clinical, metabolic, and pharmacological findings. *Arch Gen Psychiatry* 1980;37:685–690.
173. Freedman R: Interactions of antipsychotic drugs with norepinephrine and cerebellar neuronal circuitry: Implications for the psychobiology of psychosis. *Biol Psychiatry* 1977;12:181–197.
174. Lake CR, Sternberg DE, van Kammen DP: Schizophrenia: Elevated cerebrospinal fluid norepinephrine. *Science* 1980;207:331–333.
175. Sternberg DE, van Kammen DP, Lake CR, et al: The effect of pimozide on CSF norepinephrine in schizophrenia. *Am J Psychiatry* 1981;138:1045–1051.
176. Farley IJ, Price KS, McCullough E, et al: Norepinephrine in chronic paranoid schizophrenia: Above-normal levels in limbic forebrain. *Science* 1978;200:456–458.
177. Kleinman JE, Bridge P, Karoum F, et al: Chronic schizophrenia: Postmortem studies, in Baxter C, Melnechuk T (eds): *Perspectives in Schizophrenia Research.* New York, Raven Press, 1980.
178. Sternberg DE, Charney DS, Heninger GR, et al: Impaired presynaptic regulation of norepinephrine in schizophrenia: Effects of clonidine in schizophrenic patients and normal controls. *Arch Gen Psychiatry* 1982;39: 285–289.
179. Jimerson DC, Post RM, Stoddard FJ, et al: Preliminary trial of the noradrenergic agonist clonidine in psychiatric patients. *Biol Psychiatry* 1980;15: 45–57.
180. Snyder SH, Banerjee SP, Yamamura HI, et al: Drugs, neurotransmitters, and schizophrenia. *Science* 1974;184:1243–1253.
181. Challacombe DN: 5-Hydroxytryptamine metabolism in coeliac disease, in Hemmings G, Hemmings WA (eds): *Biological Basis of Schizophrenia.* Baltimore, University Park Press, 1978.
182. Bender DA: Tryptophan and serotonin in schizophrenia: A clue to biochemical defects?, in Hemmings G, Hemmings WA (eds): *Biological Basis of Schizophrenia.* Baltimore, University Park Press, 1978.
183. Bender BA, Cockcroft PM: Increase in brain tryptophan and 5-hydrotryptamine on administration of phenothiazines to rats. *Biochem Soc Transact* 1977;15:155.
184. von Hungen K, Roberts S, Hill DF: Serotonin-sensitive adenylate cyclase activity in immature rat brain. *Brain Res* 1975;84:257–267.

185. Creese I, Snyder SH: ^{3}H-spiroperidol labels serotonin receptors in rat cerebral cortex and hippocampus. *Eur J Pharmacol* 1978;49:201–202.
186. Manowitz P, Gilmour DG, Racevskis J: Low plasma tryptophan levels in recently hospitalized schizophrenics. *Biol Psychiatry* 1973;6:109–118.
187. Gilmour DG, Manowitz P, Frosch WA, et al: Association of plasma tryptophan levels with clinical change in female schizophrenic patients. *Biol Psychiatry* 1973;6:119–128.
188. Wyatt RJ, Vaughan T, Galanter M, et al: Behavioral changes of chronic schizophrenic patients given L-5-hydroxytryptophan. *Science* 1972;177: 1124–1126.
189. Chouinard G, Annable L, Young SN, et al: A controlled study of tryptophan-benserazide in schizophrenia. *Commun Psychopharmacol* 1978;2: 21–31.
190. Sardesai VM, Ward V, Provido H, et al: The effect of schizophrenic factor on liver tryptophan oxygenase. *Commun Psychopharmacol* 1977;1: 439–446.
191. Trulson ME, Jacobs BL: Long-term amphetamine treatment decreases brain serotonin metabolism: Implications for theories of schizophrenia. *Science* 1979;205:1295–1297.
192. Freedman DX, Belendiuk K, Belenkiuk GW, et al: Blood tryptophan metabolism in chronic schizophrenics. *Arch Gen Psychiatry* 1981;38: 655–659.
193. Bennett JP Jr, Enna SJ, Bylund DB, et al: Neurotransmitter receptors in frontal cortex of schizophrenics. *Arch Gen Psychiatry* 1979;36:927–934.
194. Whitaker PM, Crow TJ, Ferrier IN: Tritiated LSD binding in frontal cortex in schizophrenia. *Arch Gen Psychiatry* 1981;38:278–280.
195. Bird ED, Barnes J, Iversen LL, et al: Increased brain dopamine and reduced glutamic acid decarboxylase and choline acetyl transferase activity in schizophrenia and related psychoses. *Lancet* 1977;2:1157–1159.
196. Levy R: Brain biochemistry in schizophrenia. *Lancet* 1978;1:35.
197. Perry EK, Blessed G, Perry RH, et al: Brain biochemistry in schizophrenia. *Lancet* 1978;1:35–36.
198. Crow TJ, Owen F, Cross AJ, et al: Brain biochemistry in schizophrenia. *Lancet* 1978;1:36–37.
199. Bird ED, Spokes EG, Barnes J, et al: Glutamic-acid decarboxylase in schizophrenia. *Lancet* 1978;1:156.
200. Scheel-Kruger J, Cools AR, Honig W: Muscimol antagonizes the ergometrine-induced locomotor activity in nucleus accumbens: Evidence for a gaba-dopaminergic interaction. *Eur J Pharmacol* 1977;42:311–313.
201. Perry TL, Buchanan J, Kish SJ, et al: Gamma-aminobutyric-acid deficiency in brain of schizophrenic patients. *Lancet* 1979;1:237–239.
202. Marco E, Mao CC, Revuelta A, et al: Turnover rates of gamma-aminobutyric acid in substantia nigra, n. caudatus, globus pallidus and n. accumbens of rats injected with cataleptogenic and non-cataleptogenic antipsychotics. *Neuropharmacology* 1978;17:589–596.
203. Gold BI, Bowers MB Jr, Roth RH, et al: GABA levels in CSF of patients with psychiatric disorders. *Am J Psychiatry* 1980;137:362–364.
204. Stien R: Hallucinations after sudden withdrawal of baclofen. *Lancet* 1977;2: 44–45.
205. Beckmann H, Frische M, Ruther E, et al: Baclofen (para-chlorphenyl-GABA) in schizophrenia. *Pharmakopsychiatria.* 1977;10:26–31.
206. Schopf J, Hucker H: Baclofen in the treatment of schizophrenia: A pilot study. *Pharmakopsychiatria.* 1977;10:89–91.

207. Tamminga CA, Crayton JW, Chase TN: Muscimol: GABA agonist therapy in schizophrenia. *Am J Psychiatry* 1978;135:746–747.
208. Schulz SC, van Kammen DP, Buchsbaum MS, et al: Gamma-hydroxybutyrate treatment of schizophrenia: A pilot study. *Pharmakopsychiatria.* 1981;14:129–134.
209. Jimerson DC, van Kammen DP, Post RM, et al: Diazepam in schizophrenia: A preliminary double-blind trial. *Am J Psychiatry* 1982;139:489–491.
210. Murphy DL, Wyatt RJ: Reduced platelet monoamine oxidase activity in chronic schizophrenia. *Nature* 1972;238;225–226.
211. Wyatt RJ, Murphy DL, Belmaker R, et al: Reduced monoamine oxidase activity in platelets: A possible genetic marker for vulnerability to schizophrenia. *Science* 1973;179:916–918.
212. Murphy DL, Belmaker R, Wyatt RJ: Monoamine oxidase in schizophrenia and other behavior disorders. *J Psychiatr Res* 1974;11:221–247.
213. Domino EF, Khanna SS: Decreased blood platelet MAO activity in unmedicated chronic schizophrenic patients. *Am J Psychiatry* 1976;133: 323–326.
214. Murphy DL, Donnelly CH, Miller L, et al: Platelet monamine oxidase in chronic schizophrenia: some enzyme characteristics relevant to reduced activity. *Arch Gen Psychiatry* 1976;33:1377–1381.
215. Berrettini WH, Prozialeck W, Vogel WH: Decreased platelet monoamine oxidase activity in chronic schizophrenia shown with novel substrates. *Arch Gen Psychiatry* 1978;35:600–605.
216. Gruen R, Baron M, Levitt M, et al: Platelet MAO activity and schizophrenic prognosis. *Am J Psychiatry* 1982;139:240–241.
217. Owen F, Bourne R, Crow TJ, et al: Platelet monoamine oxidase in schizophrenia: An investigation in drug-free chronic hospitalized patients. *Arch Gen Psychiatry* 1976;33:1370–1373.
218. Mann JJ, Kaplan RD, Georgotas A, et al: Monoamine oxidase activity and enzyme kinetics in three subpopulations of density-fractionated platelets in chronic paranoid schizophrenics. *Psychopharmacology* 1981;74:344–348.
219. Groshong R, Baldessarini RJ, Gibson DA, et al: Activities of types A and B MAO and catechol-o-methyltransferase in blood cells and skin fibroblasts of normal and chronic schizophrenic subjects. *Arch Gen Psychiatry* 1978; 35:1198–1205.
220. Meltzer HY, Arora RC: Skeletal muscle MAO activity in the major psychoses: Relationship with platelet and plasma MAO activities. *Arch Gen Psychiatry* 1980;37:333–339.
221. Reveley MA, Glover V, Sandler M, et al: Brain monoamine oxidase activity in schizophrenics and controls. *Arch Gen Psychiatry* 1981;38:663–665.
222. Schildkraut JJ, Orsulak PJ, Schatzberg AF, et al: Platelet monoamine oxidase activity in subgroups of schizophrenic disorders. *Schizophr Bull* 1980; 6:220–225.
223. Meltzer HY, Arora RC, Jackman H, et al: Platelet monoamine oxidase and plasma amine oxidase in psychiatric patients. *Schizophr Bull* 1980;6: 213–219.
224. Schildkraut JJ, Herzog JM, Orsulak PJ, et al: Reduced platelet monoamine oxidase activity in a subgroup of schizophrenic patients. *Am J Psychiatry* 1976;133:438–440.
225. Wyatt RJ, Potkin SG, Murphy DL: Platelet monoamine oxidase activity in schizophrenia: A review of the data. *Am J Psychiatry* 1979;136:377–385.
226. Haier RJ, Buchsbaum MS, Murphy DL, et al: Psychiatric vulnerability,

monoamine oxidase, and the average evoked potential. *Arch Gen Psychiatry* 1980;37:340–345.
227. Dorus E, Pandey GN, Shaughnessy R, et al: Low platelet monoamine oxidase activity, high red blood cell lithium ratio, and affective disorders: A multivariate assessment of genetic vulnerability to affective disorders. *Biol Psychiatry* 1979;14:989–993.
228. Meltzer HY, Biochemical studies in schizophrenia, in Bellak L (ed): *Disorders of the Schizophrenic Syndrome.* New York, Basic Books, 1979.
229. Fischer E, Spatz H, Saavedra JM, et al: Urinary elimination of phenethylamine. *Biol Psychiatry* 1972;5:139–147.
230. Sandler M: The dopamine hypothesis revisited, in Hemmings G, Hemmings WA (eds): *Biological Basis of Schizophrenia.* Baltimore, University Park Press, 1978.
231. Staub RA, Gillin JC, Wyatt RJ: Monoamine oxidase inhibitors potentiate phenylethylamine effects in rhesus monkeys. *Biol Psychiatry* 1980;15: 429–436.
232. Perlow MJ, Chiueh CC, Lake CR, et al: Increased dopamine and norepinephrine concentrations in primate CSF following amphetamine and phenylethylamine administration. *Brain Res* 1980;186:469–473.
233. Angrist B, Thompson H, Shopsin B, et al: Clinical studies with dopamine receptor stimulants. *Psychopharmacologia* 1975;44:273–280.
234. Gold MS, Bowers MB Jr: Neurobiological vulnerability to low-dose amphetamine psychosis. *Am J Psychiatry* 1978;135:1546–1548.
235. Potkin SG, Karoum F, Chuang L, et al: Phenylethylamine in paranoid chronic schizophrenia. *Science* 1979;206:470–471.
236. Jeste DV, Doongaji DR, Panjwani D, et al: Cross-cultural study of a biochemical abnormality in paranoid schizophrenia. *Psychiatry Res* 1980;3: 341–352.
237. Sack RL, Goodwin FK: Inhibition of dopamine-B-hydroxylase in manic patients: A clinical trial with fusaric acid. *Arch Gen Psychiatry* 1974;31: 649–654.
238. Heath RG, Nesselhof W, Bishop MR, et al: Behavioral and metabolic changes associated with administration of tetraethylthiuram disulfide (Antabuse). *Dis Nerv Syst* 1965;26:99–105.
239. Ewing JA, Mueller RA, Rouse BA, et al: Low levels of dopamine-β-hydroxylase and psychosis. *Am J Psychiatry* 1977;134:927–928.
240. Kety SS: Biochemical hypotheses of schizophrenia, in Millon T (ed): *Theories of Psychopathology and Personality.* Philadelphia, WB Saunders Co, 1973.
241. VanderKamp H: A biochemical abnormality in schizophrenia involving ascorbic acid. *Int J Neuropsychiatry* 1966;2:204–206.
242. Herjanic M: Ascorbic acid and schizophrenia, in Hawkins D, Pauling LC (eds): *Orthomolecular Psychiatry: Treatment of Schizophrenia.* San Francisco, Freeman, 1973.
243. Wise CD, Stein L: Dopamine-β-hydroxylase deficits in the brains of schizophrenic patients. *Science* 1973;181:344–347.
244. Pfeiffer CC, Iliev V: A study of zinc deficiency and copper excess in the schizophrenias. *Int Rev Neurobiol* 1972;1(Suppl):141–165.
245. Baron M, Perlman R, Levitt M, et al: Plasma copper and dopamine-β-hydroxylase in schizophrenia. *Biol Psychiatry* 1982;17:115–120.
246. Nicolson GA, Greiner AC, McFarlane WJG, et al: Effect of penicillamine on schizophrenic patients. *Lancet* 1966;1:344–347.

247. Weiner WJ, Nausieda PA, Klawans HL: Effect of chlorpromazine on central nervous system concentrations of manganese, iron, and copper. *Life Sci* 1977;20:1181–1186.
248. Mason JW, Docherty JP: Psychoendocrine research on schizophrenia: A need for reevaluation, in Baxter C, Melnechuk T (eds): *Perspectives in Schizophrenia Research*. New York, Raven Press, 1980.
249. De La Fuente J, Rosenbaum AH: Prolactin in psychiatry. *Am J Psychiatry* 1981;138:1154–1160.
250. Kleinman JE, Weinberger DR, Rogol AD, et al: Plasma prolactin concentrations and psychopathology in chronic schizophrenia. *Arch Gen Psychiatry* 1982;39:655–657.
251. Meltzer HY, Sachar EJ, Frantz AG: Serum prolactin levels in unmedicated schizophrenic patients. *Arch Gen Psychiatry* 1974;31:564–569.
252. MacSweeney D, Timms P, Johnson A: Thyro-endocrine pathology, obstetric morbidity and schizophrenia: Survey of a hundred families with a schizophrenic proband. *Psychol Med* 1978;8:151–155.
253. Prange AJ Jr, Loosen PT, Wilson IC, et al: Behavioral and endocrine responses of schizophrenic patients to TRH (protirelin). *Arch Gen Psychiatry* 1979;36:1086–1093.
254. Inanaga K, Nakano T, Nagata T, et al: Behavioral effects of protirelin in schizophrenia. *Arch Gen Psychiatry* 1978;35:1011–1014.
255. Ferrier IN, Cotes PM, Crow TJ, et al: Gonadotropin secretion abnormalities in chronic schizophrenia. *Psychol Med* 1982;12:263–273.
256. Wolfe LS: Eicosanoids: Prostaglandins, thromboxanes, leukotrienes, and other derivatives of carbon-20 unsaturated fatty acids. *J Neurochem* 1982;38:1–14.
257. Ragheb M, and Ban TA: Prostaglandins and schizophrenia: A review. *Prog Neuropsychopharmacol Biol Psychiatry* 1982;6:87–93.
258. Hedqvist P: Basic mechanisms of prostaglandin action on autonomic neurotransmission. *Annu Rev Pharmacol Toxicol* 1977;17:259–279.
259. Abdulla YH, Hamadah K: Effect of ADP on PGE_1 formation in blood platelets from patients with depression, mania and schizophrenia. *Br J Psychiatry* 1975;127:591–595.
260. Rotrosen J, Miller AD, Mandio D, et al: Prostaglandins, platelets, and schizophrenia. *Arch Gen Psychiatry* 1980;37:1047–1054.
261. Horrobin DF: Schizophrenia as a prostaglandin deficiency disease. *Lancet* 1977;1:936–937.
262. Horrobin DF: Indomethacin, prostaglandins, and schizophrenia. *Br Med J* 1977;2:1357.
263. Horrobin DF, Ally AI, Karmali RA, et al: Prostaglandins and schizophrenia: Further discussion of the evidence. *Psychol Med* 1978;8: 43–48.
264. Abeles JH: Schizophrenia as a prostaglandin deficiency disease. *Lancet* 1977;1:1319–1320.
265. Turner P: Schizophrenia as a prostaglandin deficiency disease. *Lancet* 1977; 1:1058.
266. Tollefson GD, Garvey MJ: Indomethacin and prostaglandins: Their behavioral relationships in an acute toxic psychosis. *Brief Reports* 1982;2: 62–64.
267. Litvin Y: Prostaglandins and renin in schizophrenia. *Lancet* 1977;2:1038.
268. Feldberg W: Possible association of schizophrenia with a disturbance in prostaglandin metabolism: A physiological hypothesis. *Psychol Med* 1976; 6:359–369.

269. Mathe AA, Sedvall G, Wiesel FA, et al: Increased content of immunoreactive prostaglandin E in cerebrospinal fluid of patients with schizophrenia. *Lancet* 1980;1:16–17.
270. Falloon I, Watt DC, Lubbe K, et al: N-acetyl-p-amino-phenol (paracetamol, acetaminophen) in the treatment of acute schizophrenia. *Psychol Med* 1978;8:495–499.
271. Wolfe LS, Coceani F: The role of prostaglandins in the central nervous system. *Annu Rev Physiol* 1979;41:669–684.
272. Vincent JE, Melai A, Bonta IL: Comparison of the effects of prostaglandin E_1 on platelet aggregation in normal and essential fatty acid deficient rats. *Prostaglandins* 1974;5: 369–373.
273. Rudin DO: The major psychoses and neuroses as omega-3 essential fatty acid deficiency syndrome: Substrate pellagra. *Biol Psychiatry* 1981;16: 837–850.
274. Hughes J: Isolation of an endogenous compound from the brain with pharmacological properties similar to morphine. *Brain Res* 1975;88:295–308.
275. Hughes J, Smith TW, Kosterlitz HW, et al: Identification of two related pentapeptides from the brain with potent opiate agonist activity. *Nature* 1975; 258:577–579.
276. Watson SJ, Akil H, Berger PA, et al: Some observations on the opiate peptides and schizophrenia. *Arch Gen Psychiatry* 1979;36:35–41.
277. Jacquet YF, Marks N: The c-fragment of β-lipotropin: An endogenous neuroleptic or antipsychotogen? *Science* 1976;194:632–635.
278. Volavka J, Davis LG, Ehrlich YH: Endorphins, dopamine, and schizophrenia. *Schizophr Bull* 1979;5:227–239.
279. Davis GC, Buchsbaum MS, and Bunney WE Jr: Research in endorphins and schizophrenia. *Schizophr Bull* 1979;5:244–250.
280. Buchsbaum MS, Davis GC, van Kammen DP: Diagnostic classification and the endorphin hypothesis of schizophrenia: Individual differences and psychopharmacological strategies, in Baxter C, Melnechuk T (eds): *Perspectives in Schizophrenia Research.* New York, Raven Press, 1980.
281. van Praag HM, Verhoeven WMA: Endorphin research in schizophrenic psychoses. *Compr Psychiatry* 1981;22:135–146.
282. van Ree JM, de Wied D: Endorphins in schizophrenia. *Neuropharmacology* 1981;20:1271–1277.
283. Terenius L, Wahlstrom A, Johansson L: Endorphins in human cerebrospinal fluid and their measurement, in Usdin E, Bunney WE Jr, Kline NS (eds): *Endorphins in Mental Health Research.* New York, Oxford University Press, 1979.
284. Domschke W, Dickschas A, Mitznegg P: CSF β-endorphin in schizophrenia. *Lancet* 1979;1:1024.
285. Lindstrom LH, Widerlov E, Gunne LM, et al: Endorphins in human cerebrospinal fluid: Clinical correlations to some psychotic states. *Acta Psychiatr Scand* 1978;57:153–164.
286. Terenius L, Wahlstrom A, Lindstrom C, et al: Increased CSF levels of endorphins in chronic psychosis. *Neurosci Lett* 1976;3:157–162.
287. Rimon R, Terenius L, Kampman R: Cerebrospinal fluid endorphins in schizophrenia. *Acta Psychiatr Scand* 1980;61:395–403.
288. Naber D, Pickar D, Post RM, et al: Endogenous opioid activity and β-endorphin immuno-reactivity in CSF of psychiatric patients and normal volunteers. *Am J Psychiatry* 1981;138:1457–1462.
289. Brambilla F, Genazzani AR, Facchinetti F, et al: β-endorphin and β-lipotropin plasma levels in chronic schizophrenia, primary affective disorders and

secondary affective disorders. *Psychoneuroendocrinology* 1981;6:321–330.
290. Wagemaker H Jr, Cade R: The use of hemodialysis in chronic schizophrenia. *Am J Psychiatry* 1977;134:684–685.
291. Cohen IM, Scheiber SC, Yamamura H: Why should dialysis benefit schizophrenia? *J Nerv Ment Dis* 1979;167:475–477.
292. Weddington WW Jr: Can dialysis help the chronic schizophrenic? *Am J Psychiatry* 1977;134:1310.
293. Ferris GN: Can dialysis help the chronic schizophrenic? *Am J Psychiatry* 1977;134:1310.
294. Levy NB: Can dialysis help the chronic schizophrenic? *Am J Psychiatry* 1977;134:1311.
295. Begleiter H, Porjesz B, Chou CL: Dialysis in schizophrenia: A double-blind evaluation. *Science* 1981;211:1066–1068.
296. Hariprasad MK, Nadler IM, Eisinger RP: Hemodialysis for uremic schizophrenics: No psychiatric improvement. *J Clin Psychiatry* 1981;42:215–216.
297. Linkowski P, Vanherweghem JL, Jadot C: Hemodialysis in schizophrenia. *Lancet* 1979;2:1381–1382.
298. Scheiber SC, Cohen I, Yamamura H, et al: Dialysis for schizophrenia: An uncontrolled study of eleven patients. *Am J Psychiatry* 1981;138:662–665.
299. Kinney MJ, Varga E, Varga V, et al: Hemoperfusion for chronic schizophrenia: Preliminary psychiatric results. *J Clin Psychiatry* 1981;42: 175–178.
300. Gunne L, Lindstrom L, Terenius LM: Naloxone-induced reversal of schizophrenic hallucinations. *J Neural Transm* 1977;40:13–19.
301. Volavka J, Mallya A, Baig S, et al: Naloxone in chronic schizophrenia. *Science* 1977;196:1227–1228.
302. Davis GC, Bunney WE Jr, DeFraites EG, et al: Intravenous naloxone administration in schizophrenia and affective illness. *Science* 1977;197:74–76.
303. Janowsky DS, Segal DS, Bloom F, et al: Lack of effect of naloxone on schizophrenic symptoms. *Am J Psychiatry* 1977;134:926–927.
304. Emrich HM, Cording C, Piree S, et al: Indication of an antipsychotic action of the opiate antagonist naloxone. *Pharmakopsychiatria* 1977;10:265–270.
305. Berger PA, Watson SJ, Akil H, et al: The effects of naloxone in chronic schizophrenia. *Am J Psychiatry* 1981;138:913–918.
306. Pickar D, Vartanian F, Bunney WE Jr, et al: Short-term naloxone administration in schizophrenic and manic patients; a World Health Organization Collaborative Study. *Arch Gen Psychiatry* 1982;39:313–319.
307. Simpson GM, Branchey MH, Lee JH: A trial of naltrexone in chronic schizophrenia. *Curr Ther Res* 1977;22:909–913.
308. Mielke DH, Gallant DM: An opiate antagonist in chronic schizophrenia: A pilot study. *Am J Psychiatry* 1977;134:1430–1431.
309. Gitlin MJ, Gerner RH, Rosenblatt M: Assessment of naltrexone in the treatment of schizophrenia. *Psychopharmacology* 1981;74:51–53.
310. Kline NS, Li CH, Lehmann HE, et al: Beta-endorphin-induced changes in schizophrenia and depressed patients. *Arch Gen Psychiatry* 1977;34: 111–113.
311. Berger PA, Watson SJ, Akil H, et al: Beta-endorphin and schizophrenia. *Arch Gen Psychiatry* 1980;37:635–640.
312. Gerner RH, Catlin DH, Gorelick DA, et al: Beta-pendorphin: Intravenous infusion causes behavioral change in psychiatric inpatients. *Arch Gen Psychiatry* 1980;37:642–647.
313. Pickar D, Davis GC, Schulz SC, et al: Behavioral and biological effects of

acute beta-endorphin injection in schizophrenic and depressed patients. *Am J Psychiatry* 1981;138:160–166.
314. Verhoeven WMA, van Praag HM, van Ree JM, et al: Improvement of schizophrenic patients treated with (des-tyr[1])-gamma-endorphin (DTγE). *Arch Gen Psychiatry* 1979;36:294–298.
315. van Ree JM, deWied D, Verhoeven WMA, et al: Antipsychotic effect of gamma-type endorphins in schizophrenia. *Lancet* 1980;2:1363–1364.
316. Emrich HM, Zaudig M, Zerssen DV, et al: Des-tyr[1]-gamma-endorphin in schizophrenia. *Lancet* 1980;2:1364–1365.
317. Verhoeven WMA, Westenberg HGM, Gerritsen TW, et al: (Des-tyrosine[1])-gamma-endorphin in schizophrenia: Clinical, biochemical, and hormonal aspects. *Psychiatry Res* 1981;5:293–309.
318. van Praag HM, Verhoeven WMA, van Ree JM, et al: The treatment of schizophrenic psychoses with gamma-type endorphins. *Biol Psychiatry* 1982;17:83–98.
319. Verhoeven WMA, van Ree JM, Bentum AH, et al: Antipsychotic properties of des-enkephalin-gamma-endorphin in treatment of schizophrenic patients. *Arch Gen Psychiatry* 1982;39:648–654.
320. Versteeg DHG, Kovacs GL, Bohus B, et al: Effect of des-tyr[1]-gamma-endorphin and des-tyr[1]-alpha-endorphin on alpha-MPT-induced catecholamine disappearance in rat brain nuclei: A dose-response study. *Brain Res* 1982; 231:343–351.
321. Geffard M, Gaffori O, Chauveau J, et al: Dramatic increase in pineal melatonin levels in the rat after subcutaneous injection of des-tyrosine[1]-gamma-endorphin. *Neurosci Lett* 1981;27:329–334.
322. Palmour RM, Ervin FR, Wagemaker H, et al: Characterization of a peptide derived from the serum of psychiatric patients. *Abstr Soc Neurosci* 1977;7:32.
323. Lewis RV, Gerber LD, Stein S, et al: On B_H-leu[5]-endorphin and schizophrenia. *Arch Gen Psychiatry* 1979;36:237–239.
324. Ross M, Berger PA, Goldstein A: Plasma beta-endorphin immunoreactivity in schizophrenia. *Science* 1979;205:1163–1164.
325. Zioudrou C, Streaty RA, Klee WA: Opioid peptides derived from food proteins. *J Biol Chem* 1979;254:2446–2449.
326. Dohan FC: Cereals and schizophrenia: Data and hypothesis. *Acta Psychiatr Scand* 1966;42:125–152.
327. Dohan FC, Grasberger JC, Lowell FM, et al: Relapsed schizophrenics: More rapid improvement on a milk and cereal free diet. *Br J Psychiatry* 1969;115: 595–596.
328. Singh MM, Kay SR: Wheat gluten-schizophrenia findings. *Science* 1976; 194:449–450.
329. Levy DL, Weinreb HJ: Wheat gluten-schizophrenia findings. *Science* 1976; 194:448.
330. Smith JM: Wheat gluten-schizophrenia findings. *Science* 1976;194:448.
331. Singh MM: Some insights into the pathogenesis of schizophrenia, in Hemmings G, Hemmings WA (eds): *Biological Basis of Schizophrenia.* Baltimore University Park Press, 1978.
332. Rice JR, Ham CH, Gore WE: Another look at gluten in schizophrenia. *Am J Psychiatry* 1978;135:1417–1418.
333. Singh MM, Kay SR: Wheat gluten as a pathogenic factor in schizophrenia. *Science* 1976;191:401–402.
334. Potkin SG, Weinberger D, Kleinman J, et al: Wheat gluten challenge in

schizophrenic patients. *Am J Psychiatry* 1981;138:1208–1211.
335. Luchins D, Freed WJ, Potkin SG, et al: Gluten and haloperidol absorption. *Biol Psychiatry* 1980;15:819–820.
336. Osborne M, Crayton JW, Javaid J, et al: Lack of effect of a gluten-free diet on neuroleptic blood levels in schizophrenic patients. *Biol Psychiatry* 1982; 17:627–629.
337. Storms LH, Clopton JM, Wright C: Effects of gluten on schizophrenics. *Arch Gen Psychiatry* 1982;39:323–327.
338. Hekkens WTJM: Antibodies to gliadin in serum of normals, coeliac patients and schizophrenics, in Hemmings G, Hemmings WA (eds): *Biological Basis of Schizophrenia.* Baltimore, University Park Press, 1978.
339. Manowitz P: Amino acid levels in schizophrenia: A clue to etiology. *Biol Psychiatry* 1978;13:489–492.
340. Kinnell HG, Kirkwood E, Lewis C: Food antibodies in schizophrenia. *Psychol Med* 1982;12:85–89.
341. McGuffin P, Gardiner P, Swinburne LM: Schizophrenia, celiac disease, and antibodies to food. *Biol Psychiatry* 1981;16:281–285.
342. Boehme DH: Preplanned fasting in the treatment of mental disease: Survey of current soviet literature. *Schizophr Bull* 1977;3:288–296.
343. Dohan FC: Schizophrenia: Are some food-derived polypeptides pathogenic? Coeliac disease as a model, in Hemmings G, Hemmings WA (eds): *Biological Basis of Schizophrenia.* Baltimore: University Park Press, 1978.
344. Lycke E, Norrby R, Roos B: A serological study on mentally ill patients with particular reference to the prevalence of herpes virus infections. *Br J Psychiatry* 1974;124:273–279.
345. Laury GV: Diagnosis: Schizophrenic reaction due to or associated with intracranial viral infection. *Psychiatr Q* 1981;53:170–174.
346. Torrey EF, Peterson MR, Brannon WL, et al: Immunoglobulins and viral antibodies in psychiatric patients. *Br J Psychiatry* 1978;132:342–348.
347. Torrey EF, Yolken RH, Winfrey CJ: Cytomegalovirus antibody in cerebrospinal fluid of schizophrenic patients detected by enzyme immunoassay. *Science* 1982;216:892–893.
348. Durell J, Archer EG: Plasma proteins in schizophrenia: A review. *Schizophr Bull* 1976;2:147–159.
349. Heath RG, Krupp IM: Catatonia induced in monkeys by antibrain antibody. *Am J Psychiatry* 1967;123:1499–1504.
350. Gajdusek DC: The possible role of slow virus infection in chronic schizophrenic dementia, in Bergsma D, Goldstein AL (eds): *Birth Defects: Original Article Series,* vol XIV, no 5. New York, A.R. Liss, 1978, pp 81–87.
351. Pulkkinen E: Immunoglobulins, psychopathology and prognosis in schizophrenia. *Acta Psychiatr Scand* 1977;56:173–182.
352. Gilman SC, Schwartz JM, Milner RJ, et al: Beta-endorphin enhances lymphocyte proliferative responses. *Proc Natl Acad Sci USA* 1982;79: 4226–4230.
353. Tyrrell DAJ, Parry RP, Crow TJ, et al: Possible virus in schizophrenia and some neurological disorders. *Lancet* 1979;1:839–841.
354. Crow TJ, Ferrier IN, Johnstone EC, et al: Characteristics of patients with schizophrenia or neurological disorder and virus-like agent in cerebrospinal fluid. *Lancet* 1979;1:842–844.
355. Bock E: Immunoglobulins, prealbumin, transferrin, albumin, and alpha$_2$-macroglobulin in cerebrospinal fluid and serum in schizophrenic patients, in Bergsma D, Goldstein AL (eds): *Birth Defects: Original Article Series,* vol

XIV, no 5. New York, A.R. Liss, 1978, pp 283–295.
356. Vartanian ME, Kolyaskina GI, Lozovsky DV, et al: Aspects of humoral and cellular immunity in schizophrenia, in Bergsma D, Goldstein AL (eds): *Birth Defects: Original Article Series,* vol. XIV, no. 5. New York, A.R. Liss, 1978, pp 339–364.
357. Stevens JR: Receptor supersensitivity: Relationships to cerebral anatomy and histopathology of schizophrenia. *Biol Psychiatry* 1981;16:1119–1122.
358. Pandey RS, Gupta AK, Chaturvedi UC: Autoimmune model of schizophrenia with special reference to antibrain antibodies. *Biol Psychiatry* 1981;16: 1123–1136.
359. Goldstein AL, Rossio J, Kolyaskina GI, et al: Immunological components in schizophrenia, in Baxter C, Melnechuk T, (eds): *Perspectives in Schizophrenia Research.* New York, Raven Press, 1980.
360. Rudin DO: The choroid plexus and system disease in mental illness. II. Systemic lupus erythematosus: A combined transport dysfunction model for schizophrenia. *Biol Psychiatry* 1981;16:373–397.
361. Rudin DO: Covert transport dysfunction in the choroid plexus as a possible cause of schizophrenia. *Schizophr Bull* 1979;5:623–626.
362. Osmond H, Smythies J: Schizophrenia: A new approach. *J Ment Sci* 1952; 98:309–315.
363. Rosengarten H, Friedhoff AJ: A review of recent studies of the biosynthesis and excretion of hallucinogens formed by methylation of neurotransmitters or related substances. *Schizophr Bull* 1976;2:90–105.
364. Pollin W, Cardon PV Jr, Kety SS: Effects of amino acid findings in schizophrenic patients treated with iproniazid. *Science* 1961;133:104–105.
365. Friedhoff AJ, Van Winkle E: Isolation and characterization of a compound from the urine of schizophrenics. *Nature* 1962;194:897–898.
366. Friedhoff AJ, Van Winkle E: The characteristics of an amine found in the urine of schizophrenic patients. *J Nerv Ment Dis* 1962;135:550–555.
367. Bourdillon RE, Clarke CA, Ridges AP, et al: 'Pink spot' in the urine of schizophrenics. *Nature* 1965;208:453–455.
368. Smythies JR: The pink spot. *Lancet* 1966;1:367.
369. Masters AB: The pink spot. *Lancet* 1966;1:367.
370. Narasimhachari N, Himwich HE: The determination of bufotenin in urine of schizophrenic patients and normal controls. *J Psychiatr Res* 1972;9: 113–121.
371. Narasimhachari N, Plaut JM, Himwich HE: Indolethylamine-n-methyltransferase in serum samples of schizophrenics and normal controls. *Life Sci* 1972;2:221–227.
372. Narasimhachari N, Baumann P, Pak HS, et al: Gas chromatographic-mass spectrometric identification of urinary bufotenin and dimethyltryptamine in drug-free chronic schizophrenic patients. *Biol Psychiatry* 1974;8:293–305.
373. Saavedra JM, Axelrod J: Psychotomimetic N-methylated tryptamines: Formation in brain in vivo and in vitro. *Science* 1972;175:1365–1366.
374. Bidder TG, Mandel LR, Ahn HS, et al: Blood and urinary dimethyltryptamine in acute psychotic disorders. *Lancet* 1974;1:165.
375. Oon MCH, Murray RM, Rodnight R, et al: Factors affecting the urinary excretion of endogenous formed dimethyltryptamine in normal human subjects. *Psychopharmacology* 1977;54:171–175.
376. Gillin JC, Kaplan J, Stillman R, et al: The psychedelic model of schizophrenia: The case of N,N-dimethyltryptamine. *Am J Psychiatry* 1976;133: 203–208.
377. Baldessarini RJ, Stramentinoli G, Lipinski JF: Methylation hypothesis. *Arch*

Gen Psychiatry 1979;36:303–305.

378. Maj M, Zizolfi S, Del Vecchio M: Blood levels of S-adenosylmethionine in unmedicated schizophrenic and depressive patients. *Neuropsychobiology* 1981;7:188–191.
379. Stein L, Wise CD: Possible etiology of schizophrenia: Progressive damage to the noradrenergic reward system by 6-hydroxydopamine. *Science* 1971; 171:1032–1036.
380. Baldessarini RJ, Fischer JE: Substitute and alternative neurotransmitters in neuropsychiatric illness. *Arch Gen Psychiatry* 1977;34:958–964.
381. Horrobin DF: Schizophrenia: Reconciliation of the dopamine, prostaglandin, and opioid concepts and the role of the pineal. *Lancet* 1979;1:529–531.
382. Buscaino GA: The amino-hepato-entero-toxic theory of schizophrenia: An historical evaluation, in Hemmings G, Hemmings WA (eds): *Biological Basis of Schizophrenia.* Baltimore, University Park Press, 1978.
383. Baruk H: Psychoses from digestive origins, in Hemmings G, Hemmings WA (eds): *Biological Basis of Schizophrenia.* Baltimore, University Park Press, 1978.
384. Rosenthal R, Bigelow LB: Quantitative brain measurement in chronic schizophrenia. *Br J Psychiatry* 1972;121:259–264.
385. Randall PL: A neuroanatomical theory on the etiology of schizophrenia. *Med Hypotheses* 1980;6:645–658.
386. Randall PL: An alternative mechanism of action for neuroleptic and antidepressant drugs. *Med Hypotheses* 1981;7:251–260.
387. Riscalla LM: Blindness and schizophrenia. *Med Hypotheses* 1980;6:1327–1328.
388. Smith JA: The pineal gland: Its possible significance in schizophrenia, in Hemmings G, Hemmings WA (eds): *Biological Basis of Schizophrenia.* Baltimore, University Park Press, 1978.
389. Barker SA, Carl GF, Monti JA: Hyperformaldehydism: A unifying hypothesis for the major biochemical theories of schizophrenia. *Med Hypotheses* 1980;6:671–686.

CHAPTER 8

THE PSYCHONEURO-ENDOCRINOLOGY OF SCHIZOPHRENIA

GREGORY M. ASNIS
NEAL D. RYAN

Schizophrenia is a major psychotic disorder characterized by a combination of symptoms—Schneiderian-like delusions and hallucinations, thought disorder, bizarre behavior, and social dysfunction.[1] As a psychotic disorder, various biological studies have investigated whether there are signs of altered psychobiology (eg, reduced platelet monoamine oxidase, increased plasma creatinine phosphokinase, etc).[2]

One approach that some investigators have pursued in the biological study of schizophrenia is its psychoneuroendocrinology. The latter examines hypothalamic functioning through the assessment of easily measurable peripheral hormones (at this point measuring hypothalamic factors is impractical). The hypothalamus secretes various releasing and inhibiting factors (peptides into the portal system and hence to the pituitary) causing a cascade reaction with release or inhibition of hormones from the pituitary and subsequent hormones from peripheral target endocrine glands. The hypothalamic factors are controlled by multiple neurotransmitters (predominantly dopamine, norepinephrine, and serotonin) that are rich in the hypothalamus.[3,4] Each of these neurotransmitters, particularly dopamine, has been hypothesized to be abnormal in certain brain regions (particularly the limbic region) of schizophrenics.[5,6]

Researchers investigating the psychoneuroendocrinology of schizophrenia operate under the presumption that proposed neurotransmitter and/or receptor abnormalities in the brains of schizophrenics (mainly the mesolimbic and forebrain regions) might extend to or influence the hypothalamus.

It must be emphasized that there is no evidence directly implicating abnormalities (structural or biochemical) in the hypothalamus of schizophrenics. In addition, in contrast to major depressive disorders, the endogenous subtype, the schizophrenic syndrome (excluding schizoaffective schizophrenia and schizophrenia with superimposed depression), does not have a cluster of hypothalamic signs (such as depressed mood, decrease in appetite, psychomotor retardation, diurnal mood variation, and decrease in sexual libido). Therefore, one would not expect widespread neuroendocrine disturbances in schizophrenia as have been demonstrated in endogenously depressed patients.[7]

As recently reviewed by Sachar,[7] the neuroendocrinology of depression has a number of limitations (the latter equally applies to the neuroendocrinology of schizophrenia). In summary, although hormones can be measured accurately in the periphery, hypothalamic releasing and inhibiting factors, the major factors regulating the hormones, are not yet easily measured; each hormone is controlled by several neurotransmitters, making any interpretation of the neurotransmitter basis for a hormone disturbance speculative; many hormones are sensitive to stress and affected by age, sex, and menopausal status; and many hormones are secreted episodically, have a diurnal rhythm, and are associated with sleep.[7]

Keeping the above limitations in mind, the psychoneuroendocrinology of schizophrenia will be reviewed by summarizing the literature as well as presenting data from our own laboratory. A major focus of this review will be on prolactin (PRL) and human growth hormone (HGH) for the following reasons: (1) Most neuroendocrine studies of schizophrenia have evaluated these hormones. (2) Although most hormones are regulated by multiple neurotransmitters, PRL and HGH are predominantly controlled by dopamine, the neurotransmitter most implicated in schizophrenia. Cortisol, thyroid-stimulating hormone (TSH), and gonadotropins will also be briefly reviewed.

Prolactin (PRL)

PRL, a hormone secreted by the anterior pituitary gland, is *mainly* regulated by tonic inhibition via hypothalamic prolactin inhibiting factor (PIF) with stalk sectioning resulting in increased PRL release.[8] PIF is controlled by dopamine secreted from tuberoinfundibular dopaminergic (TIDA) neurons. There is some evidence that PIF may in fact be dopamine, with the latter being inhibitory to PRL at the level of the pituitary.[9] Agents that increase dopaminergic input (levodopa, dopamine, apomorphine) suppress PRL, whereas agents that decrease dopaminergic input (neuroleptics, reserpine, alphamethylparatyrosine [AMPT]) elevate PRL levels.[9,10] Other neurotransmitters appear not to have a major influence in the PRL secretion in humans (although serotonin and histamine [H[1] receptors] appear to be stimulatory and acetylcholine inhibitory.)[11] Thus, a PRL assessment might serve as a noninvasive means ("window of the brain") of measuring brain dopamine, particularly from TIDA neurons. The most widely accepted biochemical theory of schizophrenia is the dopamine hypothesis (summarized as an increased dopaminergic activity, whether secondary to an increase in number and sensitivity of postsynaptic receptors or a decrease in number and sensitivity of presynaptic dopamine receptors that are inhibitory to dopamine synthesis. For a review of the dopamine hypothesis, see Meltzer and Stahl).[12] Many investigators have evaluated PRL in schizophrenia with the following hypothesis: if dopamine hyperactivity extends from the mesolimbic area (the site believed to be responsible for psychosis in schizophrenia,[13] to the TIDA neurons and/or pituitary dopamine receptors, PRL levels will be abnormal.

Basal PRL Investigators have evaluated basal PRL levels in unmedicated acute/subacute and chronic schizophrenics with the hypothesis that if dopamine hyperactivity extends to the TIDA neurons and/or pituitary dopamine receptors, basal PRL levels should be lower than in normal subjects. Table 8-1 summarizes the literature. Most of these studies have presented data demonstrating *no significant group differences.*[14–21] But many of these studies did suggest that a small subgroup (10% to 20%) of schizophrenics had a slightly elevated PRL,[15–17,19] whereas one study found that 10% of schizophrenics had a low level of PRL.[14] Two studies did find that over 50% of the schizophrenics studied had a lower PRL in one study[22] and a higher PRL in another study[23] (normative data unfortunately was obtained from other laboratories).

The most striking impression of basal PRL studies in schizophrenia is that the findings have been inconsistent. The research designs in many of these studies have not been well constructed, nor have many of the studies taken into account an appropriate understanding of PRL secretion. (1) Two of the studies performed did PRL assessments of schizophrenic subjects in their own laboratory, but then used published data of PRL of normal controls from other laboratories.[18,23] PRL assays can differ significantly. Thus, suggested differences may be artifactual. In addition, some studies used their own normative data, but did not present it.[15,18,19,23] (2) *PRL is a stress-related hormone* (like cortisol and growth hormone) subject to marked fluctuations. The stress of venipuncture can cause an elevation of PRL.[7] Thus, assessment of PRL should involve an insertion of an intravenous (IV) cannula/butterfly with sampling occurring at least 30 minutes later (adaptation) for a more accurate basal PRL level. Many of the studies reviewed involved only single samples.[14,15,18,19] In addition, since PRL is a stress-related hormone, it is subject to elevations

Table 8-1
Basal PRL in Schizophrenia: A Review of the Literature

Meltzer et al, 1974[14]	22 Schizophrenics – 16 acute, 5 chronic, 1 latent (10M, 12F) 13 Normal males	No group differences; 2 of 22 schizophrenics had lower PRL than normal controls
Meltzer et al, 1976[15]	27 Schizophrenics – 16 acute, 11 chronic (12M, 15F) Normal controls, but data not presented	No group differences; 4 of 27 schizophrenics had slightly increased PRL
Kolakowska et al, 1976[23]	18 Chronic schizophrenics (4M, 7F) No normal controls	No group differences; 4 of 27 schizophrenics had slightly increased PRL
Brambilla et al, 1976[16]	18 Chronic schizophrenics (10M, 10F) 8 Normal controls (4M, 4F)	6 of 11 schizophrenics had had higher PRL than normal controls
Ettigi et al, 1976[17]	17 Chronic schizophrenic males 21 Control men – 9 alcoholics, 12 normal volunteers	No group differences; 2 of 17 schizophrenics had higher PRL than normal controls
Wode-Helgodt et al, 1977[18]	43 Schizophrenics (acute?, chronic?) (17M, 26F) No normal controls for plasma PRL Normal controls for CSF PRL, but not presented	No group differences
Johnstone et al, 1977[19]	16 Chronic schizophrenic males Normal controls, but data not presented	3 of 16 schizophrenics had higher PRL than normal controls
Gruen et al, 1978[20]	18 Schizophrenic men – acute/subacute 20 Normal men	No group differences
Brambilla et al, 1979[22]	10 Chronic schizophrenics (8M, 2F) Normal controls, but not presented	6 of 10 schizophrenics had lower PRL than normal controls
Meltzer et al, 1980[21]	35 Chronic schizophrenics (21M, 14F) 12 Acute schizophrenics (2M, 10F) 25 normal controls (13M, 12F)	No group differences
Asnis et al, 1982 (unpublished)	25 Schizophrenics – 5 acute/subacute and 20 Chronic (16M, 9F) 34 Endogenous depressives (10M, 24F) 70 Normal controls (42M, 28F)	No group differences

due to the stress of new hospitalizations. Gruen et al[24] demonstrated the PRL levels to be significantly higher in schizophrenics immediately after admission (within 36 hours) in comparison with 1 week post admission. The study by Meltzer et al[14] examined PRL levels within 48 hours of admission which may have been too soon after hospitalization. Thus, studies should wait a period of time (≥ 1 week) for patients to accommodate themselves to a hospitalization. (3) PRL secretion is episodic, with increased elevations occurring during sleep. It is clear that it takes over 1 to 1.5 hours after awakening for PRL to reach stable morning levels.[25] Although most of the studies were sampled between 8:00 AM and 10:00 AM, many of the studies fail to note how long subjects had been awake.[14–16,19,23] Thus, if PRL assessments in schizophrenics were assessed soon after awakening, PRL levels may be artifactually elevated. (4) Estrogen potentiates PRL secretion, and thus normal women have been found to have PRL levels higher than normal men.[26] Asnis et al recently demonstrated higher PRL levels in normal, depressive, and schizophrenic women in contrast to their male counterparts (unpublished data) (see Table 8-2). Most of the studies reviewed (see Table 8-1) combined data on male and female schizophrenics in comparison to normal persons without analyzing the data separately for each sex.

We evaluated the basal PRL levels of a group of chronic schizophrenics (N=25; 9F, 16M), in comparison with endogenous depressives (N=34; 24F, 10M) and normal subjects (N=70; 28F, 42M). All subjects were free of psychotropic medication for at least one week, and all patients were hospitalized for a minimum of one week before neuroendocrine testing. Basal PRL levels were assessed via an IV butterfly that was

Table 8-2
Basal Plasma Prolactin Levels in Schizophrenics, Depressives, and Normal Persons*

	Men	Women	Men versus Women
Normal persons	N=42 M=8.5 s=2.9	N=28 M=12.3 s=5.8	$t=3.62$ $P<0.001$
Schizophrenics	N=16 M=8.5 s=6.2	N=9 M=14.3 s=7.3	$t=2.10$ $P<0.05$
Depressives	N=10 M=6.8 s=3.6	N=24 M=11.0 s=5.8	$t=2.12$ $P<0.05$

*For normal versus schizophrenic versus depressive women, $F=1.02$, P is not significant; none of the subcomparisons is significant considered separately. For normal versus schizophrenic versus depressive men, $F=0.76$, P is not significant; none of the subcomparisons is significant considered separately.

inserted at 9:00 AM (1.5 hours after awakening). The baseline PRL sample was assessed 30 minutes after insertion of the butterfly needle. The data are presented separately for men and women (unpublished data) (see Table 8-2). The schizophrenics (men and women) did not differ from normal subjects or depressives ($F=0.76$ for groups of men, and $F=1.02$ for groups of women). Furthermore, there was no suggestion of a subgroup of schizophrenics having increased or decreased PRL levels.

Thus, even after controlling for sex, stress of hospitalization, and stress of venipuncture, the schizophrenics did not differ from pathological and normal controls.

In the aforementioned basal PRL studies in schizophrenia, only a small period of time (up to 60 minutes) in the morning was sampled. A more intensive evaluation (eg, from a few hours to 24 hours) is indicated. In preliminary studies, Meltzer et al[10] found that in sampling from 4 to 18 hours (with 20-minute sampling intervals), six schizophrenics did not differ from three normal controls. Further evaluations over extended periods of time are indicated in larger samples of schizophrenics.

Sleep-induced PRL secretion It is well recognized that there is an increased PRL secretion during sleep in comparison to daytime PRL levels.[25] The underlying mechanisms are unclear, although dopamine is probably unimportant. It has been noted that normal subjects given low-dose neuroleptics (30 mg of chlorpromazine) still had a nocturnal PRL rise[27]; this was also observed by Meltzer et al[10] in two chronic schizophrenics on fluphenazine decoanate. We also recently demonstrated that three chronic schizophrenics had a nocturnal PRL rise; two were on neuroleptics, and one was drug free (unpublished data). Further work should compare the nocturnal PRL increase in an adequate sample of schizophrenics in comparison to normal subjects.

Neuroleptic-PRL stimulation tests in schizophrenia Another strategy using PRL to assess the dopamine hypothesis has been to assess the PRL response to subtherapeutic doses of neuroleptics (dopamine blockers) that reliably cause an increase in PRL in humans.[28] If dopamine hyperactivity extends to the TIDA neurons and/or pituitary dopamine receptors in schizophrenia, the PRL elevation due to subtherapeutic doses of neuroleptics should be diminished in comparison to normal controls. Table 8-3 summarizes this literature. Schizophrenic men (both chronic and acute/subacute types) failed to demonstrate any significant differences in the PRL response to neuroleptic challenges in comparison to normal men.[10,20,29,30] Interestingly, Asnis et al[29] evaluated the PRL response to 0.5 mg of intramuscular (IM) haloperidol in a group of chronic schizophrenic men with tardive dyskinesia in comparison to normal men. Since tardive dyskinesia is a drug-induced neurological disorder with a hypothesized dopamine hypersensitivity in the nigrostriatal system, Asnis et al believed that this group of schizophrenics would be particularly likely to have increased dopaminergic activity in the TIDA and/or pituitary dopamine receptors with a subsequent blunted PRL response to a neuroleptic challenge. The PRL response to 0.5 mg of IM haloperidol in these chronic schizophrenic men with tardive dyskinesia was practically identical to that seen in normal men.[29] Thus, studies assessing the PRL response to neuroleptic challenges of subtherapeutic doses have found that schizophrenic men are not significantly different from normal men (Table 8-3).

The situation for chronic schizophrenic women appears to be somewhat different. Meltzer et al [31] recently found that chronic schizophrenic women (N=6) had a smaller PRL rise (trend) to 12.5 and 25.0 mg of chlorpromazine IM than did normal women (N=5) (Table 8-2).[31] We have also been interested in the PRL responses to neuroleptic challenges in chronic schizophrenic women. Much of our work investigating the PRL response to a neuroleptic challenge in women has been with haloperidol. What is most interesting is that 0.5 mg of haloperidol IM caused an unreliable PRL response (unlike that for men) with three of six normal women having a PRL increase of less than 25% above base line; and 1.5 mg caused a reliable response with no clear sign of a plateau response.[32] Thus, we decided to examine the PRL response to 1.5 mg of haloperidol IM in a group of chronic schizophrenic women (premenopausal) in comparison to normal women (premenopausal).

Five chronic schizophrenic women were hospitalized and diagnosed by the research diagnostic criteria of Spitzer et al.[33] All subjects were withdrawn from neuroleptics for seven days before being tested. Table 8-4 demonstrates the PRL response (mean PRL of 15 to 120 minutes minus PRL at time 0); the PRL response was significantly less in the schizophrenic women ($t=5.18$, $P<0.0001$; unpublished data) for five chronic schizophrenic women and six normal women. A rank order test of the PRL response in the two groups also finds that schizophrenic women had lower scores than the normal women ($P<0.01$). Thus, this preliminary data do suggest that chronic schizophrenic women have a lower PRL response to intramuscular dose (1.5 mg) of haloperidol than normal women supporting the findings of Meltzer et al.[31] In summary, these results are in contrast to the situation in schizophrenic men versus normal men where singe-dose (IM) challenges of various neuroleptics found no differences between the groups. These findings by Meltzer et al [31] and by us suggest that young schizophrenic women may have hypersensitive dopamine receptors in the hypothalamus and/or pituitary, resulting in a diminished PRL response to a neuroleptic challenge. Why this is unique for schizophrenic women is puzzling. Estrogen is known to be able to potentiate the PRL response to neuroleptics.[34] It is possible that young schizophrenic women had significantly lower estrogen levels in comparison to the young normal women, particularly since schizophrenic women often have menstrual irregularities. Further

Table 8-3
The Prolactin Responses to Neuroleptics in Schizophrenia: A Review of the Literature

Gruen et al, 1978[24]	25 mg of chlorpromazine IM	8 Schizophrenic men (acute/subacute) 10 Normal men	No group differences
Asnis et al, 1979[29]	0.5 mg of haloperidol IM	6 Chronic schizophrenic men 13 Normal men	No group differences
Meltzer et al, 1980[21]	50 mg of chlorpromazine IM	14 Chronic schizophrenic men 6 Normal men	No group differences
Meltzer et al, 1980[31]	12.5 mg or 25 mg chlorpromazine IM	6 Chronic schizophrenic women 4 Normal women	Trend for schizophrenics to have a lower PRL rise
Meltzer et al, 1981[30]	50 mg of chlorpromazine IM	14 Chronic schizophrenics 6 Normal men	No group differences
Asnis et al, 1982 (unpublished)	1.5 mg of haloperidol IM	5 Chronic schizophrenic women 6 Normal women	Schizophrenics had a significantly lower PRL rise

Table 8-4
The Prolactin Response* to Haloperidol (1.5 mg IM) in Five Schizophrenic Women and Six Normal Women

	Prolactin Response (μg/dL)
Normal Women	
Case	
1	22.7
2	24.3
3	28.6
4	45.4
5	62.7
6	71.6
Mean ± SD	42.6 ± 20.9
Schizophrenic Women	
Case	
1	3.7
2	12.0
3	13.1
4	13.4
5	43.0
Mean ± SD	17.0 ± 15.1

*Mean 15 to 120 minute posthaloperidol prolactin level minus baseline level. By the two-tailed t test, $t=5.18$ and $P<0.0001$. By the unpaired Wilcoxon test, $P<0.01$.

studies of schizophrenic women must then measure plasma estrogen levels. This also raises the question of whether the phase of the menstrual cycle must be controlled for in these studies. Preliminary data by Asnis et al[32] find that the PRL response to haloperidol in normal women was not affected by the menstrual cycle.

Agents that Affect Presynaptic Dopamine

Another strategy using PRL to assess the dopamine hypothesis in schizophrenia has utilized pharmacological agents that decrease presynaptic dopamine (and hence increase PRL) either by inhibiting dopamine synthesizing enzymes (eg, alphamethylparatyrosine [AMPT]) or depleting storage dopamine (eg, reserpine).

AMPT If dopamine hyperactivity extends to TIDA neurons in schizophrenia, it is conceivable that tyrosine hydroxylase may have increased activity; thus, administering AMPT (a tyrosine hydroxylase inhibitor) to schizophrenics might inhibit tyrosine hydroxylase less readily, resulting in a blunted PRL response in schizophrenics in comparison to normal persons. Meltzer et al recently evaluated the PRL response to AMPT (1 mg orally) in chronic schizophrenics (N=8) and normal controls (N=6); no significant differences were found.[21] In fact, the schizophrenics had a slightly greater increase in the PRL response, suggesting diminished tyrosine hydroxylase activity and thus dopamine hypoactivity.

Reserpine Reserpine causes a release of intraneuronal dopamine (as well as serotonin, norepinephrine, and histamine) from storage vesicles with subsequent deamination of these neurotransmitters intraneuronally.[35-37]

Recently, reserpine was shown to cause a marked PRL rise in humans, suggesting an important function for storage pool dopamine in PRL secretion. We found that reserpine produced a greater PRL response than did an equivalent dose of haloperidol (2.5 times more than that of haloperidol).[38] We hypothesized that if dopamine hyperactivity (dopamine hypothesis) extends to the TIDA neuron, it is possible that there is an increased amount of intraneuronal storage pool dopamine. A reserpine challenge in schizophrenics might then less effectively deplete intraneuronal dopamine, resulting in a diminished PRL rise in comparison to normal controls.

In a pilot study, we administered 0.5 mg of IM reserpine to seven chronic schizophrenic men (unmedicated for over seven days), ages 23 to 48 years and eight normal men, ages 26 to 36 years; 30 minutes after inserting an IV cannula at 9:00 AM, IM reserpine (0.5 mg) was administered. Plasma was sampled every 15 minutes up to 180 minutes for PRL (Figure 8-1). The area under the PRL curve (as well as PRL) was significantly different from 30 minutes to 180 minutes. By 90 minutes, all normal persons had a larger PRL response than did any schizophrenic tested. The PRL response was not correlated to age (of normal persons and schizophrenics), duration of illness, years of neuroleptic treatment, or drug (neuroleptic)-free period.

These are the first neuroendocrine data that clearly support the dopamine hypothesis of schizophrenia. Furthermore, these data suggest that storage pool dopamine may be increased in schizophrenia. This work must be replicated (a replication study by Asnis is in progress).

Dopamine Agonists

Another strategy exploring the dopamine hypothesis in schizophrenics has been to evaluate the PRL response to dopamine agonists. The major hypothesis has been that if dopamine hyperactivity extends to TIDA neurons and/or pituitary dopamine receptors, dopamine agonists should cause an increased suppression of PRL in schizophrenics in comparison to normal controls.

Table 8-5 summarizes this literature. These investigators utilized apomorphine, a direct dopamine agonist[17,39-41] and/or levodopa, an indirect dopamine agonist.[20,39-41] See the section on HGH-dopamine

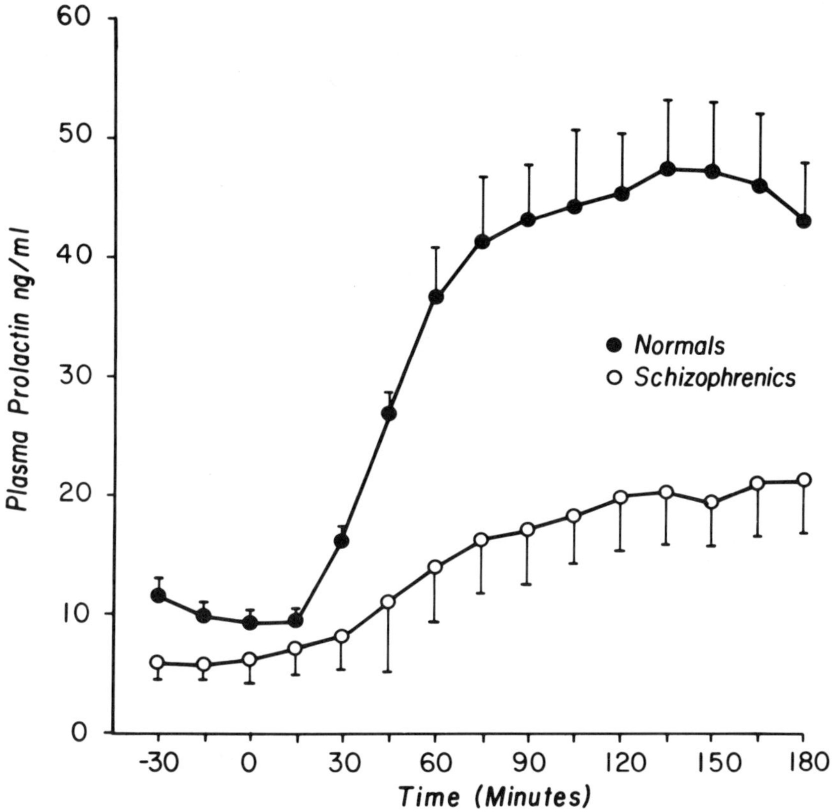

Figure 8-1 Prolactin response to 0.5 mg IM reserpine in seven schizophrenic and eight normal men.

agonist regarding problems with indirect dopamine agonist are discussed below.

Interestingly, none of the studies found data consistent with the dopamine hypothesis; in fact, a few of the studies found that PRL suppression was reduced in chronic schizophrenics, suggesting dopamine hypoactivity.[40,41]

These unusual findings need some reflection. In particular, chronic neuroleptic use may have influenced the findings. It has repeatedly been shown in the literature that chronic neuroleptic use induces dopamine hypersensitivity in the nigrostriatal region. Friend et al recently presented evidence that pituitary dopamine receptors develop subsensitivity to chronic neuroleptic treatment in contrast to nigrostriatal dopamine receptors; they treated rats for two weeks with haloperidol and found a reduced dopamine receptor binding ([^{3}H]haloperidol binding) in the pituitary.[42] If this situation occurred in schizophrenics treated with

Table 8-5
Dopamine Agonist-Induced PRL Suppression in Schizophrenia: A Review of the Literature

Ettigi et al, 1976[17]	Apomorphine, 0.75 mg SC*	17 Chronic schizophrenic men 21 Control men (9 alcoholics, 12 normal volunteers)	No group differences
Tamminga et al, 1977[40]	(1) Apomorphine, 0.75 SC (2) Levodopa, 500 mg PO†	20 Chronic schizophrenics (10M, 10F) 10 Normal controls (7M, 3F)	(1) 3 of 11 schizophrenics had a PRL suppression >20% in contrast to 5 of 5 controls ($P<0.02$) (2) 0 of 9 schizophrenics had a PRL suppression >50% versus 6 of 6 controls
Rotrosen et al, 1978[41]	(1) Apomorphine, 0.5 mg SC (2) Levodopa, 500 mg PO	17 Chronic schizophrenic men 10 Normal men, 20–30 years old	(1) Maximum suppression of PRL was decreased in schizophrenics ($P<0.04$) (2) No group differences
Gruen et al, 1978[24]	Levodopa, 500 mg PO	18 Acute/subacute schizophrenic men 20 Normal men	No group differences
Meltzer et al, 1981[30]	(1) Apomorphine, 0.75 mg SC (2) Levodopa, 500 mg PO	18 Schizophrenics (7M, 11F) 15 Normal controls (7M, 8F)	No group differences

*SC, Subcutaneously.
†PO, Orally.

neuroleptics, it might explain those reports finding a reduced PRL suppression to dopamine agonists. Ettigi et al evaluated prior neuroleptic use and the PRL response to apomorphine; they found no association.[17] Thus, there is still a need for an explanation for a decreased PRL response to dopamine agonists.

TRH-Induced PRL Secretion

Thyrotropin-releasing hormone (TRH) is a potent PRL releaser. It appears to release PRL from the pituitary by binding to receptors on the lactotrophs.[43] These receptors have not been clearly defined, but are probably dopaminergic. The PRL response to TRH has been evaluated in schizophrenics in two studies. Brambilla et al gave 500 μg of TRH IV (bolus) to 20 chronic schizophrenics (10 men, 10 women) drug free for a minimum of 10 days and 8 normal controls (4 men, 4 women). They found that the peak PRL was significantly greater than for normal controls ($P=0.05$; the statistical tests performed were not stated).[16] Since the PRL response to TRH is larger in women than in men[44] it is imperative to analyze such data separately. Brambilla et al[16] failed to analyze their data by sex (their normal controls were few in number), and thus their results may be artifactual. Prange et al[45] administered 500 μg of TRH to 17 schizophrenic patients, drug free for a minimum of six days (nine women, eight men) (nine chronic undifferentiated, five schizo-affective depressed, two catatonic withdrawn, one paranoid—subtypes made by DSM-II) and to 17 normal controls matched for age and sex. When male and female subjects were analyzed separately, the PRL response to TRH in schizophrenics did not differ from normal controls. Although Prange et al[45] analyzed their data by sex, they included five patients with the diagnosis of schizo-affective depressed; the latter may have neuroendocrine responses more like those of depressives, which may have diluted the results. Although it appears unlikely that schizophrenics differ from normal persons, further work on TRH-PRL must study schizophrenics who are not depressed (excluding schizo-affective patients). Furthermore, age and sex must be controlled.

Human Growth Hormone

Human growth hormone (HGH) is a peptide hormone secreted by the anterior pituitary gland. The control of HGH is *predominantly hypothalamic;* the major influence is excitatory (stalk section results in low HGH levels) via HGH releasing factor, but an inhibiting factor, somatostatin, also controls HGH. These hypothalamic factors in turn are controlled by various neurotransmitters. In summary, dopamine, norepinephrine, and serotonin are stimulatory to HGH in humans, with dopamine being the major influence.[46] The role of neurotransmitter regulation of HGH is complicated, for there is a suggestion of different combinations of neurotransmitters contributing to basal HGH release, sleep-induced HGH release, and stimulated HGH release (exercise, amino acids, hypoglycemia, etc).[46] We will summarize the literature as to whether schizophrenics have altered HGH levels.

Daytime basal HGH (awake) Since dopamine (as well as norepinephrine and serotonin) is stimulatory to HGH, one might hypothesize that schizophrenics who have dopamine (norepinephrine or serotonin) hyperactivity might have increased daytime basal HGH levels.

Only three studies specifically compared basal HGH levels in schizophrenia. Vigneri et al sampled HGH every 20 minutes for 24 hours (cannula study) in four unmedicated schizophrenics (three chronic, one acute) and found that the mean basal daytime HGH was 4.7 ± 4.0 ng/mL, comparable to that of normal subjects they studied in their laboratory.[47]

Ettigi et al[17] assessed basal HGH as part of another neuroendocrine assessment where subjects (17 chronic schizophrenic men) had an IV cannula inserted in the early morning (8:00 AM). With sampling one hour after the cannula insertion, the schizophrenics had a significantly higher mean basal HGH ± SEM (3.55 ± 1.08 ng/mL) in comparison to controls (1.27 ± 0.14 ng/mL) ($P < 0.05$); whereas with sampling 1.5 hours after cannula insertion, the schizophrenics had nonsignificantly higher basal HGH levels (3.72 ± 1.28 ng/mL versus 1.45 ± 0.20 ng/mL). Furthermore, 6 of the 17 schizophrenics had one or more elevated baseline HGH levels (> 6.0 ng/mL), at 1 or 1.5 hours after cannula insertion in comparison to none of the 21 controls.[17] These elevated levels may be due to a stress effect of cannula insertion. Similar to Ettigi et al,[17] Rotrosen et al[48] also examined the basal HGH in a group of chronic schizophrenics shortly after a cannula insertion (9:00 AM). The mean basal HGH (mean of samples immediately after cannula insertion, 20 minutes after insertion and 40 minutes after insertion) was similar in schizophrenics and controls (1.69 ± 0.59 ng/mL versus 1.24 ± 0.84 ng/mL, respectively; not significant).

The study of Vigneri et al is the only study that assessed a prolonged awake basal HGH (every 20 minutes for 24 hours); they found no differences in comparison to normal controls, but the sample size was extremely small.[47] In contrast, the studies by Ettigi et al[17] and Rotrosen et al[48] sampled for a maximum of 1.5 hours after cannula insertion—an inadequate sampling time for an accurate evaluation of basal HGH. Short time periods and single specimens may be confusing, for they may include spontaneous HGH peak or stress-related HGH release. In addition, normal volunteers are essential as a control group. Only Vigneri et al[47] utilized normal volunteers, whereas Ettigi et al[17] and Rotrosen et al[48] combined alcoholics and patients with nonschizophrenic character disorders with normal volunteers.

Further investigations of daytime basal HGH are indicated since the only adequately designed study (Vigneri et al[47]) examined a total of four schizophrenics.

Sleep-related HGH The release of sleep-related HGH has been highly associated with slow-wave sleep. Since slow-wave sleep has been reported to be reduced or eliminated in schizophrenics,[49] it might follow that HGH is also diminished. The problem with this reasoning is that although HGH is frequently associated with slow-wave sleep, particularly during the first half of sleep, it is not infrequently dissociated, occurring in various stages of sleep (for review of sleep and HGH release, see Parker et al[50]). A review of sleep-related HGH in schizophrenia follows.

The study by Vigneri et al found that all three chronic schizophrenics assessed failed to have an HGH release (a release was defined as a single HGH peak > 6 ng/mL), but the one acute schizophrenic studied did have an HGH release during sleep, similar to that as seen in the eight normal persons studied.[47]

The study by Syvalahlti et al, with the largest sample (N=10 chronic schizophrenics), found that 8 of 10 *medicated* chronic schizophrenics (all on neuroleptics) had an adequate HGH release[51]; of the two subjects that failed to release HGH, one had a disturbed sleep, and the other was the oldest (50 years old), which will be commented on below.

Meltzer[21] recently found that two chronic schizophrenic men treated with fluphenazine decanoate, failed to have a sleep-related HGH release.

We recently studied three chronic schizophrenics—two who were treated with neuroleptics, and one who was unmedicated; two of the three had an adequate HGH release, with the patient who was the oldest (age 50), and also unmedicated, failing to release HGH (unpublished data). Age has clearly been shown to effect sleep HGH, with increasing age causing decreased secretion and peaks.[52] Thus, age must be controlled in HGH studies.

What is most striking about the studies summarizing sleep-related HGH in schizophrenia is the extremely small sample sizes used. In the four studies reviewed, 20 patients were assessed. Thus, whatever findings are suggested are at best tentative. In addition, most of the patients studied were on therapeutic doses of neuroleptics. Although small doses of some neuroleptics have been shown not to effect sleep-related HGH,[27] it is unclear what effect large doses of neuroleptics have. A study of HGH of schizophrenics on neuroleptics and subsequently drug free would have to be done to address this question.

Although studies in this area are inconclusive, they do suggest that most chronic schizophrenics have an adequate HGH release. Future studies should have larger samples and focus on certain age decades with appropriate, matched normal controls. It is our recommendation that young adults be studied, since older normal subjects frequently fail to release HGH.

If studies do find that a subgroup of schizophrenics have an abnormality in sleep-related HGH release, what might it say about underlying neurotransmitter abnormalities? The *neurotransmitter control of sleep-related HGH release is highly confusing.* Administration of levodopa, dopamine blockers, or noradrenergic blockers does not appear to effect sleep-related HGH.[27,53,54] The role of serotonin appears to be important, although the data even here are controversial: cyproheptadine decreases whereas methylsergide increases sleep-related HGH release[55,56]; these conflictual findings are most likely secondary to the mixed properties of these serotonin blockers.

Dopamine agonists The use of dopamine agonists to assess HGH in schizophrenics versus controls has been actively pursued with the hypothesis that if dopamine hypersensitivity extended to the hypothalamus, the HGH response to dopamine agonists should be increased. Of the dopamine agonists used (Table 8-6), only apomorphine is a direct dopamine agonist. Levodopa and amphetamine are indirect dopamine agonists and are thus complicated by the following. (1) The use of levodopa brings up issues of absorption, decarboxylation, and synthesis to dopamine and its release and metabolism. Furthermore, levodopa increases norepinephrine, which is also stimulatory to HGH. (2) Amphetamine not only releases presynaptic dopamine, but also releases norepinephrine and possibly serotonin, all of which are stimulatory to HGH. With these limitations in mind, we will review this literature.

As can be seen from Table 8-6, the overwhelming majority of the studies did not find an increased HGH response to dopamine agonists, contrary to what was hypothesized.[17,39,48,57,58] Focusing on the apomorphine results, Pandey et al did find the expected increase in HGH to apomorphine, but it was limited to acute schizophrenics and not chronic schizophrenics.[59] Meltzer et al failed to replicate this finding in acute schizophrenics, which may be a function of the small sample size assessed, N=5.[39] The majority of the studies with apomorphine focused almost exclusively on *chronic schizophrenics.* In summary, they found that chronic schizophrenics as a group either were not different from normal controls[39,48,57-59] and acute schizophrenics[39] or actually had a decreased HGH response in comparison to normal controls[17,40] and acute schizophrenics.[59]

The study by Meltzer et al found that although chronic schizophrenics as a group were not different from normal persons, the HGH response was correlated with the years since the onset of illness ($r=0.67$; $df=11$; $P<0.05$).[39] The latter finding is similar to that of Ettigi et al

Table 8-6
HGH Release to Dopamine Agonists in Schizophrenia: A Review of the Literature

Tamminga et al, 1977[40]	(1) Apomorphine, 0.75 mg SC (2) Levodopa, 500 mg PO	9 Chronic schizophrenics 11 Normal controls	(1) No group differences for apomorphine, but (2) 7 of 9 schizophrenics had an abnormally low response to levodopa vs. 2 of 11 normal controls ($P<0.02$)
Ettigi et al, 1976[17]	Apomorphine, 0.75 mg SC	17 Chronic schizophrenics 21 Controls (9 alcoholics, 12 normal controls)	Schizophrenics had a significantly lower response than controls ($P<0.05$)
Pandey et al, 1977[59]	Apomorphine, 0.75 mg SC	9 Acute schizophrenics 8 Chronic schizophrenics 8 Normal controls	Acute schizophrenics had a greater response than chronic schizophrenics ($P<0.01$) and normal controls ($P<0.05$), chronic schizophrenics did not differ from normal controls
Rotrosen et al, 1976[57]	(1) Apomorphine, 0.5 mg SC (2) Levodopa, 500 mg PO	10 Chronic schizophrenics 7 Normal controls	No group differences
Rotrosen et al, 1978[41]	(1) Apomorphine, 0.5 mg SC	22 Chronic schizophrenics 9 Normal controls	No group differences
Rotrosen et al, 1978[58]	Apomorphine, 0.50 mg SC	26 Chronic schizophrenics 21 Controls	No group differences
Meltzer et al, 1981[60]	Apomorphine, 0.75 mg SC	13 Chronic schizophrenics 5 Acute schizophrenics 15 Normal controls	No group differences

($r = -0.45$; df$=15$; $P < 0.1$).[17] The duration of illness in schizophrenia thus may be an important issue in the HGH response to apomorphine and could help explain those reports, suggesting an exaggerated HGH response to apomorphine in acute schizophrenia and a blunted response in chronic schizophrenics. These findings could fit the following interpretation: acute schizophrenics may have supersensitive dopamine receptors, and as they become chronic, they may develop a hyposensitive dopamine receptor state with a more blunted HGH response to dopamine agonists. This hypothesis could best be assessed by following longitudinally the HGH response to apomorphine in schizophrenics from acute to chronic stages. This has not been done yet.

A recent presentation by Meltzer highlighted his past findings of the effect of duration of illness in schizophrenia on the HGH response to apomorphine. In addition, he presented surprising new data: the HGH response to apomorphine decreased in depressives as a function of duration of illness. As a matter of fact, when duration of illness was controlled, there were no differences between depressives, schizophrenics, and normal controls.[60]

Thus, it is possible that the HGH response to apomorphine is related to nonspecific pathology—at least common to schizophrenia and depression. Furthermore, as duration of illness increases, dopamine sensitivity may decrease.

Some investigators have found that a significant factor associated with a blunted HGH response was the duration of prior neuroleptic use. Ettigi et al found a significant negative correlation between years of prior neuroleptic use and the HGH peak to apomorphine ($r=0.48$; df$=14$; $P<0.05$).[17] Rotrosen et al also found a negative correlation between years of prior neuroleptic use and the HGH peak to apomorphine (0.5 mg subcutaneously) but did not report their data or whether this finding was statistically significant.[58] Prior neuroleptic use might have induced a dopamine subsensitivity in the hypothalamus and/or pituitary, resulting in a reduced HGH response (this is reviewed above). Thus, major factors which apparently influence the HGH response to apomorphine in schizophrenia are prior neuroleptic use and duration of illness.

Even if the HGH response to apomorphine proves nonspecific to schizophrenia, as was recently suggested by Meltzer,[60] it is possible that this response may predict neuroleptic responsivity. The latter would be of major clinical importance. Two groups of investigators have suggested that although chronic schizophrenics as a group did not differ from normal controls in their HGH response to apomorphine, those schizophrenics with an adequate HGH tended to respond better to neuroleptic treatment.[39,57]

Only a few studies have utilized indirect dopamine agonists to evaluate the HGH response in schizophrenia because of difficulties mentioned earlier in this chapter. A study by Tamminga et al[40] with 500 mg of levodopa found that a significantly greater number of chronic schizophrenics had an inadequate HGH response in comparison to normal controls (7 of 9 schizophrenics versus 2 of 11 normal controls, $P<0.02$), although the mean HGH responses did not differ between the groups. Rotrosen et al, the only other investigators evaluating HGH response to levodopa in schizophrenia, found no difference in chronic/subchronic schizophrenics versus controls (which included normal volunteers as well as hospitalized alcoholics).[48,57,58]

Langer et al, the only group to evaluate the HGH response to IV dextroamphetamine (0.1 mg/kg) in schizophrenics, found that eight schizophrenics (five acute, three chronic) did not differ from normal controls (N=21).[61] Since the HGH response to amphetamine has recently been shown to be unreliable even in normal subjects,[62] further evaluations of HGH response to dextroamphetamine may be meaningless.

Since the interpretation of the HGH responses to indirect dopamine agonists are complicated by the multiple neurotransmitters affected by indirect dopamine agonist and since HGH responses to indirect agonists have been suggested to be unreliable, it seems reasonable not to pursue this line of investigation.

Insulin tolerance test Insulin, by inducing a hypoglycemic state, causes a release of HGH. This HGH release is most likely under serotonergic and not dopaminergic control, since cyproheptadine, a serotonin blocker, reduces this release[63] and haloperidol, a dopamine blocker, has no effect.[64] Only two studies have assessed the insulin tolerance test in schizophrenia. Vigneri et al gave 0.1 μ/kg to three chronic schizophrenics and one acute schizophrenic (all unmedicated) and found an adequate HGH release (range 13–26 ng/mL); this did not appear to be different from normal controls.[47] Brambilla et al studied 62 chronic schizophrenic men aged 16–62 years (unmedicated but duration drug free not stated), and found that the HGH response to the insulin tolerance test was adequate. Although normal controls were not used, none of the schizophrenics appeared to have a blunted HGH response.[65]

Noradrenergic agonists Matussek et al evaluated the HGH response to IV clonidine (0.15 mg given over 10 minutes) in a group of psychiatric patients (unmedicated for over four weeks) and normal controls. Ten schizophrenics (acute?, chronic?) were found to have similar HGH response to 32 normal controls unmatched for age and sex.[66] In view of the importance of age and menopausal status in pharmacologically provoked HGH responses, further work must analyze schizophrenics in comparison to normals *after matching for age, sex and menopausal status.* This data does suggest that postsynaptic alpha-noradrenergic receptors are normal in schizophrenics.

Miscellaneous HGH is also released in response to exercise, psychological stimuli, protein-rich meals, and certain amino acids.[46] Evaluations of schizophrenics in these situations have not occurred yet.

In summary, the most promising findings of HGH in schizophrenia is the HGH response to apomorphine. The major findings here are either that chronic schizophrenics have a blunted HGH response or that their HGH response is negatively correlated to duration of illness and/or years of neuroleptic use. Further exploration of this response, evaluating whether it is an artifact to neuroleptic use and/or duration of illness or whether it is specific to chronic schizophrenia, must be pursued.

Cortisol

Cortisol secretion (involving hypothalamic corticotropin releasing factor, pituitary adrenocorticotropic hormone, and subsequent cortisol release from the adrenal cortex), has long been recognized to be increased in the plasma in some psychiatric patients[67]; this has been felt to reflect increased hypothalamic-pituitary-adrenal cortical activity. The neurotransmitter control of cortisol is complex, but norepinephrine and gamma-amino butyric acid are inhibitory and serotonin and acetylcholine are stimulatory[68]; dopamine does not significantly affect cortisol.

Basal cortisol studies In the 1950s, preliminary studies found no differences between schizophrenics and normal persons.[69,70] A major limitation of these studies was that the cortisol metabolites assessed did not accurately reflect total cortisol secretion. As pointed out by Cope and Black, urine free cortisol is a more valid indicator of cortisol secretion rates and highly correlates with plasma 17-OHCS levels.[71] Carroll assessed 24-hour urine free cortisol of 10 schizophrenics (mean age 28.5 years, range 15–70 years) (acute?, chronic?) in comparison to 21 depressed patients (mean age 57.8 years, range 22–80 years); all patients were drug free for at least one week. The depressives had a significantly greater urine free cortisol excretion rate than did the schizophrenics; the latter had a mean 24-hour urine free cortisol of 39.0 ng/mL, similar to that of normal persons.[72] These findings by Carroll (72) were recently replicated by Diebold et al in eight endogenous depressives (median age 58 years, range 41–73 years) versus nine acute schizophrenics (median age 26 years, range 18–37 years).[73]

Carroll evaluated cerebrospinal fluid cortisol in five schizophrenics and 14 depressives; the schizophrenics had a significantly smaller cerebrospinal fluid cortisol level with a mean cortisol level of 3.9 ng/mL, similar to that of normal persons.[72] Jimerson et al also evaluated the cerebrospinal fluid cortisol in a group of schizophrenics (N=14, mean age 26 years) versus depressives (N=8, mean age 38 years) and patients with personality disorders (N=6, mean age 23 years)—all unmedicated for two weeks; they found no differences among the groups.[74] The disparity between the data of Jimerson et al[74] and that of Carroll[72] may be related to the fact that only a *single sample* of cerebrospinal fluid was assessed in both studies. Furthermore, Jimerson et al[72] included three schizo-affective depressives, which may have contributed to the lack of difference in the schizophrenics versus the other groups.

We recently evaluated the plasma cortisol in schizophrenics (N=18, mean age 29.6 years, SD 8.9 years), endogenous depressives (N=58, mean age 41.7 years, SD 14.4 years), and normal controls (N=43, mean age 35.2 years, SD 13.7 years). All subjects had a butterfly needle inserted in the antecubital vein and kept patent with heparinized saline with sampling for plasma cortisol every 30 minutes; since the mean 1:00 to 4:00 PM plasma cortisol has been shown to highly correlate with the mean 24-hour plasma cortisol, the mean 1:00 to 4:00 PM plasma cortisol was used as a comprehensive measure of basal plasma cortisol.[75,76] A level of > 11 μg/dL was used to define cortisol hypersecretion, since this value defined ⅓ of depressives while ill, none after recovery, and only a few normal persons. Our study found that 31% of the depressives, 11% of schizophrenics, and 4% of normal persons were cortisol hypersecretors. Depressives had a significantly higher frequency of hypersecretors than did normal controls ($\chi^2 = 9.23$, $P < 0.005$) as expected; schizophrenics did not differ significantly from depressives ($\chi^2 = 1.88$) or normal persons (Fisher exact test, $P = 0.338$). Interpretation of this data must be cautious. Why did schizophrenics not differ from depressives as many prior studies have demonstrated? We recently found that in endogenous depressives, the mean 1:00 to 4:00 PM plasma cortisol was positively correlated with age,[77] which has not been demonstrated in schizophrenics (unpublished data). Thus, if prior studies examined depressives very much older than schizophrenics, an age effect might have created a significant cortisol differences between the groups.

In summary, for the most part, schizophrenics are cortisol normosecretors. The meaning of infrequent cortisol hypersecretors (11%) among schizophrenics must be further explored.

Dexamethasone suppression test (DST) Dexamethasone is a potent synthetic steroid that normally suppresses the endogenous secretion of adrenocorticotropic hormone and cortisol by affecting feedback receptors. Dexamethasone typically fails to suppress (dexamethasone resistance) endogenous cortisol in Cushing's syndrome.[78] Interestingly, dexamethasone resistance has also been demonstrated to occur frequently (40% to 70%) in endogenous depressives.[79-83] Carroll et al found that the 2-mg DST is sensitive (occurring in 40%) for endogenomorphic depression and highly specific (occurring in less than 5% of neurotic depressives and nondepressed patients).[79] Carroll et al state that one of the 30 nondepressed patients (consisting of 15 schizophrenics—acute? chronic?) was dexamethasone resistant, without stating whether that person was schizophrenic.[79] Thus, one can deduce that schizophrenics had at minimum of 0% and maximum of 7% abnormal DSTs (2 mg).[79] Brown et al, also using the 2-mg DST, found 40% of major depressives (N=20) resistant in contrast to none of eight schizophrenics (acute?, chronic?, age?).[81] Thus, the literature for the 2-mg DST is consistent: schizophrenics (like normal persons) suppress cortisol in response to 2 mg of dexamethasone.

The situation for the 1-mg DST and schizophrenics is much less clear. Recently, Schlesser et al administered the 1-mg DST to 48 schizophrenics (acute?, chronic?, age?); they found that none of the 48 schizophrenics was dexamethasone resistant, although only one 8 AM postdexamethasone plasma cortisol level was assessed.[84] Since in depressives only a small number are resistant at 8 AM only,[80] Schlesser et al may be severely underestimating dexamethasone resistance among schizophrenics by limiting postdexamethasone assessment to 8 AM.

We have evaluated the 1-mg DST in 16 schizophrenics (11 chronic, 5 subchronic or acute), 12 normal controls, and 31 depressives; an abnormal DST was considered a postdexamethasone plasma cortisol of > 5 µg/dL at 4 or 11 PM; 4 of the 16 (25%) schizophrenics, none of the 12 normal persons (0%), and 15 of the 31 depressives (48%) demonstrated dexamethasone resistance. Thus, the schizophrenics had a greater frequency of dexamethasone resistance than that of normal persons ($P=0.08$) and a smaller frequency than that of depressives ($P=0.18$). The 1-mg DST may identify a sizable portion of schizophrenics (similar to that reported by Brown, personal communication), unlike the 2-mg DST. As a matter of fact, the four schizophrenics who were dexamethasone resistant in the 1-mg DST were suppressors when subsequently given the 2-mg DST.

The significance of an abnormal DST, no matter how prevalent in schizophrenia, deserves careful attention. Carman et al suggest that schizophrenics who are dexamethasone resistant may respond to thymoleptics.[85]

Amphetamine-cortisol test Dextroamphetamine (0.1 mg/kg) has recently been demonstrated to release cortisol in normal subjects and actually suppress cortisol in endogenous depressives.[86] It has been hypothesized that the amphetamine-induced cortisol response is under the control of noradrenergic receptors (with alpha-noradrenergic receptors being stimulatory and beta-noradrenergic receptors being inhibitory). In normal persons the alpha-noradrenergic receptors appear to predominate, whereas in depressives Sachar et al have suggested that alpha-noradrenergic receptors may be hyposensitive, resulting in a predominance of the beta-noradrenergic response.[86]

We decided to explore the cortisol response to dextroamphetamine in comparison to normal subjects and depressives: eight chronic schizophrenic men (27.5 ± 5.5 years old), 11 endogenous depressives (nine women, two men; 51.9 ± 11.0 years old), and 14 normal controls (eight women, six men; 36.5 ± 13.8 years old), were studied. All subjects were drug free for at least 10 days. A butterfly needle was inserted in the antecubital vein at 9 AM and kept patent with heparinized saline. After obtaining baseline samples at −30 minutes, −15 minutes and 0 time, dextroamphetamine (0.1 mg/kg) was infused at 9:30 AM over 1 minute; blood samples for cortisol were drawn every 15 minutes for 90 minutes.

As can be seen in Figure 8-2, plasma cortisol was significantly increased from 30 minutes to 75 minutes when compared with both depressives and normals (two-tailed *t* test with Bonferroni protection).

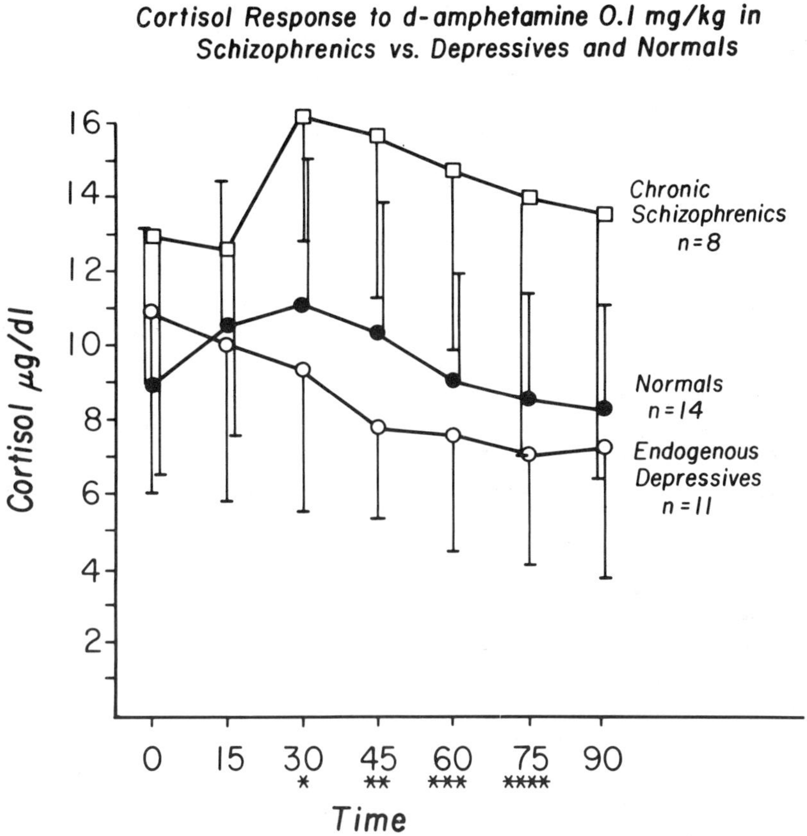

Figure 8-2 Cortisol response to dextroamphetamine (0.1 mg/kg) in schizophrenics versus depressives and normal persons.

*Schizophrenics versus normal persons, $t=3.07$, $P<0.05$; schizophrenics versus depressives, $t=3.98$, $P<0.005$.

**Schizophrenics versus normal persons, $t=3.13$, $P<0.02$; schizophrenics versus depressives, $t=5.00$, $P<0.001$.

***Schizophrenics versus normal persons, $t=3.47$, $P<0.01$; schizophrenics versus depressives, $t=3.86$, $P<0.005$.

****Schizophrenics versus normal persons, $t=2.64$, $P<0.05$; schizophrenics versus depressives, $t=3.00$, $P<0.05$.

In addition, the mean postcortisol response (mean 15- to 90-minutes cortisol level minus cortisol at time 0) was significantly different between all three groups ($F=5.7$, $P<0.025$); schizophrenics had a significantly greater mean cortisol response than did depressives ($t=2.89$, $P<0.05$) and had a trend for a greater response than normals ($t=1.46$, P not significant with Bonferroni protection).

The data suggests that schizophrenics as a group had a greater cortisol response in comparison to normal persons and depressives; in fact, the schizophrenics appeared to have a "hypernormal" cortisol release to dextroamphetamine. These preliminary findings are consistent with hyperfunction of norepinephrine in schizophrenics, as has recently been reported,[5,87] increased noradrenergic receptor sensitivity and/or decreased beta-noradrenergic receptor sensitivity. Further studies must replicate these findings as well as examine what effects age, sex, and menopausal status may have.

TRH-TSH Stimulation Test

TRH is a tripeptide, widely distributed in the brain[88] and found in other organs,[89,90] that stimulates thyrotropin (TSH) release[91,92] from the anterior pituitary.

In normal subjects, factors that may reduce the TRH-induced TSH response include the following: increasing age,[93,94] male gender,[94–96] repeated TRH administration,[97,98] thyroid hormones,[91,92,99] glucocorticoids,[100] and the infusion of dopamine.[101]

Abnormalities of the TRH-TSH test have been reported in a number of psychiatric conditions. Most noteworthy is that over 25% of depressives have a blunted TSH response to TRH.[102] In addition, manic patients (not on lithium),[103–105] alcoholics,[102,105] and anorectic subjects[102] may have a blunted TSH response to TRH. The TRH-TSH test may be of theoretical interest in schizophrenia; since a dopamine infusion decreases the TRH-induced TSH response in normal subjects,[101] one might hypothesize that dopamine hyperactivity in schizophrenia (which might extend to the pituitary) might similarly cause a blunted TSH response to TRH.

Two studies have evaluated this test in schizophrenia. Prange et al studied 17 chronic schizophrenics (medication free for eight days) (nine women, eight men; aged 23–41 years) matched for age and sex with normal controls. The ΔTSH (peak TSH minus baseline TSH) to TRH (500-μIU bolus) in schizophrenics did not differ from that of normal controls; the two groups did not have any "blunters" ($\Delta TSH < 5$ μIU/mL).[45]

Gold et al studied the TSH response to TRH (500-μg bolus) in schizophrenics (acute?, chronic?, age?, sex?, drug free for how long?); they found that none of 14 schizophrenics had a blunted response ($\Delta TSH < 7$ μIU/mL in comparison to 31 of 41 major depressives).[105] The problem with this study was that it is unclear whether the groups were matched for age and sex, factors that may be critical in the TSH response to TRH.

In summary, it does not appear that patients with schizophrenia have abnormalities in the TRH-TSH test.

Gonadotropins

Luteinizing hormone-releasing hormone (LHRH), a decapeptide hypothalamic hormone, stimulates the release of luteinizing hormone (LH) and follicle-stimulating hormone (FSH) from the anterior pituitary gland.

The neurotransmitter regulation of LHRH, LH, and FSH is unclear. Human and animal studies suggest both stimulatory and inhibitory effects of dopamine on gonadotropin secretion. Due to this unclear role of dopamine on gonadotropin secretion as well as on stimulated gonadotropin responses, a logical hypothesis of gonadotropins in schizophrenia could not be predicted.

Nonetheless, an evaluation of gonadotropins in schizophrenia is indicated. Because of a significant effect of estrogen on LH and FSH[106,107] and the overriding complications that the menstrual cycle imposes upon studies of gonadotropins, such studies in schizophrenia have been almost exclusively evaluated in men.

Most of the studies of basal levels of FSH and LH in schizophrenia have been conflictual. Basal levels of FSH and/or LH have been found to be higher,[19] lower,[108] and the same[109] compared with those in control groups. These studies are inadequate for the following reasons. Controls in all of these were taken from normative data published in the literature, except for Brambilla et al, who used mentally retarded persons as controls.[108] All of the studies except that of Siris et al[109] used single samples. Thus, an accurate statement about basal gonadotropins cannot be made in schizophrenia.

Only one study in the literature has reported on the FSH and LH response to LHRH (the hypothalamic-pituitary axis). Brambilla et al found that chronic schizophrenic men had an augmented response of both FSH and LH to LHRH in comparison to mentally retarded, age-matched men.[108] Thus, no study has evaluated the LHRH-gonadotropin test in schizophrenia in comparison to *normal controls* evaluated in the same laboratory. In summary, gonadotropins (both basal levels as well as gonadotropin levels in response to LHRH) in schizophrenia have not been adequately studied.

Conclusions

This review of the literature and presentation of our data suggest that *neuroendocrine abnormalities are not widespread in schizophrenia;*

there is not a diffuse involvement of the hypothalamopituitary-adrenal axis leading to multiple neuroendocrine abnormalities as is the case with endogenous depressive illness.

As best as can be seen, four neuroendocrine tests may be of value to pursue in schizophrenia: the PRL response to reserpine, the PRL response to haloperidol, the apomorphine-HGH test, and the dextroamphetamine-cortisol test. Two of these tests specifically suggest dopamine hypersensitivity in schizophrenia (dopamine receptor hypersensitivity for haloperidol-PRL test in chronic schizophrenic women and increased storage pool dopamine for reserpine-PRL test in chronic schizophrenic men); one of these tests suggests a dopamine hypersensitivity in acute schizophrenics and dopamine hyposensitivity in chronic schizophrenics (apomorphine-HGH test); and one of these tests suggest norepinephrine hyperactivity (dextroamphetamine-cortisol test). Since chronic schizophrenia is probably a heterogeneous disorder, each of these tests may be identifying a subgroup. Administering all four tests to the same schizophrenic patient will help clarify this issue.

The findings of the reserpine-PRL test, haloperidol-PRL test, and dextroamphetamine-cortisol test are based on *preliminary data and must be replicated* in larger samples, whereas the results of the apomorphine-HGH test appear firm, being based on multiple studies of large sample sizes.

A major consideration in the neuroendocrine findings of schizophrenia is whether a prior history of neuroleptics contributed to the results. The apomorphine-HGH test in schizophrenia has been found to be highly correlated to the duration of prior neuroleptics. This must be evaluated with the other neuroendocrine tests. If prior neuroleptic use proves important, this must be controlled to assess the specificity of each test for schizophrenia.

In addition, although all the schizophrenics were drug (neuroleptic) free for over seven days, the question of whether this is enough time drug free for an adequate neuroendocrine assessment is of importance. First, it is well known that chronic neuroleptics can induce microsomal enzymes (which are responsible for its metabolism).[110] What is unknown is just how long after drug withdrawal it takes for microsomal enzyme activity to return to normal. If, at the end of seven days, microsomal enzyme activity was still increased, challenges with a medication (reserpine, haloperidol, apomorphine, and dextroamphetamine) might be metabolized more quickly than normal. Thus, lower blood levels might explain some of the above neuroendocrine findings in schizophrenia: ie, reduced levels of reserpine and haloperidol would result in blunted PRL response; reduced apomorphine levels would result in a blunted HGH response; a reduced amphetamine level would not explain a heightened cortisol response found for schizophrenics. Measuring drug blood levels would help answer this. Second, it is unclear whether neuroendocrine responsiveness returns to normal after only seven days neuroleptic free. Recently, Brown et al demonstrated that PRL elevation in schizophrenics on chronic neuroleptics diminished over time, despite no change in neuroleptic blood level. It is suggested that dopamine receptors became hyposensitive with chronic neuroleptic treatment.[111] Whether this persists for longer than seven days after neuroleptic withdrawal and might affect neuroendocrine challenges is unclear.

Many of the above questions can best be answered by studying schizophrenics who have never been medicated or who have been medication free for at least a few months. Further study of schizophrenia with psychoneuroendocrinological strategies is clearly warranted. Such studies might help clarify the psychobiology of schizophrenia as well as possibly identify the use of particular neuroendocrine tests that might be helpful in the diagnosis of schizophrenia.

REFERENCES

1. Endicott J, Nee J, Fleiss J, et al: Diagnostic criteria for schizophrenia. *Arch Gen Psychiatry* 1982;39:884–889.
2. Bowers MB: Biochemical processes in schizophrenia. *Schizophr Bull* 1980; 5:27–37.
3. Palkovitz M, Brownstein M, Saavedra JM, et al: Norepinephrine and dopamine content of hypothalamic nuclei of the rat. *Brain Res* 1974;77: 137–149.
4. Saavedra JM, Palkovitz M, Brownstein MJ, et al: Serotonin distribution in the nuclei of the hypothalamus and preoptic region. *Brain Res* 1974;77: 157–165.
5. Bird ED, Spokes EG, Iversen LL: Brain norepinephrine and dopamine in schizophrenia. *Science* 1979;204:93–94.
6. DeLisi LE, Neckers LM, Weinberger DR, et al: Increased whole blood serotonin concentrations in chronic schizophrenic patients. *Arch Gen Psychiatry* 1981;38:647–650.
7. Sachar EJ: Endocrine abnormalities in depression, in Paykel ES (ed): *Handbook of Affective Disorders.* New York, Guilford Press, 1982.
8. Kanematsu S, Sawyer CH: Elevation of plasma prolactin after hypophyseal stalk section in the rat. *Endocrinology* 1973;93:238–241.
9. MacLeod RM: Regulation of prolactin secretion, in Martini L, Ganong WF (eds): *Frontiers in Neuroendocrinology.* New York, Raven Press, 1975.
10. Meltzer HY, Goode DJ, Fang VS: The effect of psychotropic drugs on endocrine function. I. Neuroleptics, precursors, and agonists, in DiMascio A, Lipton M (eds): *A Review of Progress.* New York, Raven Press, 1978.
11. Lal S, Martin JB: Neuroanatomy and neuropharmacological regulation of neuroendocrine function, in van Praag HM, Lader MH, Rafaelson OJ, et al (eds): *Part II Brain Mechanisms and Abnormal Behavior.* New York, Marcel Dekker, Inc, 1980.
12. Meltzer HY, Stahl S: The dopamine hypothesis: A review. *Schizophr Bull* 1976;2:19–76.
13. Stevens JR: An anatomy of schizophrenia. *Arch Gen Psychiatry* 1973;

29:117–129.
14. Meltzer HY, Sachar EJ, Frantz AG: Serum prolactin levels in unmedicated schizophrenic patients. *Arch Gen Psychiatry* 1974;31:564–569.
15. Meltzer HY, Fang VS: The effect of neuroleptics on serum prolactin in schizophrenic patients. *Arch Gen Psychiatry* 1976;33:279–286.
16. Brambilla F, Guaslalla A, Guerrini A, et al: Prolactin secretion in chronic schizophrenia. *Acta Psychiatr Scand* 1976;54:275–286.
17. Ettigi P, Nair NPV, Lal S, et al: Effect of apomorphine on growth hormone and prolactin secretion in schizophrenic patients with or without oral dyskinesia, withdrawn from chronic neuroleptic therapy. *J Neurol Neurosurg Psychiatry* 1976;39:870–876.
18. Wode-Helgodt B, Eneroth P, Fyro B, et al: Effect of chlorpromazine treatment on prolactin levels in cerebrospinal fluid and plasma of psychotic patients. *Acta Psychiatr Scand* 1977;56:280–293.
19. Johnstone EC, Crow TJ, Mashiter K: Anterior pituitary secretion in chronic schizophrenia—an approach to neurohumoral mechanisms. *Psychol Med* 1977;7:223–228.
20. Gruen PH, Sachar EJ, Altman N, et al: Relation of plasma prolactin in normal and schizophrenic subjects. *Arch Gen Psychiatry* 1978;35:108–116.
21. Meltzer HY, Busch D, So R, et al: Neuroleptic-induced elevations in serum prolactin levels: Etiology and significance, in Baxter C, Melnechuk T (eds): *Perspective in Schizophrenia Research.* New York, Raven Press, 1980.
22. Brambilla F, Bellodi L, Negri F: Dopamine receptor sensitivity in the hypothalamus of chronic schizophrenics after haloperidol therapy: Growth hormone and prolactin response to stimuli. *Psychoneuroendocrinology* 1979;4:329–339.
23. Kolakowska T, Wiles DH, Gelder MG, et al: Clinical significance of plasma chlorpromazine levels. III. Plasma levels of the drug, some of its metabolites and prolactin in patients receiving long-term phenothiazine treatment. *Psychopharmacology* 1976;49:101–107.
24. Gruen PH, Sachar EJ, Altman N, et al: Relation of plasma prolactin to clinical response in schizophrenic patients. *Arch Gen Psychiatry* 1978; 35:1222–1227.
25. Parker DC, Rossman LG, Vanderlaan EF: Relation of sleep entrained human prolactin release to REM-non REM cycles. *J Clin Endocrinol Metab* 1974; 38:646–651.
26. Vekemans M, Robyn E: The influence of erogenous estrogen on the circadian periodicity of circulating prolactin in women. *J Clin Endocrinol Metab* 1973;40:886–889.
27. Takahashi Y, Kipnis DM, Daughaday WH: Growth hormone secretion during sleep. *J Clin Invest* 1968;47:2079–2090.
28. Langer G, Sachar EJ, Halpern FS: Human prolactin responses to neuroleptic drugs correlate with antischizophrenic potency. *Nature* 1977;266:639–640.
29. Asnis GM, Sachar EJ, Langer G, et al: Normal prolactin responses in tardive dyskinesia. *Psychopharmacology* 1979;66:247–250.
30. Meltzer HY, Busch DA, Creese IR, et al: Effect of intramuscular chlorpromazine on serum prolactin levels in schizophrenic patients and normal controls. *Psychiatry Res* 1981;5:95–105.
31. Meltzer HY, Busch D, Young M, et al: Prolactin and growth hormone studies in schizophrenic patients and normal controls, in Brambilla F, Racagni G, de Wied D (eds): *Progress in Psychoneuroendocrinology.* Amsterdam, Elsevier-North Holland Biomedical Press, 1980.
32. Asnis GM, Sachar EJ, Langer G, et al: Prolactin responses to haloperidol in

normal young women. *Psychoneuroendocrinology,* in press.
33. Spitzer RL, Endicott J, Robins E: Research diagnostic criteria: Rationale and reliability. *Arch Gen Psychiatry* 1978;35:773–782.
34. Buckman MT, Peake GT: Estrogen potentiation of phenothiazine-induced prolactin secretion in man. *J Clin Endocrinol Metab* 1973;37:977–980.
35. Holzbauer M, Vogt M: Depression by reserpine of the noradrenaline concentration in the hypothalamus of the cat. *J Neurochem* 1956;1:1–21.
36. Pletscher A, Shore PA, Brodie BB: Serotonin as a mediator of reserpine action in brain. *J Pharmacol Expt Therapeut* 1956;116:84–96.
37. Carlsson A, Rosengren E, Bertler A, et al: Effect of reserpine on the metabolism of catecholamines, in Garattini S, Ghetti V (eds): *Psychotropic Drugs.* Amsterdam, Elsevier Publishing Co, 1957.
38. Asnis GM, Sachar EJ, Halbreich U, et al: The prolactin-stimulating potency of reserpine in man. *Psychiatry Res* 1981;5:39–45.
39. Meltzer HY, Busch D, Fang VS: Hormones, dopamine receptors, and schizophrenia. *Psychoneuroendocrinology* 1981;6:17–36.
40. Tamminga CA, Smith RC, Pandey G, et al: A neuroendocrine study of supersensitivity in tardive dyskinesia. *Arch Gen Psychiatry* 1977;36: 1199–1203.
41. Rotrosen J, Angrist B, Clark C, et al: Suppression of prolactin by dopamine agonists in schizophrenics and controls. *Am J Psychiatry* 1978;135:949–951.
42. Friend WC, Brown GM, Jawaki G, et al: Effect of haloperidol and apomorphine treatment on dopamine receptors in pituitary and striatum. *Am J Psychiatry* 1978;135:839–841.
43. Hinkle PM, Tashjian AH: Receptors for thyrotropin-releasing hormone in prolactin producing rat pituitary cells in culture. *J Biol Chem* 1973; 248:6180–6186.
44. Jacobs LS, Snyder PJ, Utiger RD, et al: Prolactin response to thyrotropin-releasing hormone in normal subjects. *J Clin Endocrinol Metab* 1973;36: 1969–1973.
45. Prange AJ, Loosen PT, Wilson IC, et al: Behavioral and endocrine responses of schizophrenic patients to TRH (protirelin). *Arch Gen Psychiatry* 1979; 36:1086–1093.
46. Martin JB: Brain regulation of growth hormone secretion, in Martini L, Ganong WF (eds): *Frontiers in Neuroendocrinology,* vol 4. New York, Raven Press, 1976.
47. Vigneri R, Pezzino V, Squatrit S, et al: Sleep-associated growth hormone (GH) release in schizophrenia. *Neuroendocrinology* 1974;14:356–361.
48. Rotrosen J, Angrist B, Gershon S, et al: Neuroendocrine effects of apomorphine: Characterization of response patterns and application to schizophrenia research. *Br J Psychiatry* 1979;135:444–456.
49. Caldwell DF, Domino EF: Electroencephalographic and eye movement patterns during sleep in chronic schizophrenics. *Electroenceph Clin Neurophysiol* 1967;22:414–419.
50. Parker DC, Sassini JF, Mace JW, et al: Human growth hormone release during sleep: Electroencephalographic correlation. *J Clin Endocrinol Metab* 1969;19:871–874.
51. Syvalahlti E, Pekkarainen A: Serum growth hormone levels in schizophrenic patients during sleep. *J Neurol Transm* 1977;40:221–226.
52. Finkelstein JW, Roffwarg J, Boyar RM, et al: Age-related change in the twenty-four hour spontaneous secretion of growth hormone. *J Clin Endocrinol* 1972;35:665–670.
53 Lucke C, Glick SM: Experimental modification of the sleep-induced peak of

growth hormone secretion. *J Clin Endocrinol* 1971;32:729–736.
54. Chihara K, Kato K, Maeda K, et al: Suppressive effects of L dopa on human prolactin release during sleep. *Acta Endocrinol (Kbl)* 1976;81:19–27.
55. Mendelson WD, Jacobs LS, Reichman FD, et al: Methylsergide suppression of sleep related prolactin secretion and enhancement of growth hormone secretion. *J Clin Invest* 1975;56:690–692.
56. Smythe GA, Luzarus L: Suppression of human growth hormone secretion by melatonin and cyproheptadine. *J Clin Invest* 1974;54:116–121.
57. Rotrosen J, Angrist BM, Gershon S, et al: Dopamine receptor alteration in schizophrenia: Neuroendocrine evidence. *Psychopharmacology* 1976;51: 1–7.
58. Rotrosen J, Angrist B, Paquin J: Neuroendocrine studies with dopamine agonists in schizophrenia. *Psychopharmacol Bull* 1978;14:14–16.
59. Pandey GN, Garver DL, Tamminga C, et al: Post-synaptic supersensitivity in schizophrenia. *Am J Psychiatry* 1977;134:518–522.
60. Meltzer HY: Neuroendocrinology and schizophrenia. Presented at Psychoneuroendocrinology Symposium—NIMH. Neuroscience Research Branch. Ontario, Canada, June 23, 1981.
61. Langer G, Heinze G, Rerin B, et al: Reduced growth hormone responses to amphetamine in "endogenous" depressive patients. *Arch Gen Psychiatry* 1976;33:1471–1475.
62. Halbreich U, Sachar EJ, Asnis GM, et al: Growth hormone response to dextroamphetamine. *Arch Gen Psychiatry* 1982;39:189–192.
63. Bivens CH, Lebovitz HE, Feldman JM: Inhibition of hypoglycemia-induced growth hormone secretion by the serotonin antagonists cyproheptadine and methylsergide. *New Engl J Med* 1973;289:236–239.
64. Nathan RS, Sachar EJ, Ostrow L, et al: Failure of dopaminergic blockade to affect prolactin growth hormone, and cortisol responses to insulin-induced hypoglycemia in schizophrenics. *J Clin Endocrinol Metab* 1981;52:807–809.
65. Brambilla F, Guerrini A, Guastalla A: Neuroendocrine effects of haloperidol therapy in chronic schizophrenia. *Psychopharmacology (Berlin)* 1975; 44:17–22.
66. Matussek N, Ackenheil M, Hippius H, et al: Effect of clonidine on growth hormone release in psychiatric patients and controls. *Psychiatry Res* 1980;2:25–36.
67. Mason JW: A review of psychoendocrine research on the pituitary-adrenal cortical system. *Psychosom Med* 1968;30:576–607.
68. Jones MT, Hillhouse E, Burden J: Secretion of corticotropin releasing hormone in vitro, in Martini L, Ganong WF (eds): *Frontiers in Neuroendocrinology*, vol. 4. New York, Raven Press, 1976.
69. Smith F, Simon A, Lingoes J: Excretion of urinary corticoids in mental patients. *J Nerv Ment Dis* 1956;124:381–391.
70. Romanoff L, Rodriguez R, Stelle J, et al: Determination of tetrahydrocortisol and tetrahydrocortisone in the urine of normal and schizophrenic men. *J Clin Endocrinol* 1958;17:777–785.
71. Cope CL, Black EG: The reliability of some adrenal function tests. *Br Med J* 1959;2:1117–1122.
72. Carroll BJ: Limbic system-adrenal cortex regulation in depression and schizophrenia. *Psychosom Med* 1976;38:106–121.
73. Diebold K, Kick H, Schmidt G: Urinary free cortisol excretion in endogenously depressed and schizophrenic patients. *Psychiatr Clin (Basel)* 1981;14:43–48.

74. Jimerson DC, Post RM, van Kamen DP, et al: Cerebrospinal fluid cortisol levels in depression and schizophrenia. *Am J Psychiatry* 1980;137:979–980.
75. Halbreich U, Sachar EJ, Asnis GM, et al: Studies of cortisol diurnal rhythm and cortisol response to d-amphetamine in depressed patients. *Psychopharmacol Bull* 1980;17:114–116.
76. Halbreich U, Zumoff B, Kream J, et al: The mean 1 to 4 PM plasma cortisol concentration as a diagnostic test for hypercortisolism. *J Clin Endocrinol Metab* in press.
77. Asnis GM, Sachar EJ, Halbreich U, et al: Cortisol secretion in relation to age in major depression. *Psychosom Med* 1981;43:235–242.
78. McHardy-Young S, Harris PWR, Lessoff MH, et al: Single-dose dexamethasone suppression test for Cushing's syndrome. *Br Med J* 1967; 1:740–744.
79. Carroll BJ, Curtis GC, Mendels J: Neuroendocrine regulation of depression. II. Discrimination of depressed from non-depressed patients. *Arch Gen Psychiatry* 1976;33:1051–1057.
80. Carroll BJ, Feinberg M, Greden JF, et al: A specific laboratory test for the diagnosis of melancholia: Standardization, validation and clinical utility. *Arch Gen Psychiatry* 1981;38:15–22.
81. Brown WA, Johnston R, and Mayfield D: The 24-hour dexamethasone suppression test in a clinical setting: Relationship to diagnosis, symptoms and response to treatment. *Am J Psychiatry* 1979;136:543–547.
82. Stokes PE, Pick GR, Stoll PM, et al: Pituitary-adrenal function in depressed patients: Resistance to dexamethasone suppression. *J Psychiatr Res* 1975;12:271–281.
83. Asnis GM, Halbreich U, Nathan RS, et al: The dexamethasone suppression test in depressive illness: Clinical correlates. *Psychoneuroendocrinology*, in press.
84. Schlesser MA, Winokur G, Sherman BM: Hypothalamic-pituitary-adrenal axis activity in depressive illness. *Arch Gen Psychiatry* 1980;37:737–743.
85. Carman JS, Wyatt E, Crews EL, et al: Dexamethasone suppression test: Predictor of thymoleptic response in catatonic, paranoid, hebrephrenic and schizoaffective patients, in Perris C, Struwe G, Jansson B (eds): *Biological Psychiatry: 1981.* Amsterdam, Elsevier-North Holland Biomedical Press, 1981, pp 1189–1193.
86. Sachar EJ, Halbreich U, Asnis GM, et al: Paradoxical cortisol responses to dextroamphetamine in endogenous depression. *Arch Gen Psychiatry* 1981; 38:1113–1117.
87. Carlsson A: Introduction, in Usdin E, Kopin IJ, Barchas JD (eds): *Catecholamines: Basic and Clinical Frontiers.* New York, Pergamon Press, 1979, pp 1845–1847.
88. Lal S, Martin J: Neuroanatomy and neuropharmacological regulation of neuroendocrine function, in van Praag H (ed): *Handbook of Biological Psychiatry, Part III.* New York, Marcel Dekker, Inc, 1980.
89. Morley JE, Garvin TJ, Pekary AE, et al: Thyrotropin releasing hormone in the gastrointestinal tract. *Biochem Biophys Res Commun* 1977;79:314–318.
90. Gibbons JM Jr, Mitnick M, Chieffo V: In vitro biosynthesis of TSH- and LH-releasing factors by the human placenta. *Am J Obstet Gynecol* 1975; 12:127–131.
91. Sawin CT, Hershman JM: Clinical use of thyrotropin-releasing hormone. *Pharmacol Ther (Oxford):* 1976;1:351–366.
92. Hershman JM: Clinical application of thyrotropin-releasing hormone. *N Engl*

J Med 1974;290:886–890.
93. Snyder PJ, Utiger RD: Response to thyrotropin releasing hormone (TRH) in normal man. *J Clin Endocrinol* 1972;34:380–385.
94. Wenzel KW, Meinhold H, Herpich M: TRH-Stimulationstest mit alters-und geschlechtsabhangigem TSH-Anstieg bei Normalpersonen. *Klin Wochenschr* 1974;52:722–727.
95. Haigler ED Jr, Pittman JA Jr, Hershman JM, et al: Direct evaluation of pituitary thyrotropin reserve utilizing synthetic thyrotropin-releasing hormone. *J Clin Endocrinol Metab* 1971;33:573–581.
96. Noel GL, Dimond RC, Wartofsky L, et al: Studies of prolactin and TSH secretion by continuous infusion of small amounts of thyrotropin-releasing hormone (TRH). *J Clin Endocrinol Metab* 1974;39:6–17.
97. Snyder PJ, Utiger RD: Repetitive administration of thyrotropin-releasing hormone results in small elevations of serum thyroid hormones and in marked inhibition of thyrotropin response. *J Clin Invest* 1973;52:2305–2312.
98. Rabello MM, Snyder PJ, Utiger RD: Effects on the pituitary-thyroid axis and prolactin secretion of single and repetitive oral doses of thyrotropin-releasing hormone (TRH). *J Clin Endocrinol Metab* 1974;39:571–578.
99. Burger HG, Patel YC: TSH and TRH: Their physiological regulation and the clinical application of TRH, Martini L, Blesser GM (eds): *Clinical Neuroendocrinology.* New York, Academic Press, 1977.
100. Otsuki M, Dakoda M, Baba S: Influence of glucocorticoids on TRH induced TSH response in man. *J Clin Endocrinol Metab* 1973;36:95–102.
101. Burrow GN, May PB, Spaulding SW: TRH and dopamine interactions affecting pituitary hormone secretion. *J Clin Endocrinol Metab* 1971; 45:65–75.
102. Loosen PT, Prange AJ Jr: Serum thyrotropin response to thyrotropin-releasing hormone in psychiatric patients: A review. *Am J Psychiatry* 1982;139:4.
103. Takahashi S, Kondo H, Yoshimura M, et al: Thyrotropin responses to TRH in depressive illness: Relation to clinical subtypes and prolonged duration of depressive episode. *Folia Psychiatr Neurol Jpn* 1974;28:355–365.
104. Kirkegaard C, Bjorum N, Cohn D, et al: TRH stimulation test in manic depressive disease. *Arch Gen Psychiatry* 1978;35:1017–1023.
105. Gold MS, Pottash, ALC, Extein I, et al: The TRH test in the diagnosis of major and minor depression. *Psychoneuroendocrinology* 1981;6:159–169.
106. Santen RJ: Is aromatization of testosterone to estrodial required for inhibition of luteinizing hormone secretion in men? *J Clin Invest* 1975;56: 1555–1563.
107. Yen SSC, Tasai GC, VandenBerg G, et al: Gonadotropin dynamics in patients with gonadal dysgenesis: A model for the study of gonadotropin regulation. *J Clin Endocrinol Metab* 1972;35:897–904.
108. Brambilla F, Revere C, Guastalla A, et al: Gonadotropin response to synthetic gonadotropin hormone-releasing hormone (GnRH) in chronic schizophrenia. *Acta Psychiatr Scand* 1976;54:131–145.
109. Siris SG, Siris ES, Van Kammen DP, et al: Effects of dopamine blockade on gonadotropins and testosterone in men. *Am J Psychiatry* 1980;137:211–214.
110. Conney AH: Pharmacological implications of microsomal enzyme induction. *Pharmacol Rev* 1967;19:317–366.
111. Brown WA, Laughren TP: Tolerance to the prolactin-elevating effect of neuroleptics. *Psychiatry Res* 1981;5:317–322.

CHAPTER 9

DRUG TREATMENT OF ACUTE SCHIZOPHRENIA

SAMUEL G. SIRIS
ARTHUR RIFKIN

The advent of effective psychopharmacologic treatment for psychoses in the 1950s triggered the most enormous revolution in the management of psychotic patients since Pinel. Before these drugs were introduced, the chronically hospitalized population in the United States, for example, was approaching 600,000. By the 1980s this figure is closer to 150,000—despite an increase in overall population.

In addition to the very obvious issues of patient care, the revolution spawned by pharmacotherapy has had numerous ramifications in the scientific understanding of psychoses. Drug responsiveness has become a tool in the teasing apart of syndromes of affective and schizophrenic psychosis. To be sure, there would be many logical and practical shortcomings to using the results of pharmacological treatment as a sole criterion for a diagnostic nosology, and these data certainly must be integrated with phenomenological, genetic, biochemical, physiological, epidemiological, and other information for the proper categorization of disease. On the other hand, treatment response, particularly relatively acute treatment response, has become not only a diagnostic validator of great utility, but also a most potent impetus to further diagnostic clarifications—since a variety of specific potent interventions is now at our disposal.

This chapter will be a clinically based formulation of acute drug treatment in schizophrenia. Discussion of the biological bases of acute schizophrenic psychoses, with which this treatment chapter interdigitates, may be found elsewhere in this volume.

PSYCHOTIC DECOMPENSATION IN SCHIZOPHRENIA

Most descriptions of drug use in schizophrenia and well-designed studies of medication efficacy approach psychosis as a unitary phenomenon: either the patient is psychotically decompensated or the patient is not, and the research documenting the substantial efficacy of antipsychotic medication is generally based on patients who are quite grossly disorganized. Clinically, of course, the phenomenology of psychosis is not dichotomous in this way. Psychotic decompensation is a process of shifting and progressively less adaptive mental equilibrium. Whether this process is continuous or discontinuous and whether the observed clinical changes precede, follow, or occur simultaneously with biologically observed manifestations of illness await future clarification. In practice, however, these issues are crucial. Presumably (and this is admittedly an assumption, but one that seems eminently reasonable and is consistent with clinical experience), the sooner we intercede and begin treatment during the course of a psychotic decompensation, the better our chances of success and the less morbidity will be suffered by the patient, his family, and his community. But how soon can the clinician know, with confidence, that an episode of psychosis is occurring? This can be a very sophisticated judgment, at times confounding the most astute clinician. No doubt the patient's past history can be an invaluable clue in this regard. Take, for example, the patient who on four separate occasions has begun to suspect, and then be obsessed with, the idea that his father is having an affair a week before a florid decompensation. When these thoughts begin to occur again, one can presume that another psychotic episode has begun to unfold and act accordingly with appropriate interventions. Although such a clear-cut prodrome is often not apparent, a general understanding of the phenomenology of decompensation is of considerable value to the clinician – and can be quite helpful to insightful patients as well in the ongoing management of their disorders.

In their review of the literature, Docherty et al[1] discerned several more or less distinct and identifiable "stages" in psychotic disorganization.

The first of these is the stage of "overextension." During this stage the patient subjectively feels pushed beyond his capacity to cope. He may feel overwhelmed or feel that he has to "run faster just to stay in the same place." Indeed, the patient may be speeded up, and it may be unclear, in this as in all stages, which effects are primary and which effects are secondary attempts at compensation or at explaining away biologically determined phenomena in an attempt to retain the reassuring subjective sense of mastery. In this stage, the patient is often anxious, irritable and/or distractible. Relationships and productivity begin to suffer. The patient's habitual methods of managing stresses and anxiety may begin to fail, and the patient begins to adopt less familiar and frequently less satisfactory modes of coping. Those who know the patient may report a "change of personality" at this stage.

The change in personality may become even more noticeable in the next stage. This is the stage of "restricted consciousness." In this stage the patient dramatically reduces his range of thought – attempting to maintain compensation through a narrowing of his attention to a restricted focus which is still within his capacity to manage. Obsessive preoccupations may appear or become more intense and tightly held. Avoidances, including phobically justified avoidances, occur as the patient becomes more and more withdrawn. For those patients with good social contacts, their friends may say "I just can't seem to reach him anymore," although the patient himself may speak of loneliness and dependency. Subjective feelings of depression are common at this stage, in conjunction with the self-centered concerns which so often accompany this type of dysphoria. The self-centered dysphorias of boredom, hypochondriasis, and somatization are also frequently seen at this stage—all restricting the field of awareness and limiting the range of issues with which the individual is willing to cope. Naturally, this circumstance very often leads to an accelerating deterioration of the patient's situation unless the patient's environment has made supportive adjustments. And often, despite such adjustments, the deterioration proceeds anyway.

The next state is "disinhibition." Impulses begin to emerge unchecked by the usual constraints of the patient's personality. These include aggressive impulses which may lead to arguments, fights, reckless driving, sexual impulses that may lead to promiscuity or exhibiting, and more general manifestations of disinhibition such as loudness, overeating or overdrinking, drug abuse, and risk taking. (Obviously the downhill slope for the patient now becomes more and more slippery.) At this point various dissociative phenomena may appear, and material which the patient ordinarily holds out of his awareness may intrude on his conscious mental life. Mood swings become less well modulated, less appropriate to the situational context, and less well integrated.

These phenomena run over into the next stage of decompensation, which is "psychotic disorganization." At this point the capacity for Aristotelian logic may degenerate, leading to grossly impaired judgment and illogicality. Linguistic functions may become impaired, leading to a disruption in the fundamental semantic connectedness of language (ie, thought disorder). Additionally, the patient often loses the fundamental exercise of the boundary sense of where his self ends and the outside world begins. Thus, internal fantasies may be misperceived as external realities (ie, delusions and notions of thought broadcast) or perceptions (ie, hallucinations). In the other direction, segments of mental content may seem as if they originated external to the person (ie, thought insertion and/or delusions of passivity and being controlled).

Finally, a stage of "psychotic resolution" may be attained. Although generally quite maladaptive, this stage is more stable than that of "psychotic disorganization." Here, psychotic phenomena become more fixed and organized. Delusions may become systematized, and patterns of behavior are developed which may tend to reify perceptions that were disjointed and unsupported at the previous stage. Anxiety may be reduced in this stage, but efforts to disrupt the psychotic equilibrium may be greeted with the most intense modes of refusal. In many ways, this final stage confirms the notion of a dissociation of activation and disorganization in the schizophrenic psychotic process—a dissociation which may ultimately be found to have a meaningful implication for understanding pathophysiology and treatment.[2]

It is important to bear these stages of decompensation, and the concept of these stages, in mind during the pharmacologic considerations that follow, since so much of what we currently know has been validated entirely with patients in the final two stages of decompensation (psychotic disorganization and psychotic resolution). This is a necessity, of course, because it is only among patients who are substantially psychotic that the diagnosis of schizophrenia can be made with reliability and confidence. However, it is also our clinical impression, among patients whose schizophrenic diagnosis has been established during a previous psychotic episode, that early intervention with neuroleptic medication during prepsychotic stages of decompensation may "nip an episode in the bud," reducing both its severity and its duration. It is also an unproven clinical impression that early intervention may reduce the overall dosage requirement of neuroleptic. Certainly, then, astute clinical judgment is vitally important to differentiate minor and insignificant perturbations in a fundamentally stable clinical course from the early stages of a true psychotic decompensation.

THE CHOICE OF A NEUROLEPTIC

Antipsychotic efficacy is not a factor in the choice of a neuroleptic agent. With the exception of promazine, which may be less efficacious, but is generally no longer used, all neuroleptics are equivalent in their capacity to interrupt the schizophrenic psychosis,[3] and none has been found to have specific advantages over others in the various schizophrenic syndromes which have so far been described.[4] This does not mean, however, that there may not be idiosyncratic differences between drugs in terms of an individual patient's responsiveness. This is not infrequently observed to be the case,[5] and a schizophrenic patient who fails to respond to the first chosen neuroleptic agent after a trial of adequate dosage for adequate duration merits a course of a second antipsychotic drug—generally chosen from another class. At times, a third or fourth neuroleptic drug may be tried. There is no general rationale, however, for combining two or more different antipsychotics. There is no evidence that antipsychotic effects are any more additive under this circumstance than would be the case with an equipotent dosage of a single neuroleptic, and multiplying drugs can lead to more compliance problems, more mistakes with dosage, more chance for side effects, and more general confusion about what is due to what in the patient's treatment. On the other hand, it is generally very appropriate to select an antipsychotic drug to which the patient has responded well in the past, since such patients have frequently been observed to respond well to the same agent upon subsequent administration.[6]

Potency, or relative strength of the medication per milligram, of course, is a separate consideration than efficacy, the therapeutic usefulness of the drug when used at its own optimal dose. Neuroleptic drugs vary considerably in potency, and the dose prescribed should reflect the potency of the particular agent chosen. As a guideline, the relative potencies of commonly used neuroleptics are shown in Table 9-1.[7,8] There is, approximately, a 50-fold range of potency among the commonly used neuroleptic drugs, from chlorpromazine, chlorprothixine, and thioridazine on the lower end to fluphenazine and haloperidol on the upper end.

The main differences among the neuroleptics which create differential considerations for their choice in treatment concern their side effects. Here there are important differences between the low-potency antipsychotic drugs (principally chlorpromazine and thioridazine) and the other

Table 9-1
Equipotent Doses of Neuroleptic Drugs

Generic Name	Brand Name(s)	Equipotent Dose*
Chlorpromazine	Thorazine	100 mg PO
Chlorprothixene	Taractan	100 mg PO
Thioridazine	Mellaril	100 mg PO
Mesoridazine	Serentil	50 mg PO
Carphenazine	Proketazine	25 mg PO
Triflupromazine	Vesprin	25 mg PO
Acetophenazine	Tindal	20 mg PO
Prochlorperazine	Compazine	15 mg PO
Butaperazine	Repoise	10 mg PO
Loxapine	Loxitane	10 mg PO
Molindone	Lidone	10 mg PO
	Moban	10 mg PO
Piperacetazine	Quide	10 mg PO
Perphenazine	Trilafon	8 mg PO
Trifluoperazine	Stelazine	5 mg PO
Thiothixine	Navane	4 mg PO
Haloperidol	Haldol	2 mg PO
Fluphenazine	Permitil	2 mg PO
	Prolixin	2 mg PO
Fluphenazine—Depot	Prolixin Enanthate	1/15 cc IM every 2 weeks
	Prolixin Decanoate	1/15 cc IM every 2 weeks

*PO, oral; IM, intramuscular.

more high-potency compounds. The low-potency neuroleptics tend to result in much more sedation and autonomic side effects, such as orthostatic hypotension, blurry vision, dry mouth, constipation, and propensity for urinary retention. These side effects may be particularly problematic in outpatients (ie, in patients being managed acutely without hospitalization or in patients discharged from the hospital), because these patients are not then under close medical supervision. Lack of continuous medical supervision increases the risk of urine retention or severe constipation, leading to medical complications. Additionally, side effects which patients find bothersome predispose to drug noncompliance. Away from close medical supervision, medication noncompliance is perhaps the leading cause of apparent lack of drug responsiveness. Another feature which must not be overlooked is that sedation, blurry vision, and orthostatic hypotension may present much greater risks to patients who are away from the more protected hospital setting and who are climbing stairs, driving cars, or operating machinery.

The side effect of orthostatic hypotension is most likely due to a blockade of peripheral alpha-adrenergic receptors. Chlorpromazine is most active in this blockade and results in the greatest degree of orthostatic hypotension. Thioridazine leads to less, but still substantial, hypotension. The side effect of sedation is probably due to central alpha-adrenergic blockade. Again, chlorpromazine has the greatest degree of sedative side effects, and thioridazine is the second most sedating neuroleptic. Dry mouth, blurry vision, constipation, and urine retention, on the other hand, are the result of the drugs' peripheral anticholinergic spectrum of activity. In terms of these latter effects, thioridazine is most potent and chlorpromazine is second to that. In terms of both of these two families of side effects, haloperidol and fluphenazine, the most potent of the high-potency neuroleptics, are the least likely to lead to noticeable clinical effects.

Certainly, the patient's overall medical condition must also be taken into account with the choice of a neuroleptic. A patient with coronary artery disease or cerebrovascular disease has extra reasons to avoid drugs that could lead to orthostatic hypotension. Other medications which the patient is taking, also, could reinforce or add to these effects on a pharmacokinetic or a pharmacodynamic basis. Older patients are also at greater risk vis-à-vis the autonomic side effects of antipsychotic drugs, since they tend to have less functional compensatory reserve in general and since, specifically with regard to the issues of orthostatic hypotension, falling, and injury, older people tend to break when they fall rather than bounce, as younger people might.

On the other hand, the sedative properties of the low-potency phenothiazines may be an advantage in certain situations. Highly overactive patients may be slowed down by these nonspecific effects, and particularly patients with problematic insomnia may be benefited. It is true that even high-potency neuroleptics have some soporific qualities, which may be adequate to the task in less extreme cases, and that the same effects of low-potency phenothiazines can be gained by the combined use of a sedative agent with a high-potency neuroleptic. But the use of a low-potency antipsychotic instead reduces polypharmacy and diminishes the need for other agents that can be habituating. Under these circumstances, it is convenient that the entire daily neuroleptic regimen can be administered as a bedtime dose. This is because the half-life of the medication and its effects are sufficiently long that multiple daily dosages are not required. Still in all, the sedative effects of the medication, as well as some of the other effects that may be bothersome during waking hours, are concentrated during the six to eight hours after drug ingestion. Nevertheless, lethargy and fatigue during the day often result more from the low-potency drugs, even in those patients who do not complain of manifest drowsiness. Furthermore, the use of thioridazine in doses greater than 800 mg/day is inadvisable due to the risk of a pigmentary retinopathy.[9]

There is also variability in the form of common extrapyramidal side effects between the low- and high-potency neuroleptics. The use of chlorpromazine is frequently associated with the occurrence of akinesia, tremor, and parkinsonian rigidity. Thioridazine, however, although fairly sedating, tends to be associated with fewer extrapyramidal side effects—presumably because it has such strong anticholinergic properties that these effects may be blocked.

High-potency neuroleptics more frequently lead to dystonias, especially among younger men, and akathisia as extrapyramidal side effects. Acute dystonias and akathisia are particularly disturbing side effects to patients. Dystonias, with their abrupt onset and peculiar or disfiguring contortions become emergencies to patients and their families, who may rush to an emergency room in great distress and then mistrust their doctor or medication in general on the basis of this bad experience. This occurrence can be softened or avoided by beginning patients on anticholinergic antiparkinsonian medication prophylactically, especially when high-potency neuroleptics are used, and by warning patients, in a non-threatening way, that occasionally people develop stiff neck muscles with these drugs. They should further be told that if this happens, not to be alarmed—if they come to the office, or to an emergency room, another medication can be given (a parenteral anticholinergic, such as benztropine or diphenhydramine) which will rapidly relieve these symptoms.

Akathisia, at times, can be a difficult side effect because it can superficially resemble psychotic agitation. This is particularly so if an otherwise psychotic patient describes his subjective experience of the akathisia as being one in which he is being controlled by an outside force. The danger here is that if the akathisia is mistaken as psychosis, the makings of a vicious circle are present, with increased doses of drugs then being used to treat a condition that has been caused by the drug in the first place. This mistake can be avoided by a careful appraisal of the agitation. Most patients can distinguish the sensation of akathisia as being distinctly physical if a proper inquiry is made for this. Concomitantly, the clinician will note that, with akathisia, the positive symptoms of psychosis are not exacerbated. Although the patient may be pacing around, and be rationalizing this pacing, the general basic sense is that the moving about, or constant urge to move about, is ego dystonic. The patient does not want to be moving restlessly. Rather, it is something uncomfortable which is happening to him. Often, but not always, akathisia will abate with the use of anticholinergic antiparkinsonian agents. When these are ineffective, lowering the neuroleptic dose can be attempted. Above all, recognizing the side effect of akathisia is crucial because the experience of it is extremely disagreeable to the patient and its existence is just the sort of occurrence that can preclude the development of trust and lead to the patient abruptly discontinuing needed antipsychotic medication as soon as he gets away from constant direct supervision.

A final extrapyramidal side effect that can all too easily escape detection is akinesia.[10–12] Akinesia is an insidious extrapyramidal reaction that can resemble anergia, anhedonia, lack of motivation, withdrawal, or demoralization. Hence, it can be very easy to confuse clinically with either postpsychotic depression[13,14] or the so-called negative symptoms of schizophrenia. The patient with akinesia typically sits around "like a bump on a log." The patient may either take to bed or simply sit quietly uninvolved in activity without interest or engagement. There is a lack of spontaneity in speech and gesture; on questioning, most often, the patient will report a subjective sense of drowsiness. Motor slowness may be easily confused with psychomotor retardation, and the patient may accurately report that his existence is generally pleasureless. Confirmation that this state was akinesia occurs when the patient's clinical state rapidly changes with the institution of anticholinergic antiparkinsonian medication. Within a day or two the patient "wakes up," feels more alive, and becomes spontaneous and involved. Unlike other extrapyramidal side effects that have more obvious motor manifestations and are somewhat less likely to occur after a patient has received medication for a substantial time, akinesia may occur at any time and develop gradually and nondramatically, so as not to be noticed. It therefore is a prime reason for the continuation of antiparkinsonian drug treatment past the acute stages of treatment and indefinitely into the maintenance phase.

An additional potential neurological complication of neuroleptic medication is increased risk of epileptic seizures. Seizures have been reported in conjunction with a variety of neuroleptics, most frequently in patients with organic abnormalities,[15] and the issue of which antipsychotic medication might be least likely to predispose to seizures is still unresolved. A relatively low incidence of seizures was reported in epileptics who were treated by thioridazine, so that may be a drug of choice in this situation.[16] However, an in vitro technique involving guinea pig hippocampal slices has more recently suggested that molindone may be the most advantageous neuroleptic to use when there is a risk of seizure.[17] In that study, molindone may actually have reduced neuronal excitability, whereas almost all other neuroleptics increased it to a greater or lesser extent. Also of interest was the observation that the greatest excitability induced by chlorpromazine and thioridazine occurred at relatively low concentrations, probably less than therapeutic tissue level concentrations, with the implication that the greatest risk for seizure with these drugs may occur when treatment is just beginning or when the drug is being discontinued—although no incidence of seizures on this latter occasion has been clinically reported. In all cases, the increased electrical excitability resulting from the introduction of neuroleptics was removed by benzodiazepines in the in vitro preparation.

Molindone has also been reported to be unique, as well, in the area of weight gain. Whereas a number of patients are plagued by the side effect of weight gain (not just fluid, but flesh) when undergoing treatment with neuroleptics, this has not been observed to be the case with molindone,[18-20] so this drug may be particularly indicated in those schizophrenic patients prone to corpulence.

STRATEGIES OF DOSAGE

As was the case with the choice of drug, the best initial choice for dose is the dose of that drug which led to that patient's getting better from a previous similar episode of illness. If historical precedent is not available as a guide, the general norm is that acutely psychotic patients will generally respond to a neuroleptic regimen in the dosage range of 400–1200 mg of oral chlorpromazine per day or its equivalent.[4,21]

Within this range, and even in cases outside it, the dosage must be individualized, because patients will vary widely in terms of their tolerance of various side effects and in terms of pharmacokinetic factors. In this latter regard, what the body does to the drug can become just as much an issue in treatment as what the drug does to the body. Even assuming that willful noncompliance is not an issue (which it certainly may well be, unless the patient is under close medical supervision), somatic compliance is always a factor in dosing. Oral medications, the most common form of dosing, in particular, have a torturous obstacle course to run before arriving at their locus of action. Once swallowed, they first pass into the acid environs of the stomach, where neuroleptics are gradually broken down. Some stomachs are considerably more acid, of course, than others, and gastric emptying times also vary considerably. Concomitant medications may play a role here as well. For example, anticholinergic agents delay gastric emptying. Simultaneous administration of an anticholinergic agent is not harmful, but it could result in the delivery of a smaller amount of neuroleptic to the intestine and a delay in this delivery in acute treatment.[22] This effect of an antiparkinsonian agent has been reported to be substantial.[22,23] However, a well-designed, double-blind crossover study by Simpson and colleagues has more recently clearly refuted the concept that contemporaneous oral administration of antiparkinsonian medication and a neuroleptic lowers the blood level of neuroleptic, at least in the case of chlorpromazine and trihexyphenidyl.[24] Two earlier reports had also failed to find this effect with benztropine and either butaperazine or perphenazine.[25,26] So the best assumption, currently, is that coadministration of an anticholinergic probably does not interfere with neuroleptic absorption in most patients.

The same consideration with regard to delayed gastric emptying may be at play with antispasmodics and sympathomimetic compounds[27] and may also occur with lithium coadministration,[28] although with lithium a mechanism other than anticholinergic activity is involved. Also in the stomach, colloidal antacids such as aluminum hydroxide gel may absorb neuroleptics, so that they become unavailable to the body.[29] The same unavailability through physical absorption can also occur with cholestyramine and kaolin-containing products.[27]

Once the neuroleptics get into the small intestine, absorption can begin, but enzymes in the gut wall can break them down. Similarly, all the portal circulation passes to the liver, where the "first pass" effect takes place. The liver is the locus of metabolic breakdown for neuroleptic drugs, and the oral route of administration requires that they must pass through the liver first before attaining the general circulation. Liver disease may influence neuroleptic metabolism, although the cytochrome P450 system, which is the metabolizing agent involved, is present in diseased as well as healthy liver. Probably considerable liver disease is necessary to lead to any meaningful impairment in neuroleptic metabolism, but exact relationships in this regard have not been worked out and it is possible that idiosyncratic situations may exist. What is clear is that, considering the "first pass" effect, orally administered medications would be more influenced by variations in liver physiology than parenterally administered compounds. With oral compounds, an overactive liver not only is more rapid in eliminating drugs from the general circulation, but also renders the effective dose reaching the general circulation smaller. For an underactive or impaired liver, of course, the effects would be the opposite. More frequent than liver disease is the influence on hepatic metabolism caused by the induction of liver enzymes through previous exposure to drugs and other substances. Barbiturates are probably the most famous nonspecific enzyme inducers, but it should be remembered that a number of substances, including nicotine from cigarettes, can serve this function. On the other hand, certain other coadministered drugs, such as tricyclic antidepressants, can effectively compete for the same enzyme system and slow neuroleptic metabolism.[30] Allowing for substantial variability due to these above-stated factors, a fair first approximation is that the equivalent parenteral dose of a neuroleptic is half of the oral dose.

Once in the general circulation, neuroleptics exist in an equilibrium of drug bound to plasma protein and unbound. Typically, 95% to 98% of the drug is bound, so that minor shifts of pH or other factors affecting plasma binding can result in disproportionate changes in the absolute amount of unbound drug present. This can be quite important, since it is only the unbound drug that is available to cross the blood-brain barrier and exert the antipsychotic effects. Hypoalbuminemia, or for that matter variations in the concentration of plasma proteins within the normal range, can also influence the ratio of bound to unbound drug. This important issue has been generally overlooked in studies of the relationship of plasma drug level to efficacy (see below).

In addition to the interindividual variabilities which probably exist in the permeability of the blood-brain barrier to antipsychotic drugs and in the modes of transit they must still then make to their putative loci of action within certain crucial dopaminergic synapses, the body variably offers different places for these drugs to go as well. Much of the neuroleptic drug gets tied up in other body spaces such as adipose stores and never gets into the brain at all. Hepatic metabolism contributes more variability than habitus and overall body mass, but these factors contribute to variability in drug dosage requirements as well.

So, with all of the above provisos, we generally look for the equivalent of 400–1200 mg of oral chlorpromazine per day for the treatment of the acute psychosis in schizophrenia. The question had been raised as to whether heroic doses of neuroleptics, administered acutely, might foreshorten a psychotic episode and bring about a more rapid control of symptoms. Indeed, some early open noncontrolled trials had seemed to support such a notion.[31–34] A tabulation of the more recent double-blind controlled studies, investigating the question of high acute doses in acute rather than chronic patients, is shown in Table 9-2.

As is seen in Table 9-2, there have been eight double-blind studies in acute patients in which two or more doses of the same neuroleptic were compared. All of these studies involved high-potency neuroleptics, and in five of the eight cases, that neuroleptic was haloperidol. In only one of these studies[35] was a small dose of neuroleptic employed as the lower dose which would be below the recommended initial dosage range. That

Table 9-2
Double-Blind, Controlled Studies of Acute Treatment with High-Dose Neuroleptics*

Study	Patients	Lower Dose	Higher Dose	Duration	Result and Comment
Reschke, 1974[35]	N=50 "Schizophrenics" Acutely ill hospital admissions with severe agitation or assaultiveness	CPZ 25 mg IM HPD 1 mg IM PBO Injections every 30 minutes until remission or total of four injections	HPD 2 mg IM HPD 5 mg IM	2 hours Plus later follow-up on open oral medication	2- and 5-mg doses of HPD showed significantly more improvement
Anderson et al, 1976[37]	N=19 8 were schizophrenic, the rest manic by RDC	HPD 5 mg IM each hour until remission or 15 mg; X=13 mg IM	HPD 5 mg IM, then 10 mg IM each 30 minutes until remission or 55 mg; X=33 mg IM	3 hours	No significant differences between groups in symptoms or side-effects; 11 patients had marked improvement
Ericksen et al, 1978[38]	N=42 Acutely decompensated "schizophrenic" patients	HPD 15 mg PO per day	HPD 60 mg IM per day for 5 days, then 45 mg/day tapering to 15 mg/day	18 days	No difference between groups for treatment effects; more side effects in high-dose group.
Donlon et al, 1980[39]	N=63 Acutely ill, newly admitted schizophrenics	HPD 10 mg PO per day	HPD 20 mg PO on day 1 increasing to 100 mg PO on day 5; (X=90 mg/day)	10 days	All 3 treatment groups had similar therapeutic efficacy, similar cognitive improvements, and similar side effects
and			or		
Wahba et al, 1981[40]	(criteria given)		HPD 10 mg PO on day 1 increasing to 100 mg PO on day 10; (X=77 mg/day)		

Neborsky et al, 1981[41]	N=20 Men with acute psychotic symptomatology	HPD 2 mg IM each hour up to 4 hours	HPD 10 mg IM each hour up to 4 hours	7 days	No difference between groups in improvement; both groups improved substantially, mostly in initial period
		until oral compliance possible			
	(criteria given)	then			
	19 were schizophrenic or schizo-affective	2 mg HPD PO	10 mg HPD PO		No differential in side effects between the two groups
		As often as once an hour until previously defined target item improved satisfactorily; then that amount of HPD was repeated each day for the next 6 days			
		X=10 mg for initial period	X=41 mg for initial period		
		X=12.5 mg/day subsequently	X=48 mg/day subsequently		
Wijsenbeek et al, 1974[42]	N=26 "schizophrenics" newly admitted with acutely psychotic paranoid symptoms	TFP 60 mg PO per day	TFP 600 mg PO per day	6 weeks	No meaningful differences between groups on clinical effects or side effects, except that patients with severe conceptual disorganization improved more on that parameter with low doses
Donlon et al, 1978[43]	N=32 acutely decompensated hospitalized schizophrenic patients (criteria given)	FLU 20 mg PO per day	FLU 80 mg PO per day	1 week	No between group differences on improvement or side effects

Table 9-2 (continued)

Study	Patients	Lower Dose	Higher Dose	Duration	Result and Comment
Escobar et al, 1982[44]	N=14 acutely ill schizophrenics (N=13) or schizo-affective patients by DSM-III	FLU 2.5 mg PO three times daily X=5.7 mg/day	FLU 5 mg IM each hour for 6 hours; (X=5.2 injections), then equal number of 5-mg pills PO in next 6 hours	24 hours blind Rating to 1 week	No meaningful differences between groups in clinical improvement; at 24 hours only, high-dose group had statistically significantly more EPS
		Then open FLU 10 mg/day increasing to 35 mg PO per day over one week			
Man and Chen, 1973[50]	N=30 Acutely disturbed psychotic patients	CPZ 50 mg IM	HPO 5 mg IM	0.5 up to 7.5 hours X=2.5 hours	Antipsychotic results of the two treatments were similar: marked or moderate response in 14/15 HPD patients and 11/13 CPZ patients;
		Up to 7 injections at 30-min intervals, or until patient was no longer assaultive or manic, or until it was clear there would be no further benefit (most patients received 2 or 3 injections)			two CPZ patients developed severe hypotension and one CPZ patient developed status epilepticus; Therefore, it was concluded that HPD was safer.
Gerstenzang and Krulisky, 1977[51]	N=58 Patients brought to emergency room with disruptive behavior; half were "apparently schizophrenic"	CPZ 50 mg IM (N=28)	HPD 5 mg IM (N=30)	30–60 min following a single injection	Half the HPD patients became calm, cooperative and alert; another 8 improved; only 3 CPZ patients were successfully controlled and 11 were partly controlled; covariant analysis favored HPD for conceptual disorganization, tension, hostility, uncooperativeness, and excitement; no adverse reactions noted

Levenson et al 1976[52]	N=12 Schizophrenic by RDC	HPD 2.5 mg IM per day FLU 2.5 mg IM per day TTX 5 mg IM per day All doses tripled by day 4, then maintained		21 days	No statistically significant differences between drugs, though sample size is small and chance of type II error is large; drugs were used in equipotent doses; rapid response rate was high
Stotsky, 1977[53]	N=30 Acutely excited, agitated psychotic patients 24 "schizophrenics," 4 "psychotic depressions," 2 "manics"	TTX 4 or 8 mg IM each hour, prn for 4 hours (X=10.1 mg)	HPD 4 or 8 mg IM each hour, prn for 4 hours (X=15 mg)	6 hours	Groups did not improve differentially over time, although both groups improved significantly; no statistically significant differences in side effects
Paprocki and Versiani, 1977[54]	N=35 Acutely and severely ill newly hospitalized "schizophrenic" women	HPD 8.8–12.5 mg IM per day (X=11.5 mg) (N=18)	LOX 87.5–125 mg IM per day (X=115 mg) (N=17)	4 days	Similar results; in analysis of covariance LOX showed some superiority in agitated behaviors; subsequent improvement on oral medication was equivalent between groups; adverse effects were similar between groups
Lerner et al, 1979[36]	N=40 Newly admitted psychotic patients 14 "schizophrenic" 9 "schizo-affective" 5 "manic" 2 "paranoid state"	Diazepam 30–40 mg IV over 3 hours	HPD 20–35 mg IV over 3 hours	24 hours	Definite improvement occurred in both groups, but no statistically significant group differences

*Abbreviations: CPZ, chlorpromazine; EPS, extrapyramidal symptoms; FLU, fluphenazine; HPD, haloperidol; LOX, loxitane; PBO, placebo; RDC, Research Diagnostic Criteria[35]; TFP, trifluoperazine; TTX, thiothixine; IM, intramuscular; PO, oral.

was also the only study to employ a placebo group. Other studies found patients to be generally improved by the treatments provided, but Reschke, with the use of the placebo group, presents conclusive evidence that this improvement was on the basis of a pharmacological effect, rather than a nonspecific acute situational factor, such as all the attention that was paid to patients by virtue of being in such a protocol.[35] The utility of neuroleptics in reducing psychotic symptoms has been established beyond doubt over longer periods, such as days and weeks, but acute effects over hours remain in some degree of doubt with regard to their specific antipsychotic nature.[36]

The other comparative studies of a "standard" versus a "high" loading dose of neuroleptic found no advantage to megadose in acutely psychotic patients when a substantial dose, either oral or parenteral, was used as the standard.[37–44] Although specific diagnostic criteria were not stated for all of the studies, and affectively ill patients were definitely included in some trials, the results of these varied studies are sufficiently similar that the issue in acute treatment is fairly well established. (Megadose, on the other hand, may have a role in chronic refractory patients,[45–48] but a discussion of that aspect of treatment goes beyond the scope of this chapter.)

A further item of interest observable in the studies cited in Table 9-2 is that, in most, no difference was observed in side effects between the standard and the high dose. In only two of the eight studies that were straight dosage comparisons did side effects appear to be greater in the high-dose group. As a whole, this group of studies would stand to confirm the safety, if not the efficacy, of high doses of high-potency neuroleptics, a safety that received further testament in the open trial conducted by Quitkin et al[49] in which patients received oral fluphenazine in doses up to 1200 mg per day without apparent adverse effect.

The final six studies listed in Table 9-2 involve double-blind comparisons of different agents, often at megadose, in the acute treatment of schizophrenia.[36,50–54] No therapeutic differences were apparent between the high-potency neuroleptics tested in these trials. The low-potency phenothiazine chlorpromazine, however, did produce problematic side effects when an attempt was made by Man and Chen to utilize it in the megadose situation.[50] Among 15 patients treated with 50-mg intramuscular injections of chlorpromazine, at half-hour intervals for up to seven injections, two patients suffered severe hypotension and one developed status epilepticus. No such complications arose in comparable patients treated with intramuscular haloperidol, and it was concluded that chlorpromazine might be a less safe drug to give in this manner. Additionally, the one study that suggested a difference in efficacy between neuroleptics[51] found that the patients acutely treated with 50 mg of chlorpromazine intramuscularly did not seem to do as well as patients treated with 5 mg of haloperidol intramuscularly. In this study, of course, the drug comparison is also confounded by the fact that the doses employed were not equipotent and that the chlorpromazine dose (even allowing for the approximately 2:1 advantage which arises from parenteral as opposed to oral administration) falls short of the 400–1200 mg per day range considered to be necessary for acute treatment.

The last study listed on Table 9-2, that of Lerner et al,[36] raises an interesting issue about which debate has not yet concluded. This is the only study that does not compare two neuroleptic regimens, but rather acutely compares haloperidol with high intravenous doses of a minor tranquilizer, diazepam. Diazepam, of course, is not an antipsychotic agent or used for the acute treatment of schizophrenia (although the possibility does exist that, in high doses, benzodiazepines may have antipsychotic properties—see section on nonstandard treatments, below). The point of this study, though, was to test the notion that very rapid improvements seen during the first day or so with acute administration of high doses of neuroleptic may not really be the result of specific antipsychotic effects, but might rather be the result of the nonspecific sedation which results, even with high-potency neuroleptics, with these acute high doses. Lerner et al contend that their finding a lack of statistical significance in the outcome of their two treatment groups supports this hypothesis. It must also be noted, however, that their global rating measure, although not statistically significant, favored haloperidol after 24 hours with $P=0.12$, two tailed (equivalent to trend-level significance one tailed), and their modest sample size (20 patients in each group) leaves ample room for a type II error in this case. Furthermore, data were available for only half the patients at the four-hour rating point—presumably due to the degree of sedation. It may be hard for a patient to manifest psychosis, or to have it rated, if he or she is asleep or nearly so. Nevertheless, their point is well taken about the sedative properties of neuroleptic "loading," and a number of authors agree that there may indeed, therefore, be a role for rapid administration of larger than usual doses of neuroleptics in acutely agitated, belligerent, or destructive schizophrenic patients whose behavior is a danger to themselves or others. In such a situation, it is advisable to choose a high-potency neuroleptic and to administer it intramuscularly for the most rapid onset of action. The rapid onset of action will not only quiet the patient most quickly, but will protect the patient from the risks of needing to make the next (oral) dosing decision before the effect of the previous dose has become fully manifest.

Patients may be built up to their maximum neuroleptic dosage (equivalent of 400–1200 mg of chlorpromazine per day) over just a few days to a week. Again, side effects and clinical factors provide the guidelines. Sedation, hypotension, or severe anticholinergic effects will limit the increments and ceiling dose, particularly with the low-potency neuroleptics, although sedation not infrequently occurs as well with high-potency antipsychotics, more often in the higher dosage ranges. Clinical factors of assaultiveness, belligerence, or self-destructive behavior suggest maximizing the dose, even if this may be benefiting the patient only through the nonspecific sedative actions of the drugs. High doses are maintained for the length of time it takes to control the acute psychotic symptomatology. Although the interval involved may well be shorter, often six to eight weeks is required to quell the acute psychosis in schizophrenia. By this time it is expected that 95% of patients will show some signs of improvement,[55] and more than half will have improved moderately or markedly.[56]

In some patients, clinical response to the neuroleptic is associated temporally with an increase in side effects. It is as if, clinically at least, the patient has become less tolerant to the effects of the medication. The observer may get the impression that after having "soaked up" the medication for a while, with precious little evidence that it was having any effect at all, patients then suddenly appear to be "snowed by it." This was a clinical observation which had led to studies (Table 9-2) of the possibility that rapid "neuroleptization" might help psychiatric patients much as digitalization has been used for cardiac patients. Those studies, of course, showed rapid neuroleptization with high doses to be of no special benefit to acute schizophrenic patients beyond that provided by rapid administration of standard doses. Nevertheless, when patients respond in terms of positive psychotic symptoms and then appear to become "snowed," it is a signal to begin gradually reducing the dose. Ten percent dose reduction per day is a conservative pace if side effects are not severe. More rapid reduction may be required in cases of more extreme adverse effects. It should be borne in mind that steady state is not attained pharmacokinetically for four to seven days at a given dose. Thus, even though a recently increased dose is being held steady, the amount of medication in a patient's system is increasing over that length of time. By the same token, with a newly lowered dose, the amount of available medication is decreasing for the same interval. During the decreasing dosage phase, the patient should be carefully observed for the reemergence of psychotic symptoms on his way to a maintenance dose. The progression of phenomena outlined above under the rubic stages of psychotic decompensation may be helpful; in particular, the inability to sleep properly may be an important danger sign.

Needless to say, in light of the long-term danger of tardive dyskinesia, the maintenance medication dose should be adjusted to the lowest level at which the remission can be continued. This topic is further discussed in the chapter concerning the long-term drug treatment of schizophrenia.

There are no particular advantages to the use of divided doses in neuroleptic administration. As noted above, the half-lives of antipsychotic drugs are sufficiently long that a substantial fraction of the initial dose will still be circulating in the patient's blood stream 24 hours after a daily dose, and there is no evidence of any diurnal antipsychotic decrement in patients who have been managed in this way. In fact, efficacy has been reported to be superior for a single daily dose than for the same daily dose administered in a divided way two, three, or four times per day.[57] It is not entirely clear why that would be the case, although it is possible that when these drugs are administered in a single large oral bolus that a greater percentage of the compound is able to escape degradation in the gut wall and/or liver and thus survive these "first pass" effects.

Fortunately, on the other hand, a number of neuroleptic side effects may not last for more than a few hours after oral dosage. Sedation side effects fall into this category and clearly taper off after several hours, whereas the antipsychotic effects do not. Obviously, this factor can be of positive advantage in promoting sleep when medication is administered in a single nighttime dose. But even for patients who have no trouble with insomnia, it is an advantage for the soporific effect of medication to play itself out while the patient is asleep anyway. The same can be said about dry mouth, which will go unnoticed during sleep, and certainly blurry vision is minimized as a problem when the eyes are shut. There is even some evidence that administration by a single nighttime dose results in fewer extrapyramidal side effects than do other dosage schedules.[58] Recumbency is also a benefit during hours when a patient would be most prone to orthostatic hypotension – although a caveat should be observed here: should the patient arise at night, there might be an increased risk for dizziness or falling, especially in a groggy state in the dark, and the patient should be specifically warned about this. Here, of course, the same conservative countermeasures can be applied as would be used in any patient with orthostatic hypotension: advise the patient to "dangle" his legs, sitting on the side of the bed for several minutes before arising, not to get up from a bed or chair without a firm hand hold, not to use the stairs immediately upon arising, to "sit down" rather than fall down if he becomes dizzy in an open space while standing, etc.

There is a final additional advantage to a single daily dose strategy of oral neuroleptic medication which is far from insignificant. That is the issue of medication compliance. Among outpatients, the rate of noncompliance can be enormous,[59,60] with some reports indicating that the rate of noncompliance can be as great as 80% or more. Some of this noncompliance may be due to accidental forgetting. Another component results from intentionally not taking the medication. In either case, once a day dosing is an advantage. In terms of simple forgetting, certainly a once a day routine is the least likely pattern to get missed or for the patient to become confused about. In the case of intentional avoidance, the reluctance to ingest medication may not always be due solely to the patient's denial or embarrassment. The patient may feel stigmatized or ostracized, rightly or wrongly, if others know that he takes antipsychotic medication. A once a day regimen simplifies the patient's task of maintaining his medication as a private affair—allowing the patient not to take the medication to work during the day or, perhaps, on the other hand, allowing the patient to spend the night with someone without having to bring these pills along. These considerations make it quite expectable that the more often drug dosage is divided, the more problematic compliance is found to be.[61]

Many times, the issue of compliance is resolved through the use of long-acting intramuscular depot preparations of neuroleptics: in this country fluphenazine decanoate or fluphenazine enanthate. This is a very appropriate use for these depot drugs, and they certainly can have a role in acute as well as maintenance treatment. Since there is often a vicious cycle of reduced medication compliance coincident with the early and intermediate stages of psychotic decompensation or relapse, the use of depot medication is often the most efficient way to attempt to avert hospitalization. The long-acting intramuscular medication requires very little compliance, approximately one minute of compliance every two weeks, and all interpersonal and/or intrafamilial stops can be let out, if necessary, to generate this brief hiatus of drug acceptability—therapeutic pressure which, most often, does not have to be reexerted the subsequent fortnight when the patient's excitement is reduced and reality testing is more intact. It is more prudent, however, not to make the depot administration the patient's first exposure to fluphenazine. True allergic reactions are extremely rare, but they still are possible—in which case a depot preparation would be problematic in taking so long to clear. More of a risk is that the usual side effects could be intolerable, and short-term flexibility in dosing will have been lost. The most conservative course, therefore, is to give at least one short-acting dose of fluphenazine before switching over to a depot form. Once the depot form has been administered, however, there is no further need for any more doses of the short-acting form of the drug. Fluphenazine begins to be released immediately from the injection site, and no other "tapering" oral or short-acting intramuscular doses are required. In fact, by far the greatest daily amount of fluphenazine is released from an enanthate- or decanoate-based injection during the first 24 hours. After that, medication release becomes much more strictly dependent on fatty acid metabolism and becomes consequently much more steady. The enanthate and decanoate preparations of fluphenazine are quite similar, except that the decanoate is somewhat longer lasting. The enanthate-bound fluphenazine will be almost entirely released after 10 days to two weeks. On the other hand, the decanoate formulation can be administered every three weeks, although biweekly injections are still the therapeutic norm.

Since many of the so-called "allergic" reactions to neuroleptics are extrapyramidal, typically acute, dystonic reactions, and since these can be markedly unpleasant occurrences for the patient, engendering subsequent compliance difficulties, it is sensible to administer antiparkinsonian medication right from the start of neuroleptic treatment. In fact, when the initial neuroleptic treatment is going to be parenteral, it may be reasonable, if the clinical situation permits, to administer the oral anticholinergic antiparkinsonian medication beforehand, realizing that the oral medication may take 30–45 minutes to get into the general circulation in significant amounts, whereas intramuscular medication may take only one-third to one-half as long.

BLOOD LEVELS OF ANTIPSYCHOTIC MEDICATIONS

In light of the tortuous route which antipsychotic medications must take to reach their ultimate locus of pharmacodynamic action and the multiplicity of pharmacokinetic variables which are, at best, difficult to predict, a logical thought is that measuring the blood concentrations of these drugs might provide a crude measure of their bioavailability and a potentially worthwhile index of their therapeutic activity. Such investigations are now possible because of technical advances, represented by the radioreceptor assay and gas chromatography/mass spectrometry, which allow the measurement of nanogram quantities of these substances in the plasma or serum. These studies have also been spurred by the discovery that plasma drug levels are meaningful correlates of treatment response for at least some tricyclic antidepressants.[62]

Unfortunately, however, many of the plasma neuroleptic studies have been complicated by methodological flaws. In addition to the ever-present difficulties of diagnosis of schizophrenia, even when modern operationalized criteria are employed (and some of the blood-level studies freely admitted all psychotic patients whether schizophrenic, affective, or "other"), there is the necessity in blood level work to include patients who are capable of getting better. Inclusion of chronically refractory patients or others unlikely to show a positive clinical response into a study sample can rapidly render the results uninterpretable. This sort of methodological difficulty is much more bothersome with schizophrenia than it is with depression because schizophrenia is more polymorphous in its presentation and often involves less clear remissions with more residual symptoms. On the other hand, the newest cases of schizophrenia are often the most suspect diagnostically. A major difficulty also is that, clinically, antipsychotic drugs sometime take two to three months to have their fullest therapeutic effects, but the maintenance of such a long drug trial at a constant dose in a substantial number of these patients can become extremely problematic.

This brings us to a very serious methodological flaw which befalls many of the studies which purport to find a "therapeutic window" of efficacy for plasma concentrations of neuroleptics. That a lower end of such a window would exist is intuitively obvious—at some point the medication dose and blood concentration become too small to affect the illness meaningfully. It is the upper end of this window which may be the artifact of a flawed study design. This is the case in any study which does not have a fixed-dose paradigm.[63] "Fixed dose" means that a patient is assigned to dosage schedule of medication at the start of a study without regard to his clinical status either at that point or subsequently. Usually, this means that every patient in the study receives the same dosage schedule. But this need not be the case as long as the dosage schedules are assigned randomly among the patients. Also, the dosage does not need to be held constant for the entire protocol, so long as the dosage schedule followed is predetermined. Any schedule that is regulated in relationship to the patient's clinical response, however, is not a fixed-dose design. The flaw in this latter approach is that patients who are nonresponsive repeatedly have their dosage raised in a vain attempt to attain a remission. Consequently, plasma levels in this nonresponsive group wind up being quite high, creating the spurious appearance of an upper end to the therapeutic window—that high plasma concentrations are associated with poor clinical response. Indeed, in such studies, high plasma levels are associated with poor clinical response, but this is because poor response leads to high plasma levels by virtue of the study design, not vice versa.

In some instances, the fixed-dose concept seems to have been confused with the steady-state concept in the study design. What is meant by steady state is that the daily dose of medication is held constant for a sufficient period of time that the plasma concentration has reached a reasonable approximation of the asymptote it would have achieved had that dose been administered indefinitely. Operationally, this is usually taken as being a time equal to at lease five half-lives of the drug (for neuroleptics, generally five to seven days). Steady state, of course, is actually an unsteady state, with the plasma level increasing after each new dose and then falling again in saw-toothed fashion. It is thus quite important that blood samples be taken at standard intervals after the drug administration—in most studies this has been taken to be approximately 12 hours after the bedtime medication. In studies of prolonged drug administration, there is definite value in achieving a steady state as well as in having a fixed-dose study design.

The term therapeutic window has also been incorrectly used in discussions of the concept of therapeutic ratio.[63] In the case of a true therapeutic window, the actual desired clinical effect of the drug decreases or disappears at the upper end of the window as well as at the lower end. Although colloquially employed, the use of this term is not strictly correct to describe the situation in which higher levels of the drug are undesirable clinically because side effects supervene in that range, either obscuring the desired clinical effect or making the drug use in that range intolerable to the patient even though the desired clinical benefit is still apparent. This relationship between the range of benefit through drug effect versus the range where undesirable side effects limit drug use is properly referred to as the therapeutic ratio. For example, if an extrapyramidal side effect such as akathisia limited neuroleptic use in a certain patient above a specified range, this would be a consideration of therapeutic ratio. Only if the antipsychotic efficacy of the medication were lost in the higher range would a true therapeutic window exist.

With these provisos in mind, existing studies can be considered.

There is evidence that serum levels of neuroleptic which are less than the equivalent of 50 ng of chlorpromazine per mL are associated with poor antipsychotic response. Tune et al reached this conclusion in a study of 30 patients, diagnosed by the research diagnostic criteria[64] as suffering from schizophrenia, who were treated with either haloperidol, fluphenazine hydrochloride, chlorpromazine, molindone, thiothixene, or trifluoperazine.[65] The paradigm in this protocol was not fixed dose, but samples were collected at a fair approximation of steady state: four to six hours after the last oral dose when the patients had been maintained on a consistent dosage regimen for at least four days. The timing of the serum collection and the clinical assessment was after 14 to 28 days of neuroleptic treatment. Although the drawbacks of a lack of fixed-dose design are recognized, the critique involving the risk of finding a spurious upper end to a therapeutic window do not apply in this study, since it is a study of the threshold of efficacy (or the lower end of the therapeutic window, assuming that one would, in fact, exist). The variation in time to response and the use of as many as six neuroleptics in 30 patients, of course, are limitations. The reporting of this result also involves the essentially untested assumption that therapeutic serum levels can be meaningfully related in terms of chlorpromazine equivalencies as we now compute them. However, this study represents the best approximation we currently have of a clinical serum or plasma neuroleptic concentration threshold. The nonfixed-dose study of Rivera-Calimlim et al, which purports to find a therapeutic window for plasma chlorpromazine, can be taken as corroborating evidence for this threshold since, in that study as well, the lower end of the window was found to be 50 ng/mL.[66]

There has been no fixed-dose study confirming an acute treatment therapeutic window for blood concentrations of chlorpromazine as reported by Rivera-Calimlim et al,[22,66] and two fixed-dose studies with chlorpromazine have failed to find any evidence of a relationship between blood levels of this drug and clinical response. The first of these was a 15-week study by Loga et al in which 12 schizophrenic patients were given 300 mg of oral chlorpromazine per day.[67] The diagnostic criteria were not given, the number of patients was small, and the dosage would be considered low, but the duration of this study was sufficient to get a full response to the dose employed. More recently, May et al studied 48 newly admitted patients with functional psychoses of the schizophrenic type (diagnosed by four different sets of operationalized criteria) and treated for 28 days with a fixed-dose regimen of chlorpromazine—1 mg/lb on the first day and then 3 mg/lb for the rest of the study.[68] In this rigorous study as well no relationship was found between plasma drug level and clinical response. Nonfixed-dose studies of chlorpromazine blood levels, when patients were receiving oral doses in the 75–400 mg per day range[69] and the 150–600 mg per day range,[70] also have shown no relationship with clinical response.

The blood level relationship that does seem to emerge from studies such as these, however, is that patients with higher concentrations of demethylated chlorpromazine and chlorpromazine sulfoxide seem to have a less favorable clinical response than patients with lower levels of these metabolites.[69–71] Chlorpromazine, of course, has an enormous number of metabolites, many of which are active in one way or another. This makes chlorpromazine—and many of the other phenothiazines as well—very difficult drugs to study in terms of blood level-clinical response relationships.

A much more favorable drug to study from the standpoint of blood concentrations is haloperidol. This is because haloperidol is not metabolized by hydroxylation and demethylation—metabolic pathways destined to lead to a multiplicity of metabolites with various degrees of activity. Instead, the first metabolic step for haloperidol severs the molecule in half, and all further metabolites are nonpsychoactive. Some preliminary data have been presented consistent with a hypothesis that a therapeutic window exists for haloperidol, with blood concentrations of 5–8 ng/mL on the lower end and 15–20 ng/mL on the upper end,[72–74] but these findings cannot yet be considered to be conclusive inasmuch as two studies were of a nonfixed-dose design.[72,73] The largest study with the most rigorous design had the greatest favorable response in the midrange of plasma concentrations (10 out of 11 patients), but also had a greater than 50% response rate at both the lower (6 of 11 patients) and upper (7 of 11 patients) ranges.[74] If a therapeutic window of blood haloperidol concentrations were to be found, it would seem to be at variance with observations from the aforementioned acute high-dose studies. These observations were that, although high haloperidol doses offer no special advantage in the acute treatment of schizophrenic psychosis, there also was no indication that high doses—which could be expected to result in a high range of blood levels—resulted in a less advantageous antipsychotic effect.[35,37-41]

A fixed-dose study of butaperazine[75] and nonfixed-dose studies of thiothixene[76] and flupentixol[77] have not found any relationship between blood levels and clinical response. In the thiothixine study, however, the data suggest that increases or decreases in the cis isomer, among the eight Research Diagnostic Criteria schizophrenic patients involved, correlated with improvement or deterioration, respectively, in the clinical course after 15 days.[76] This is a finding which deserves replication of the study with a larger sample.

An intriguing possibility, which could be of substantial potential clinical value, is that blood levels of neuroleptics measured after the initial doses at the start of treatment could be prognostic of the later extent of clinical response. Gottschalk et al found that the plasma levels of thioridazine after one day of treatment with 4 mg/kg correlated significantly with certain measures of clinical response in 25 initially medication-free acute schizophrenic patients.[78] This study had the advantage of a fixed-dose design. Yesavage et al found a similar relationship between serum levels of thiothixine 2.5 hours after a 20-mg oral test dose and clinical improvement one to three weeks later in 30 men diagnosed as having schizophrenia by DSM-III criteria.[79] Although this study did not have a fixed-dose design and the timing of the endpoint was somewhat variable, the treatment regimen paralleled what would be vigorous high-dose neuroleptic treatment in an inpatient setting, with final doses of thiothixene in nonresponding patients reaching 160 mg/day. In this study, acute serum levels were also found to correlate positively with age, leading the authors to speculate that this relationship could be linked with the observation that older patients may require lower doses of neuroleptic agents and be prone to a higher incidence of side effects. The previously mentioned chlorpromazine metabolite study of Sakurai et al, finding poorer clinical response in patients with higher relative levels of sulfoxide and demethylated metabolites, should be mentioned in this section as well, since these metabolite results were measured three hours after the initial 50-mg dose of chlorpromazine.[70] Finally, in the aforementioned well-designed study of May et al, although plasma chlorpromazine concentrations did not bear a relationship to clinical responses later, the plasma concentrations after the first day's treatment with chlorpromazine (1 mg/lb) did correlate with the four-week clinical response to the 3-mg/lb dose.[68] Furthermore, saliva chlorpromazine levels were measured in that same study. The 24-hour saliva concentrations also correlated with the later clinical response. In fact, saliva concentrations correlated more strongly than did the plasma concentrations. However, neither the plasma nor the saliva concentrations correlated with either the patients' initial subjective responses to the medication[80] or the appearance of the extrapyramidal side effect of akinesia.[81] Although provocative, of course, and apparently to at least some extent prognostic, those early blood level studies do not establish the utility of adjusting dosage on the basis of early blood levels. Any such development would entail extensive further clinical research.

A new technical and conceptual advance is represented in the work of Casper et al in a study that measured the concentration of butaperazine in red blood cells as well as in the plasma.[75] The authors reasoned that the concentration of neuroleptic functionally free in the plasma, and hence free to cross the blood-brain barrier, would be more accurately represented by the drug concentration to be found in erythrocytes than by the total plasma concentration. As hypothesized, whereas no relationship was found between clinical response and plasma butaperazine levels among 24 newly hospitalized patients diagnosed as having schizophrenia by research diagnostic criteria treated for two weeks with butaperazine in a fixed-dose design, a significant inverted U-shape relationship was found between clinical response and red cell concentrations (ie, a therapeutic window). This technique of assessment of neuroleptic concentrations represents another promising avenue for future research.

In conclusion, the full story is not yet in on the usefulness of neuroleptic drug levels in clinical work, although there are several attractive leads. Useful information certainly exists, however, in those cases where blood levels are far too low—indicating compliance problems, poor absorption, or unusually rapid metabolism; in those cases where blood levels are far too high—suggesting overdose; or in evaluating other situations such as problematic side effects.

CLINICAL PREDICTORS OF DRUG RESPONSE

A number of important predictors have emerged for good or poor outcome, in general, for schizophrenia. These prognostic items have held up through drug treatment, but it has not been demonstrated that they are, indeed, predictors of favorable or unfavorable neuroleptic response per se.[82] It may well be that they are simply general predictors. That is, the predictions they make are valid whether or not patients are treated with drugs. Thus, these predictors may have a lot to do with the patients' disorders and/or their coexisting recuperative resources, and little or nothing to do with drug response itself. For example, a patient with a good premorbid history of adjustment is more likely to make a good recovery with neuroleptic treatment than is a patient with a poor premorbid history. But a patient with a good premorbid history would also probably have a better chance of improvement without drugs than would a patient with a poor premorbid history. This, of course, is not to say that drugs should not be used. Either patients' chance of recovery is improved with the use of drugs. The issue is that differential phenomenological predictors of drug responsiveness, if they exist at all, have not been teased out. This would require large-scale placebo-controlled studies which, for the most part, have not been done.

Certainly, a knowledge of the general predictors is of value to clinicians. Many of these were summarized from the earlier literature by Robins and Guze.[83] Good prognostic indicators include good premorbid adjustment, acute onset of the episode (less than six months of symptoms), presence of precipitating factors, and confusion. Other observed prognostic factors, weighing in the direction of prediction a good response, seem related to the issue of presence of (or differential diagnosis with) affective disorder. These include prominent depressive symptoms at the time of the psychotic episode, guilty concerns, thoughts of death, family history of affective disorder, and lack of a family history of schizophrenia. Since that time, there have been considerable refinements in definitions and subcategories of these predictors, particularly in the area of premorbid psychosocial adjustment,[82,84–87] but little has emerged that is specifically an indication or a contraindication for the use of neuroleptics among acute schizophrenia patients, or as a basis for choosing among the neuroleptics for any other reason than on the basis of their particular side effects.

One constellation of symptoms, though, is less likely to respond to neuroleptic administration. These are the so-called "negative" symptoms of schizophrenia. This includes the "burned-out," withdrawn, apathetic syndrome which may afflict patients, especially in the chronic stages of their illnesses. Such symptoms are unlikely to respond to neuroleptic medication. However, care should be exercised to differentiate these negative symptoms of schizophrenia from the neuroleptic-induced akinesia side effect.[10–12] Akinesia can be treated by the addition of antiparkinsonian medication and possibly also by reducing the neuroleptic dosage. In fact, akinesia can look sufficiently like this negative symptom constellation clinically that these negative symptoms should never be written off as untreatable without a thorough trial of antiparkinsonian treatment. Thus, predominance of negative symptoms at the acute clinical presentation may constitute an unfavorable prognostic indicator of neuroleptic response in comparison to such "positive" psychotic symptoms as hallucinations, delusions, or thought disorder. Indeed, a DSM-III diagnosis of acute schizophrenia requires the presence of these positive symptoms at the time of the episode.[88] Further consideration of negative symptoms in schizophrenia, therefore, takes us beyond the scope of this chapter and is more sensibly considered as an issue in the management of chronic schizophrenia.

There is one final set of predictors to drug response in schizophrenia which is intriguing and which is of potential clinical usefulness. This involves the response of patients at the very start of treatment—both the patients' subjective response and the antipsychotic response in the first hours and days of treatment.

Van Putten and May, following up on other work,[89] reported that the subjective responses of patients to an initial test dose of chlorpromazine, as measured on the euphoric-dysphoric dimension, was significantly correlated with measures of subsequent clinical outcome.[90] This held up for the subjective response among the 48 schizophrenic patients studied at all three intervals measured—4, 24, and 48 hours after the initial test dose of 1 mg/lb. In the second day, an additional 3-mg/lb dose was administered. Thus, the patients who complain that the medication is making them feel bad and that it is not going to help may have more than just casual accuracy in their statements—although it is not entirely clear whether this was based on pharmacological effect, the patients' own "self-fulfilling prophesy," or the patients' early evidence of positive response to helpful ambient psychosocial factors. Teasing these issues apart would have required a placebo control group (ie, subjective response to placebo) in this study of acutely psychotic patients. Clinical experience, however, would tempt us to believe that more than placebo response is involved, and initial subjective response is a provocative prognostic lead. Even if physicians don't follow up on it, presumably patients do, since it is most reasonable to suppose that many of the patients who stop their medication as soon as they are discharged from the hospital are among those who feel that the antipsychotic drugs make them feel dysphoric.

A related finding by the same group of investigators was that the clinical response after 48 hours to 1 mg of chlorpromazine per lb in the first day and 3 mg/lb in the second day was consistently correlated with all 10 clinical outcome measures tested after four weeks of treatment at the fixed dose of 3 mg of chlorpromazine per lb.[91] One can only conclude from the results of this study that a patient not showing any favorable clinical response at 48 hours is less likely to get better after four weeks of that dose of chlorpromazine than other patients who show a more favorable initial reaction. We do not know whether those patients should have their dose raised or be switched to an alternative neuroleptic (which might be rational to attempt) or whether these are patients who somehow will not do better in any case on neuroleptics, or, perhaps, will not do better with any form of treatment. Again, there are many caveats and more information is needed, but the lead is an exciting one.

NONSTANDARD TREATMENT OF SCHIZOPHRENIA

Where standard treatments for schizophrenia have failed, a variety of nonstandard interventions have been attempted. In this section, several of those most commonly tried will be reviewed.

ECT in Schizophrenia

The early literature compared electroconvulsive therapy (ECT) with no other somatic treatment; later studies compared ECT with antipsychotic drugs. Of the early studies, most are not helpful because of small sample sizes. The best is that of Brill and his associates,[92] who studied 67 patients with schizophrenia, randomly assigned to ECT or simulated ECT. There were no significant differences in outcome; 40% of the ECT group improved versus 45% of the control group. Until recently this study was the only reasonable protocol that used double-blind techniques.

A study by May[93] compared ECT with antipsychotic medication, psychotherapy, and ward milieu therapy alone, in patients in a state hospital with "intermediate" prognosis. ECT was more effective than psychotherapy and milieu therapy alone, but less effective than antipsychotic drugs.

Childers[94] divided 80 patients into four groups; ECT, fluphenazine (20 mg per day), chlorpromazine (1000 mg per day), and chlorpromazine with ECT. Childers did not do a statistical analysis, but Siris and coworkers[95] performed chi square analyses and showed that the combination of ECT plus chlorpromazine was superior to either drug ($P < 0.05$), although not superior to ECT alone.

The most recent study by Taylor and Fleminger[96] was double blind. All subjects received antipsychotic drugs for at least two weeks before random assignment. The drugs were continued while 10 received ECT and 10 received simulated ECT. Those given ECT had greater improvement ($P = 0.004$).

Remaining studies used patients with very chronic schizophrenia who were long-term residents in hospitals—not an appropriate group to demonstrate the efficacy of ECT versus drug treatment.

The evidence to date is mildly encouraging that ECT is effective in schizophrenia, but there is enormously more evidence to support the use of antipsychotic drugs. Much further research is required to determine whether the combination of ECT and drugs is advantageous.

The most relevant clinical question is whether ECT is useful in patients who have not responded to adequate treatment with antipsychotic drugs. Unfortunately, no controlled clinical trials have been done in reference to this question. Anecdotal reports are published of patients who have done well. A recent example is Ries and associates[97] who describe nine patients with schizo-affective disorder as diagnosed by the Research Diagnostic Criteria,[64] five depressed and four excited, who had not responded to drug treatment and yet did well with subsequent ECT. This is a less convincing anecdote than it would be had the patients had schizophrenia, since the relationship of schizo-affective disorder to schizophrenia remains controversial. These nine patients were different from usual patients with mania or major depression, however, not only because of the presence of "first-rank symptoms," which is how the Research Diagnostic Criteria defines schizo-affective disorder, but they were younger and mental confusion was common. This gives some support to the idea that these patients were not typical patients with mania or depression, for whom a response to ECT would not be as remarkable.

Nevertheless, only anecdotal evidence supports the value of ECT in such drug-unresponsive patients, leaving the clinician in the uncomfortable position of having to turn to a treatment that has not been proven. Yet in appropriately selected cases a trial of ECT is rational, since ECT is a safe treatment and it seems less acceptable to not try all avenues of treatment for such a serious disorder. Clinicians most experienced in using ECT for schizophrenia usually recommend that 20 treatments be given, even if improvement occurs early, to get the maximum response and avoid relapse.

Other less-than-established treatments also should be considered for such patients, such as propranolol, high-dose benzodiazepines, and lithium.

Propranolol in Schizophrenia

Uncontrolled anecdotal reports have been frequent about the efficacy of high doses of propranolol in schizophrenia, but only recently have controlled clinical trials been reported.

The first was done by Yorkston and co-workers,[98] who studied hospitalized patients who had not responded to adequate doses of chlorpromazine. They were placed for 12 weeks on continued chlorpromazine plus propranolol, up to 200 mg twice a day, or chlorpromazine with placebo. The group with combined treatment did better to a statistically significant degree.

Lindstrom and Persson[99] studied 12 patients who had been treated without full response with flupentixol decanoate, 20 to 60 mg every two weeks, and who were then given adjunctive propranolol openly, to a daily dose of 1920 mg, for several weeks. (Flupentixol decanoate is a depot antipsychotic not currently marketed in the United States.) Then, under double-blind conditions the patients were randomized to enter two two-week periods of propranolol or propranolol placebo, ie a discontinuation study. To a statistically significant degree the patients did better during the propranolol period.

Myers and associates[100] studied 20 patients with schizophrenia who had not responded to antipsychotic medication. All were treated with fluphenazine decanoate 25 mg or flupentixol decanoate, 40 mg every two weeks, and randomized to receive propranolol up to 1920 mg per day or placebo for three months. No difference was seen between the two groups.

These three foregoing studies were of propranolol with concomitant antipsychotic medication. The generally encouraging results may have been due, some said, to propranolol's ability to increase the blood level of the antipsychotic. For example, Peet and associates[101] gave chlorpromazine alone or with propranolol to 10 hospitalized patients with chronic schizophrenia for two seven-week crossover periods. Plasma levels of chlorpromazine, chlorpromazine sulfoxide, prolactin, and total neuroleptic level (as measured by the radioreceptor assay) were statistically significantly elevated during the period of combined treatment.

Three studies have examined the effect of propranolol in schizophrenia when given alone. King and co-workers,[102] in patients with chronic disorders, found propranolol no different from placebo. Yorkston and associates[103] compared propranolol (670 mg per day) with chlorpromazine (300 mg per day) in 46 newly admitted patients. Both groups improved equally. Only 18 of 46 (39%) had good results during the 12-week trial, a rather low figure for newly admitted patients. Perhaps the doses were too low, and the two treatments were not adequately tested. But, even though 300 mg of chlorpromazine per day is considered a low dose in most centers,[55] there are few studies showing dose-response relationships. The apparently necessary custom of using higher dosage has not as yet been very well justified.

Peet and co-workers[104] took patients with a diagnosis of chronic schizophrenia from four hospitals. They were then "washed out" with placebo for two weeks (four if they had been receiving depot antipsychotics) and then randomized to receive chlorpromazine (400 mg per day) propranolol (640 mg per day), or placebo for the next three months. The authors found no differences among the three groups and concluded that propranolol is ineffective in schizophrenia. This conclusion, it appears to us, should be tempered for two reasons: (1) during the washout period, which averaged 30 days, no worsening was described; and (2) chlorpromazine was not found to be better than placebo. This suggests that these patients were too refractory to treatment to be an adequate group in which to test a new treatment. This study, probably, should be considered a trial of propranolol as a second treatment in patients resistant to standard treatment and who are chronically ill, rather than as a test of the hypothesis of whether propranolol has an antipsychotic property.

It appears to us that it is too early to reach conclusions about the role of propranolol in schizophrenia. However, we think that there are sufficient data to justify a trial of its use, probably with concomitant standard antipsychotics, in appropriately selected treatment-resistant patients.

Benzodiazepines in Schizophrenia

To date, double-blind studies, with one exception, have not shown benzodiazepines to be effective in schizophrenia.[105-109] The exception is the study of Kellner and associates.[110] Using a model of intensive design, they studied three patients who were repeatedly switched from chlordiazepoxide to placebo, while an antipsychotic drug was continued; statistically significant improvement was associated with the chlordiazepoxide at doses much higher than those used to treat anxiety, ie, 150–300 mg per day. The overall subject of the use of benzodiazepines in schizophrenia has been reviewed recently by Nestoros.[111]

The rationale for using benzodiazepines in schizophrenia is based on the following: (1) schizophrenic symptoms may be associated with a hyperactivity in dopaminergic transmission[112,113] and/or hypoactivity in gamma-amino butyric acid (GABA)-ergic neurotransmission[112,114]; (2) enhancement of GABA-ergic neurotransmission decreases dopaminergic neurotransmission in many systems, including the limbic system[115]; (3) GABA-mimetic drugs suppress dopamine agonist-induced behaviors in monkeys[116]; and (4) benzodiazepines stimulate the GABA system.[117]

Perhaps the negative results from double-blind controlled studies have been the result of low dosage.[111] Anecdotal reports are encouraging. Beckmann and Haas[118] treated 15 patients with doses of diazepam between 200 and 400 mg per day. All nine patients diagnosed as paranoid-hallucinatory subtype of schizophrenia improved; whereas only one of six patients subtyped as schizo-affective improved. What seems remarkable is that sedation was seen, except for one patient, only after the first dose of 50 mg. Three patients had a marked loss of inhibitions of sexual and social behavior.

Nair and co-workers[119] gave diazepam up to 200 mg/day for 12 weeks to 12 inpatients with schizophrenia who had not responded to standard antipsychotic drug treatment given for six months. The antipsychotic drugs were continued. Nair et al reported marked improvement in seven patients and mild improvement in one. Again, remarkably, the only adverse reaction reported was confusion and disorientation in one patient while receiving 160 mg/day.

These tantalizing results suggest that double-blind controlled studies should be done with high-dose benzodiazepines, and until then such treatment might be considered in patients who are not responding to standard treatment.

Lithium in Schizophrenia

Unfortunately, we tend to consider drugs by the names given them when they first appear. We forget that these compounds do not appear naturally with labels attached to them proclaiming their category and that it requires clinical trials to establish the bounds of a drug's efficacy and not the label we attach. Lithium is a case in point. For many years since its introduction in 1949 it was considered axiomatic that it was a "thymoleptic," active only in affective disorders. In fact, a response to lithium was considered by some to be evidence that the patient had affective disorder and not schizophrenia.

Consequently, little research has been done to investigate the value of lithium in schizophrenia. The chapter on the treatment of mania has reviewed the evidence for lithium treatment of schizo-affective states. Prien and co-workers[120] showed that in excited schizo-affective patients lithium was as effective as chlorpromazine for those with mild excitement, whereas chlorpromazine was superior in those with more than mild excitement. This study is not relevant, perhaps, unless we consider schizo-affective disorder to be related to schizophrenia, and patterns of response to schizo-affective disorder are the same as for schizophrenia. These considerations are controversial at present. Certainly, the evidence is far from definitive. In our opinion, it is best to consider the place of schizo-affective disorder unknown and investigate it as a separate diagnosis.

The study by Biederman and associates[121] is quite relevant because in their comparison of lithium and haloperidol versus haloperidol alone they included a spectrum of newly admitted inpatients diagnosed as having schizophrenia or schizo-affective disorder. Their definition of schizo-affective disorder was purposely very broad. A patient with typical schizophrenia without any features of excitement was considered a number one. A patient with typical mania without any features of schizophrenia was given number six. Patients given numbers two through five had gradations of schizophrenic and manic symptoms, and were put into the study. The expectation was that patients toward the manic end of the spectrum would show more of an advantage to the combination of haloperidol plus lithium, compared with haloperidol alone, than would those near the schizophrenic end.

The result was that all groups showed a statistically significant advantage to the lithium plus haloperidol group, and the advantage was equal throughout the groups: the patients with just a tinge of excitement were as benefited by the combination as those with a manic-like state and just a tinge of schizophrenia. This suggests that lithium as adjunctive treatment to an antipsychotic is effective in schizophrenia, but it is not a definitive test of the hypothesis.

Small et al[122] also tested the value of lithium in schizophrenia by comparing a four-week period of lithium plus an antipsychotic with a four-week period of the antipsychotic alone. The periods were alternated several times under double-blind conditions. There was a statistically significant advantage to the periods of combined treatment. This was a particularly impressive finding because the subjects were long-term inpatients who would be expected to be unresponsive to drug treatment.

The most that can be said for the use of lithium in schizophrenia is that its use is supported by research data to a limited degree and that it should be considered in patients who have not responded to standard treatment with antipsychotic agents.

Unfortunately, no clear scientific statements can be made on the subject of which nonstandard treatment of schizophrenia to attempt first or in whom. Research on this topic is in its early stages, and appropriate comparisons have not yet been made. In fact, the majority of the studies cited in this section on nonstandard treatments have not used operational criteria to substantiate their diagnoses of schizophrenia, which limits the interpretability of the findings. Certainly, however, when standard treatments have been exhausted, nonstandard treatments should be attempted as an effort to bring relief to very ill patients who are otherwise nonresponsive. But in choosing among these treatments the clinician is left, for the present time at least, to his own experience and his own judgment in balancing the chances for success against the risks and side effects of the different available modalities.

THE TREATMENT OF SCHIZO-AFFECTIVE DISORDERS

Any consideration of the treatment of schizo-affective disorders is, of necessity, confounded by uncertainty with regard to the definition of schizo-affective disorder and what its diagnostic criteria should be. This uncertainty even extends to DSM-III.[88] Whereas the diagnoses of all other psychiatric disorders are concretized through operational criteria in DSM-III, the uncertainty over the diagnosis of schizo-affective disorder is concretized by the absence of operationalized criteria.

Kasanin originally introduced the term "schizo-affective psychosis" in 1933 to describe patients who had an apparent mixture of schizophrenic and manic-depressive symptoms.[123] Since that time a number of other terms have also been employed in attempts to describe what is probably a heterogenous grouping of psychotic disorders, at least some of which are very closely related to major affective disorders, if not identical with them altogether.[124–126] Regardless of the terms of definitions employed, many patients definitely exist who have a composite of symptoms traditionally associated with both schizophrenia and affective disorders. The definitional confusion, however, makes it even more difficult than usual to interpret the results of past treatment studies.

A number of early studies, mostly anecdotal, reported that lithium was useful in treating patients with excited schizo-affective states.[127–133] More recently, under double-blind conditions, Alexander et al found that three out of three schizo-affective manic patients improved with three weeks of lithium treatment in comparison with placebo and that all three of these patients had shown improvement at one week as well.[134] However, all three of these patients were still substantially psychotic at the end of three weeks, with residual ratings of 6 or 7 on the 15-point Bunney-Hamburg psychosis rating scale[135] following improvements of 4 or 5 points. After double-blind discontinuation of the lithium, two of these patients became substantially more psychotic again, whereas one continued to improve.

There have been one large and two smaller double-blind studies comparing the efficacy of lithium and chlorpromazine in excited schizo-affective patients. The large study was that of Prien et al, which was an 18-hospital collaborative study including 83 patients.[120] Lithium and chlorpromazine doses were adjusted clinically, but blindly, for the three-week trial, the plasma level range of the former turning out to be 0.6–2.0 mEq/mL and the oral dose of the latter finally being 200–3000 mg per day. Although most patients were still not symptom free at the end of the trial, in general completers in both treatment groups showed improvement. Of interest was the observation that both groups showed improvement in both manic and schizophrenic symptoms. By rank order, lithium was not as rapid in controlling the excited behavior, although this difference was not statistically significant. The authors further divided this series of patients into those who were "highly active" (ie, poor control of hostile aggressive behavior) (N=42) and those who were only "mildly active" (N=41). Among the highly active group, chlorpromazine treatment was superior to lithium. Six out of the 17 lithium treated patients in this group were dropped from the study because of poor treatment response or lack of further cooperation. Additionally, 3 of these 17 left the hospital against advice, and one was dropped due to toxicity. Thus, only 7 of 17 highly active patients assigned to lithium even completed the trial. Only 1 of the 25 patients in the highly active group randomized to chlorpromazine failed to complete the trial. On the other hand, differences in response to lithium and chlorpromazine in the mildly active group were much smaller, and it was concluded that the two treatments were of similar utility in the less activated cohort of patients.

Brockington et al's small double-blind series (11 completers) comparing lithium and chlorpromazine in patients with schizo-affective mania found no evidence of differential therapeutic effect after one month between lithium and chlorpromazine.[136] Almost half of the patients completing that study were rated as recovered, and most of the rest improved. The results reported by Johnson et al, however, were quite different.[137–139] In that double-blind series of patients treated for three to four weeks, less than half got a good response with chlorpromazine, although none did worse with that drug, whereas most patients receiving lithium (with blood levels in the range 1.16–1.97 mEq/L) got worse. Although one lithium-treated patient had a partial remission, five were found to develop early signs of neurotoxicity. The discrepancy of this finding with the absence of neurotoxicity as a frequent problem in other studies of lithium in schizo-affective disorder is not easily explained, although the relatively high blood lithium concentrations may be partially responsible.

In summary, then, although lithium may well be useful in the acute treatment of many schizo-affective manic patients, particularly the less highly activated ones, in no series was lithium found to be superior to chlorpromazine; the neuroleptic seemed to be the drug choice for most hostile and agitated patients. This may have been due in part to the sedative properties of chlorpromazine, which could be very beneficial in the management of irritable, accelerated patients. Other neuroleptics have not been compared, in a double-blind controlled trial, with lithium or chlorpromazine in schizo-affective manic patients.

Since there was some usefulness to lithium, though, and since there seems to be a relationship between at least some excited schizo-affective states and mania,[124–126] the question then naturally follows as to whether combining lithium with a neuroleptic might be more beneficial in excited schizo-affective patients than the neuroleptic used alone. Biederman et al[121] undertook just such a study in 36 patients diagnosed as schizo-affective disorder, manic type, according to the Research Diagnostic Criteria.[64] All patients were treated with an individually adjusted dose of haloperidol (range 8–70 mg per day orally). In addition, either lithium or placebo was added for a five-week trial. The blood levels of lithium were controlled in the range of 0.67–1.55 mEq/L. A modest but statistically significant difference was found between the treatment groups, favoring lithium. The advantage did not seem to be restricted to affective symptoms such as euphoria or talkativeness, but appeared to extend to more traditionally "schizophrenic" symptoms as well. Furthermore, although "more affective" schizo-affective patients tended to make better recoveries, the benefit of adjunctive lithium was found to apply to the "more schizophrenic" schizo-affective patients as well as the "more affective" ones. The important advantages of lithium seemed to take effect after the acute phase of treatment for the psychosis in terms of helping patients attain a qualitatively superior remission. This leaves open the question of whether patients might have achieved just as good a result had the lithium been added later, perhaps in the third or fourth week, avoiding the risks of venipuncture or of missing manifestations of toxicity in acutely excited psychotic patients.

Similar results regarding the potential usefulness of adjunctive lithium in schizo-affective manic patients diagnosed by the Research Diagnostic Criteria were found in five patients under double-blind conditions by Carman et al.[140] These patients had been stabilized for eight weeks on their optimal dose of neuroleptic and then, double-blind, had lithium (0.75–1.3 mEq/L) added for either the first or second four weeks out of the next eight. Arousal was clinically and statistically reduced in four of the five patients for their lithium versus their placebo period.

Notably, in the studies of Biederman et al[121] and Carman et al,[140] there was no observation of any manifestation of neurotoxicity with the combination of neuroleptic and lithium as had been described for haloperidol and lithium by Cohen and Cohen.[141] Baastrup et al have also reviewed 245 cases of combined treatment without adverse effect,[142] so we may conclude that there is probably not a special danger in combining lithium with haloperidol or other neuroleptics. However, this issue is still controversial, and since there is also probably not an advantage to beginning lithium treatment from the very outset, we recommend considering its use a bit later in treatment. (See also the discussion of this question in Chapter 4.)

Among patients with schizo-affective depressions, there is one well-designed double-blind study which compared amitriptyline (mean 182 mg per day), chlorpromazine (mean 600 mg per day), and combined amitriptyline and chlorpromazine (means 150 and 450 mg per day respectively) over one month in 36 patients.[136] Although none of the groups did very well in this study, the chlorpromazine group did the best with 4 patients out of 11 remitting. In the amitriptyline group, only 1 out of 13 remitted and only 2 out of 12 in the combined group remitted. One possible drawback to this study was that chlorpromazine and amitriptyline are both sedating drugs and both are relatively anticholinergic in their pharmacological activity. Another potentially confounding factor was that some patients were included on the basis of having a paranoid psychosis in the absence of any distinctly "schizophrenic" feature. It may then be that some patients with psychotic depressions, rather than schizo-affective disorder (at least according to the Research Diagnostic Criteria), were included in this sample. Even so, the poor treatment response was striking, given that a 20% overall response rate is lower than would be expected in either well-treated depressed patients or schizophrenic patients with affective features (ordinarily considered to be a positive prognostic feature during the acute illness).

In two of the aforementioned lithium studies, a small number of schizo-affective depressed patients were also included.[134,140] In these and in another study,[143] there is little evidence that lithium helps the schizo-affective depressed state in the way that it seems to be of potential benefit in the schizo-affective manic state.

A further issue concerns the treatment of postpsychotic depressions as a course-related phenomenon in at least some schizophrenic patients.

This topic is addressed separately in Chapter 10.

Acknowledgment

Research for this chapter was partially supported by a grant number 1R01-MH 34309 from the National Institute of Mental Health.

REFERENCES

1. Docherty JP, van Kammen DP, Siris SG, et al: Stages of onset of schizophrenic psychosis. *Am J Psychiatry* 1978;135:420–426.
2. Klein DF, Gittleman R, Quitkin F, et al: *Diagnosis and Drug Treatment of Psychiatric Disorders: Adults and Children.* Baltimore, The Williams & Wilkins Co, 1980, pp 798–806.
3. Davis JM: Recent developments in the treatment of schizophrenia. *Psychiatr Ann* 1976;6:71–106.
4. Klerman GL: Drug therapy of schizophrenia: I. Nature of the disorder and the drugs used in treatment. *Drug Ther* Jan 1973;3:94–106.
5. Hollister LE: Clinical use of psychotherapeutic drugs: Current status. *Clin Pharmacol Ther* 1969;10:170–198.
6. Appleton WS: Third psychoactive drug usage guide. *Dis Nerv Syst* 1976;37: 39–51.
7. AMA Department of Drugs: *AMA Drug Evaluations* ed 4. New York, John Wiley & Sons, Inc, 1980, pp 163–186.
8. Schooler NR, Levine J, Severe JB, et al: Prevention of relapse in schizophrenia: An evaluation of fluphenazine decanoate. *Arch Gen Psychiatry* 1980;37:16–24.
9. Potts AM: Agents which cause pigmentory retinopathy. *Dis Nerv Syst* 1968; 29(Suppl):16–18.
10. Rifkin A, Quitkin F, Klein DF: Akinesia: A poorly recognized drug-induced extrapyramidal behavioral disorder. *Arch Gen Psychiatry* 1975;32:672–674.
11. Rifkin A, Quitkin F, Kane J, et al: Are prophylactic antiparkinson drugs necessary? A controlled study of procyclidine withdrawal. *Arch Gen Psychiatry* 1978;35:483–489.
12. Van Putten T, May PRA: 'Akinetic depression' in schizophrenia. *Arch Gen Psychiatry* 1978;35:1101–1107.
13. McGlashan TH, Carpenter WJ Jr: Post-psychotic depression in schizophrenia. *Arch Gen Psychiatry* 1976;33:231–239.
14. Siris SG, Harmon GK, Endicott J: Post-psychotic depressive symptoms in hospitalized schizophrenic patients. *Arch Gen Psychiatry* 1981;38: 1122–1123.
15. Logothetis J: Spontaneous epileptic seizures and electroencephalographic changes in the course of phenothiazine therapy. *Neurology* 1967;17:869–877.
16. Remick PA, Fine SH: Antipsychotic drugs and seizures. *J Clin Psychiatry* 1979;40:78–80.
17. Oliver AP, Luchins DJ, Wyatt RJ: Neuroleptic-induced seizures: An in vitro technique for assessing relative risk. *Arch Gen Psychiatry* 1982;39:206–209.
18. Gallant DM, Bishop MP, Steele CA, et al: Molindone: A cross-over evaluation of capsule and tablet formulations in severely ill schizophrenic patients. *Curr Ther Res* 1973;15:915–918.
19. Gardos G, Cole JO: Weight reduction in schizophrenics by molindone. *Am J Psychiatry* 1977;134:302–304.

20. Clark ML, Haber WK, Sakata K, et al: Molindone in chronic schizophrenia. *Clin Pharmacol Ther* 1970;11:668–688.
21. Davis JM: Overview: Maintenance therapy in psychiatry. I. Schizophrenia. *Am J Psychiatry* 1975;132:1237–1245.
22. Rivera-Calimlim L, Castaneda L, Lasagna L: Effects of mode of management on plasma chlorpromazine in psychiatric patients. *Clin Pharmacol Ther* 1973;14:978–986.
23. Gautier J, Jus A, Villeneuve A, et al: Influence of the antiparkinsonian drugs on the plasma levels of neuroleptics. *Biol Psychiatry* 1977;12:389–399.
24. Simpson GM, Cooper TB, Bark N, et al: Effect of antiparkinsonian medication on plasma levels of chlorpromazine. *Arch Gen Psychiatry* 1980;37:205–208.
25. El-Yousef MK, Manier DH: The effect of benztropine mesylate on plasma levels of butaperazine maleate. *Am J Psychiatry* 1974;131:471–472.
26. Hanlon TE, Schoenrich C, Freinek W, et al: Perphenazine benztropine mesylate treatment of newly admitted psychiatric patients. *Psychopharmacologia* 1966;9:328–339.
27. Hollister LE: Interactions of psychotherapeutic drugs with other drugs and with disease states, in Lipton MA, DiMascio A, Killam KF (eds): *Psychopharmacology: A Generation of Progress.* New York, Raven Press, 1978, pp 987–992.
28. Kerzner B, Rivera-Calimlim L: Lithium and chlorpromazine (CPZ) interaction. *Clin Pharmacol Ther* 1976;19:109.
29. Forrest FM, Forrest SI, Serra MT: Modification of chlorpromazine metabolism by some other drugs frequently administered to psychiatric patients. *Biol Psychiatry* 1970;2:53–58.
30. El-Yousef MK, Manier DH: Tricyclic antidepressants and phenothiazines. *JAMA* 1974;229:1419.
31. Polak P, Laycob L: Rapid tranquilization. *Am J Psychiatry* 1971;128:640–643.
32. Oldham AJ, Bott M: The management of excitement in a general hospital psychiatric ward by high dose haloperidol. *Acta Psychiatr Scand* 1971;47:369–376.
33. Feldman PE, Bay AP, Baser AN, et al: Parenteral haloperidol in controlling patient behavior during acute psychotic episodes. *Curr Ther Res* 1969;11:362–366.
34. Sangiovanni F, Taylor MA, Abrams R, et al: Rapid control of psychotic excitement states with intramuscular haloperidol. *Am J Psychiatry* 1973;130:1155–1156.
35. Reschke RW: Parenteral haloperidol for rapid control of severe, disruptive symptoms of acute schizophrenia. *Dis Nerv Syst* 1975;35:112–115.
36. Lerner Y, Lwow E. Levitin A, et al: Acute high-dose parenteral haloperidol treatment of psychosis. *Am J Psychiatry* 1979;136:1061–1064.
37. Anderson WH, Kuehnle JC, Catanzano DM: Rapid treatment of acute psychosis. *AM J Psychiatry* 1976;133:1076–1078.
38. Ericksen SE, Hurt SW, Chang S, et al: Haloperidol dose, plasma levels, and clinical response: A double-blind study. *Psychopharmacol Bull* 1978;14:15–16.
39. Donlon PT, Hopkin JT, Tupin JP, et al: Haloperidol for acute schizophrenic patients: An evaluation of three oral regimens. *Arch Gen Psychiatry* 1980;37:691–695.
40. Wahba M, Donlon PT, Meadow A: Cognitive changes in acute schizophrenia with brief neuroleptic treatment. *Am J Psychiatry* 1981;138:1307–1310.

41. Neborsky R, Janowsky D, Munson E, et al: Rapid treatment of acute psychotic symptoms with high and low dose haloperidol. *Arch Gen Psychiatry* 1981;38:195–199.
42. Wijsenbeek H, Steiner M, Goldberg SC: Trifluoperazine: A comparison between regular and high doses. *Psychopharmacologia (Berlin)* 1974;36: 147–150.
43. Donlon PT, Meadow A, Tupin JP, et al: High vs. standard dosage fluphenazine HCl in acute schizophrenia. *J Clin Psychiatry* 1978;39:800–804.
44. Escobar JI, Barron A, Kiriakos R: Serum levels of fluphenazine: Effect of dosage and route of administration, and relation to side effects and clinical response. *Psychopharm Bull* 1983;19:131–134.
45. Prien RF, Cole JO: High dose chlorpromazine therapy in chronic schizophrenia. *Arch Gen Psychiatry* 1968;18:482–495.
46. Gardos G, Cole JO: The importance of dosage in antipsychotic drug administration—a review of dose-response studies. *Psychopharmacologia (Berlin)* 1973;29:211–230.
47. Donlon PT, Hopkin J, Tupin JP: Overview: Efficacy and safety of the rapid neuroleptization method with injectable haloperidol. *Am J Psychiatry* 1979; 136:273–278.
48. Aubree JC, Lader MH: High and very high dosage antipsychotics: A critical review. *J Clin Psychiatry* 1980;41:341–350.
49. Quitkin F, Rifkin A, Kaplan JH, et al: Treatment of acute schizophrenia with ultra-high-dose fluphenazine: A failure at shortening time on a crisis-intervention unit. *Compr Psychiatry* 1975;16:279–283.
50. Man PL, Chen CH: Rapid tranquilization of acutely psychotic patients with intramuscular haloperidol and chlorpromazine. *Psychosomatics* 1973;14: 59–63.
51. Gerstenzang ML, Krulisky TV: Parenteral haloperidol in psychiatric emergencies: Double-blind comparisons with chlorpromazine. *Dis Nerv Syst* 1977;38:581–583.
52. Levenson AJ, Burnett GB, Nottingham JD, et al: Speed and rate of remission in acute schizophrenia: A comparison of intramuscularly administered fluphenazine HCl with thiothixene and haloperidol. *Curr Ther Res* 1976; 20:695–700.
53. Stotsky BA: Relative efficacy of parenteral haloperidol and thiothixene for the emergency treatment of acutely excited and agitated patients. *Dis Nerv Syst* 1977;38:967–973.
54. Paprocki J, Versiani M: A double-blind comparison between loxapine and haloperidol by parenteral route in acute schizophrenia. *Curr Ther Res* 1977; 21:80–100.
55. Kessler KA, Waletzky JP: Clinical use of the antipsychotics. *Am J Psychiatry* 1981;138:202–209.
56. Cole JO: Phenothiazine treatment in acute schizophrenia. *Arch Gen Psychiatry* 1964;10:246–261.
57. DiMascio A, Shader RI: Drug administration schedules. *Am J Psychiatry* 1969;126:796–801.
58. Polvan N, Akpinar S, Ahmed BM, et al: Different effects of trifluoperazine when administered daytime or night. *Br J Psychiatry* 1971;119:601–602.
59. Blackwell B: Treatment adherence. *Br J Psychiatry* 1976;129:513–531.
60 Stewart RB, Cluff LE: Commentary: A review of medication errors and compliance in ambulant patients. *Clin Pharmacol Ther* 1972;13:463–468.
61. Ayd FJ Jr: Once-a-day neuroleptic and tricyclic antidepressant therapy. *Int Drug Ther Newsl* 1972;7:35.

62. Siris SG, Glassman AH, Stetner F: The value of plasma concentrations in assessing the effects of tricyclic antidepressants, in Schoolar JC, Claghorn, JL (eds): *The Kinetics of Psychiatric Drugs.* New York, Brunner/Mazel, 1979, pp 215–223.
63. Davis JM, Erickson S, Dekirmenjian H: Plasma levels of antipsychotic drugs and clinical response, in Lipton MA, DiMascio A, Killam KF (eds): *Psychopharmacology: A Generation of Progress.* New York, Raven Press, 1978, pp 905–915.
64. Spitzer RL, Endicott J, Robins E: Research Diagnostic Criteria (RDC) for a selected group of functional disorders. New York, Biometrics Division, New York State Psychiatric Institute, 1978.
65. Tune LE, Creese I, DePaulo JR, et al: Clinical state and serum neuroleptic levels measured by radioreceptor assay in schizophrenia. *Am J Psychiatry* 1980;137:187–190.
66. Rivera-Calimlim L, Nasrallah H, Strauss JJ, et al: Clinical response and plasma levels: Effect of dose, dosage schedules, and drug interactions on plasma chlorpromazine levels. *Am J Psychiatry* 1976;133:646–652.
67. Loga S, Curry S, Lader M: Interactions of orphenadrine and phenobarbitone with chlorpromazine: Plasma concentrations and effects in man. *Br J Clin Pharmacol* 1975;2:197–208.
68. May PRA, Van Putten T, Jenden DJ, et al: Chlorpromazine levels and the outcome of treatment in schizophrenic patients. *Arch Gen Psychiatry* 1981; 38:202–207.
69. Sakuri Y, Nakahara T, Takahashi R: Prediction of response to chlorpromazine treatment in schizophrenics. *Psychopharmacologia (Berlin)* 1975; 44:195–203.
70. Sakurai Y, Takahasi R, Nakahara T, et al: Prediction of response to and actual outcome of chlorpromazine treatment in schizophrenic patients. *Arch Gen Psychiatry* 1980;37:1057–1062.
71. Wiles DH, Kolakowska T, McNeilly AS, et al: Clinical significance of plasma chlorpromazine levels: Plasma levels of the drug, some of its metabolites, and prolactin during acute treatment. *Psychol Med* 1976;6:407–415.
72. Magliozzi JR, Hollister LE, Arnold KV, et al: Relationship of serum haloperidol levels to clinical response in schizophrenic patients. *Am J Psychiatry* 1981;138:365–367.
73. Extein I, Augusthy A, Gold M, et al: Plasma haloperidol levels and clinical response in acute schizophrenia. *Psychopharm Bull* 1982;18:156–158.
74. Javaid JI, Davis JM, Dysken MW, et al: Neuroleptic concentrations in schizophrenic patients: Measurement by radioreceptor assay and gas chromotography. *Psychopharm Bull* 1982;18:72–74.
75. Casper R, Garver DL, Dekirmenjian H, et al: Phenothiazine levels in plasma and red blood cells. *Arch Gen Psychiatry* 1980;37:301–305.
76. Reifler BV, Ward N, Davis CM, et al: Thiothixene plasma levels and clinical response in acute schizophrenia. *J Clin Psychiatry* 1981;42:207–211.
77. Johnstone EC, Bourne RC, Cotes PM, et al: Blood levels of flupenthixol in patients with acute and chronic schizophrenia. *Ciba Found Symp* 1980; 74:99–114.
78. Gottschalk LA, Biener R, Nobel EP, et al: Thioridazine plasma levels and clinical response. *Compr Psychiatry* 1975;16:323–337.
79. Yesavage JA, Becker J, Werner PD, et al: Serum level monitoring of thiothixene in schizophrenia: Acute single-dose levels at fixed doses. *Am J Psychiatry* 1982;139:174–178.
80. Van Putten T, May PRA, Jenden DJ, et al: Plasma and saliva levels of

chlorpromazine and subjective response. *Am J Psychiatry* 1980; 137:1241–1242.

81. Van Putten T, May PRA, Wilkens JN: Importance of akinesia: Plasma chlorpromazine and prolactin levels. *Am J Psychiatry* 1980;137:1446–1448.
82. May PRA, Goldberg SC: Prediction of schizophrenia patients' response to pharmacotherapy, in Lipton MA, DiMascio A, Killam KF, (eds): *Psychopharmacology: A Generation of Progress.* New York, Raven Press, 1978, pp 1139–1153.
83. Robins E, Guze S: Establishment of diagnostic validity in psychiatric illness: Its application to schizophrenia. *Am J Psychiatry* 1970;126:983–987.
84. Klein DF, Rosen B: Premorbid asocial adjustment and response to phenothiazine treatment among schizophrenic inpatients. *Arch Gen Psychiatry* 1973;29:480–485.
85. Keniston K, Boltax S, Almond R: Multiple criteria of treatment outcome. *J Psychiatr Res* 1971;8:107–118.
86. Strauss JS, Carpenter WT Jr: The prediction of outcome in schizophrenia. I. Characteristics of outcome. *Arch Gen Psychiatry* 1972;27:739–746.
87. Strauss JS, Carpenter WT, Jr: The prediction of outcome in schizophrenia. II. Relationships between predictor and outcome variables. *Arch Gen Psychiatry* 1974;31:37–42.
88. American Psychiatric Association: *Diagnostic and Statistical Manual of Mental Disorders.* ed 3. Washington, DC, American Psychiatric Association, 1980.
89. Singh MM, Smith JM: Kinetics and dynamics of response to haloperidol in acute schizophrenia: A longitudinal study of the therapeutic process. *Compr Psychiatry* 1973;14:393–414.
90. Van Putten T, May PRA: Subjective response as a predictor of outcome in pharmacotherapy: The consumer has a point. *Arch Gen Psychiatry* 1978;35:477–480.
91. May PRA, Van Putten T, Yale C: Predicting outcome of antipsychotic drug treatment from early response. *Am J Psychiatry* 1980;137:1088–1089.
92. Brill NQ, Crumpton E, Eiduson S, et al: Relative effectiveness of various components of ECT. *AMA Arch Neurol Psychiatry* 1959;81:627–635.
93. May PR: *Treatment of Schizophrenia.* New York, Science House, 1968.
94. Childers RT: Comparison of four regimes in newly admitted female schizophrenics. *Am J Psychiatry* 1964;120:1010–1011.
95. Siris SG, Glassman AH, Stetner F: ECT and psychotropic medications in the treatment of depression and schizophrenia, in Essman WB, Abrams R (eds): *Electroconvulsive Therapies: Biological Foundations and Clinical Applications.* New York, Spectrum Publications, 1982.
96. Taylor P, Fleminger JJ: ECT for schizophrenia. *Lancet* 1980;1:1380–1383.
97. Ries RK, Wilson L, Bokan JA, et al: ECT in medication resistant schizoaffective disorder. *Compr Psychiatry* 1981;22:167–173.
98. Yorkston NJ, Zaki SA, Pitcher DR, et al: Propranolol as an adjunct to the treatment of schizophrenia. *Lancet* 1977;2:575–578.
99. Lindstrom L, Persson E: Propranolol in chronic schizophrenia: A controlled study in neuroleptic treated patients. *Br J Psychiatry* 1980;137:126–130.
100. Myers DH, Campbell L, Cocks NM, et al: A trial of propranolol in chronic schizophrenia. *Br J Psychiatry* 1981;139:118–121.
101. Peet M, Middlemiss DN, Yates RA: Propranolol in schizophrenia. II. Clinical and biochemical aspects of combining propranolol with chlorpromazine. *Br J Psychiatry* 1981;138:112–117.
102. King DJ, Turkson SNA, Leddle J, et al: Some clinical and metabolic

aspects of propranolol in chronic schizophrenia. *Br J Psychiatry* 1980:137; 458–468.

103. Yorkston NJ, Zaki SA, Weller MP, et al: DL-propranolol and chlorpromazine following admission for schizophrenia. *Acta Psychiat Scand* 1981;63:13–27.
104. Peet M, Bethell MS, Coates A, et al: Propranolol in schizophrenia. I. Comparison of propranolol, chlorpromazine and placebo. *Br J Psychiatry* 1981; 139:105–111.
105. Hollister LE, Bennett JJ, Kimbell I Jr, et al: Diazepam in newly admitted schizophrenics. *Dis Nerv Syst* 1963;24:746–750.
106. Maculans GA: Comparison of diazepam, chlordiazepoxide, and chlorpromazine in chronic schizophrenic patients. *Dis Nerv Syst* 1964;25: 164–168.
107. Gundlach R, Engelhardt DM, Hankoff L, et al: A double blind out-patient study of diazepam (Valium) and placebo. *Psychopharmacologie* 1966;9: 81–92.
108. Holden JMC, Itil TM, Keskiner A, et al: Thioridazine and chlordiazepoxide, alone and combined, in the treatment of chronic schizophrenia. *Compr Psychiatry* 1968;9:633–643.
109. Holden JMC, Holden UP: Weight changes with schizophrenic psychosis and psychotropic drug therapy. *Psychosomatics* 1970;11:551–561.
110. Kellner R, Wilson RM, Muldauer MD, et al: Anxiety in schizophrenia—the responses to chlordiazepoxide in an intensive design study. *Arch Gen Psychiatry* 1975;32:1246–1254.
111. Nestoros JN: Benzodiazepines in schizophrenia: A need for reassessment. *Int Pharmacopsychiatry* 1980;15:171–179.
112. Meltzer HY, Stahl SM: The dopamine hypothesis of schizophrenia: A review. *Schizophr Bull* 1976;2:19–76.
113. Carlsson A: Antipsychotic drugs, neurotransmitters and schizophrenia. *Am J Psychiatry* 1978;135:164–173.
114. van Kammen DP: GABA and the dopamine hypothesis of schizophrenia. *Am J Psychiatry* 1977;134:138–143.
115. Fuxe K, Anderson K, Ogren S-O, et al: GABA neurons and their interactions with monoamine neurons. An anatomical, pharmacological and functional analysis, in Krogsgaard-Larsen P, Scheel-Kruger J, Kofod H (eds): *GABA-Neuro Transmitters.* Copenhagen, Munksgaard, 1978, pp 74–94.
116. Casey DE, Gerlach J, Christensen E: Behavioral aspects of GABA-dopamine interrelationships in the monkey. *Brain Res Bull* 1979;4:489.
117. Costa E, Guidotti A: Malecular mechanisms in the receptor action of benzodiazepines. *Am Rev Pharmacol Toxicol* 1979;19:531–545.
118. Beckmann H, Haas S: High dose diazepam in schizophrenia. *Psychopharmacology* 1980;71:79–82.
119. Nair NPV, Nestoros JN, Schwartz G: High doses of diazepam improve neuroleptic-resistant schizophrenic patients. Presented at Annual Meeting of the Canadian Psychiatric Association, Winnipeg, Sept 23–25, 1981.
120. Prien RF, Caffey EM, Klett CJ: A comparison of lithium carbonate and chlorpromazine in the treatment of excited schizoaffectives. *Arch Gen Psychiatry* 1972;27:182–189.
121. Biederman J, Lerner Y, Belmaker RH: Combination of lithium carbonate and haloperidol in schizoaffective disorder: A controlled study. *Arch Gen Psychiatry* 1979;36:327–333.
122. Small JG, Kellams JJ, Milstein V, et al: A placebo controlled study of lithium combined with neuroleptics in chronic schizophrenic patients. *Am J*

Psychiatry 1975;132:1315–1317.
123. Kasanin J: The acute schizoaffective psychoses. *Am J Psychiatry* 1933;13: 97–126.
124. Procci WR: Schizoaffective psychosis: Fact or fiction? A survey of the literature. *Arch Gen Psychiatry* 1976;33:1167–1178.
125. Pope HG Jr, Lipinski JF Jr: Diagnosis in schizophrenia and manic-depressive illness: A reassessment of the specificity of 'schizophrenic' symptoms in the light of current research. *Arch Gen Psychiatry* 1978;35:811–828.
126. Pope HG Jr, Lipinski JF, Cohen BM, et al: "Schizoaffective disorder": An invalid diagnosis? A comparison of schizoaffective disorder, schizophrenia, and affective disorder. *Am J Psychiatry* 1980;137:921–927.
127. Zall H, Therman PG, Myers JM: Lithium carbonate: A clinical study. *Am J Psychiatry* 1968;125:549–555.
128. Aronoff MS, Epstein RS: Factors associated with poor response to lithium carbonate: A clinical study. *Am J Psychiatry* 1970;127:472–480.
129. Lipkin KM, Dyrud J, Meyer GG: The many faces of mania: Therapeutic trial of lithium carbonate. *Arch Gen Psychiatry* 1970;22:262–267.
130. Dinsmore PR, Ryback R: Lithium in schizoaffective disorders. *Dis Nerv Syst* 1972;33:771–776.
131. Carlson GA, Goodwin FK: The stages of mania: A longitudinal analysis of the manic episode. *Arch Gen Psychiatry* 1973;28:221–228.
132. Taylor MA, Abrams R: The phenomenology of mania: A new look at some old patients. *Arch Gen Psychiatry* 1973;29:520–522.
133. Taylor MA, Abrams R: Acute mania: Clinical and genetic study of responders and non-responders to treatments. *Arch Gen Psychiatry* 1975; 32:863–865.
134. Alexander PE, van Kammen DP, Bunney WE Jr: Antipsychotic effects of lithium in schizophrenia. *Am J Psychiatry* 1979;136:283–287.
135. Bunney WE Jr, Hamburg DS: Methods for reliable longitudinal observation of behavior. *Arch Gen Psychiatry* 1963;9:280–294.
136. Brockington IF, Kendell RE, Kellett JM, et al: Trials of lithium, chlorpromazine and amitriptyline in schizoaffective patients. *Br J Psychiatry* 1978;133:162–168.
137. Johnson G, Gershon S, Hekimian LJ: Controlled evaluation of lithium and chlorpromazine in the treatment of manic states: An interim report. *Compr Psychiatry* 1968;9:563–573.
138. Johnson G: Differential response to lithium carbonate in manic depressive and schizoaffective disorders. *Dis Nerv Syst* 1970;31:613–615.
139. Johnson G, Gershon S, Burdock EI, et al: Comparative effects of lithium and chlorpromazine in the treatment of manic states. *Br J Psychiatry* 1971; 119:267–276.
140. Carman JS, Bigelow LB, Wyatt RJ: Lithium combined with neuroleptics in chronic schizophrenic and schizoaffective patients. *J Clin Psychiatry* 1981; 42:124–128.
141. Cohen WJ, Cohen NH: Lithium carbonate, haloperidol, and irreversible brain damage. *JAMA* 1974;230:1283–1287.
142. Baastrup PC, Hollnagel P, Sorensen R, et al: Adverse reactions in treatment with lithium carbonate and haloperidol. *JAMA* 1976;236:2645–2646.
143. Hirschowitz J, Casper R, Garver DL, et al: Lithium response in good prognosis schizophrenia. *Am J Psychiatry* 1980;137:916–920.

CHAPTER 10

DRUG TREATMENT OF DEPRESSION IN PATIENTS WITH SCHIZOPHRENIA

SAMUEL G. SIRIS
ARTHUR RIFKIN

Even when the diagnostic issues are set aside which becloud the interface between schizophrenia and affective disorders,[1,2] a multitude of course-related "depression-like" symptoms still may occur in patients with schizophrenia. After an acute psychotic episode subsides, schizophrenic patients quite frequently may present a gloomy appearance. At times, in conjunction with this, they may complain of sadness, apathy, or boredom. They often anticipate failure or claim incompetence, and their self-esteem may be quite low. When questioned, they may feel guilt or shame. The patients then may attribute this guilt or shame to behavior which they engaged in while psychotic, to fantasies which they had at that time, or simply to the fact of having developed a serious psychiatric illness. Whatever the true cause (and it may well be possible that the explanations are coming as rationalizations after the fact in some of these cases), the affect involved is painful. Furthermore, the patients' ability to concentrate may be poor. After the resolution of an acute psychosis, schizophrenic patients also often have difficulty in mobilizing initiative. Common tasks and pastimes may seem to require great effort, and patients may present a picture of more or less generalized lack of interest in their usual activities and pleasures. Libido may be decreased, and patients may complain of fatigue. Such patients may become withdrawn and isolated and may come to feel and show little concern for their appearance or other social amenities. A reduction in motor activities may be manifest, and patients may stare a lot, creating a "wooden" appearance. Anorexia or weight loss may sometimes be present. Alternatively, some patients demonstrate an increased appetite and weight gain. Sleep disturbances may be present, including early, middle, and late insomnia, hypersomnia, or day-night reversal of the normal sleeping pattern. Such patients may also express morbid thoughts, including death fantasies, suicidal ideation, and nihilistic notions of various kinds.

Clinically, symptoms such as these have much in common with depression, although the patients are schizophrenic.

Upward of a dozen papers in the clinical literature have described these symptoms as being organized into a specific syndrome of one sort or another which evolves after the resolution of an acute psychotic episode. Eissler spoke of the "phase of relative clinical muteness" in schizophrenia,[3] Semrad spoke of the "neurasthenic phase,"[4] and McGlashan and Carpenter spoke of a "post-psychotic depression syndrome."[5] Additionally, there are many anecdotal clinical reports which, of course, do not agree exactly on the features of a depression-like syndrome that follows the acute psychosis in schizophrenia, but which do describe a syndrome that exists and that presents a difficult and stubborn clinical challenge. At times, the morbidity of the situation for these patients is rivaled only by the frustration of their families and by the exasperation of the treating clinician.

A variety of untoward events may be associated with a post-psychotic depression syndrome. First, there may be a premature termination of the treatment (initiated either by the patient, his family, or the clinician), which serves to deprive the patient of help when it is desperately needed. In this case, the patient may wind up being abandoned to a single room occupancy building, a state hospital, or simply to his family or community without sufficient follow-up care. Second, the patient may commit suicide. It is recognized that some schizophrenic patients do commit suicide;[6] although the proper studies have not been done to document this fully, general clinical experience would suggest that suicidal risk may be high during postpsychotic periods of hopelessness. A third untoward event that may take place is that the patient may become psychotic again. Discouraged by lack of improvement, the patient may discontinue medications, attempt to enter situations for which he is not yet prepared, or be pushed onto untenable ground by his impatient environment. Any of these factors could predispose to future decompensation. Fourth, the patient's situation may continue unchanged, which also is not a very desirable outcome.

There have been at least 11 well-organized studies of depression or depression-like symptoms in schizophrenia, documenting the incidence and seriousness of this disorder. Bowers and Astrachan found that half of 36 schizophrenic patients had depressive symptoms, either depressed mood, psychomotor retardation, lack of initiative, or withdrawal, during the postpsychotic period.[7] Steinberg et al examined the records of 41 schizophrenic patients who had received neuroleptics and scrutinized eight who had entered a six-week remission during the course of their hospital stay.[8] These eight patients were found to have disproportionately high scores on depression items. Of course, the question may be asked as to why these patients had not been discharged in comparison with the others. Perhaps their depressions were the reason, so that the true denominator in this study would be more likely to be 41 than to be 8. Shanfield et al followed 44 schizophrenic patients and compared them with a control group of 36 depressed patients.[9] In this series, during treatment, the depression rates decreased more slowly for the schizophrenic patients. Shanfield et al postulated that this represented evidence of a postpsychotic depression syndrome, although such a conclusion would be thrown into question by the ordinary natural history of depression (the patients in the control group), in that the natural history of depression is for many patients to get better rapidly when treated. In Shanfield's cohort the depressive ratings did not actually increase in the schizophrenic group, so this study cannot be counted as unequivocal evidence supporting the existence of a postpsychotic depression syndrome. Stern et al followed 17 schizophrenic patients and found that 2 developed severe depressions and 6 developed mild to moderate depressions.[10] This, however, was a difficult study to interpret in that 43% of the follow-up was by telephone in an overwhelmingly lower socioeconomic group of patients.

Most of the above studies have the drawback that the criteria for the diagnosis of schizophrenia were not carefully spelled out. Thus, they leave open the possibility that patients with affective disorders or other nonschizophrenic psychoses were included among the study results.

McGlashan and Carpenter[11] carefully followed the course of 30 schizophrenic patients, diagnosed according to the criteria of the International Pilot Study of Schizophrenia.[12] They found a bimodal distribution of depressive symptoms in these patients. Thirteen clearly had more depressive symptoms in the hospital after the resolution of their psychoses than did the other 17. This was despite the fact that both groups had similar depression ratings while psychotic. McGlashan and Carpenter found that these depressive symptoms predicted poorer rather than better social outcome, contrary to the usual finding that affective symptoms in schizophrenic patients, while psychotic, are a positive prognostic indicator. Unfortunately, the severity of the depression in the more depressed group of patients was not further explicated.

Montgomery used the research diagnostic criteria[13] to diagnose patients with acute schizophrenia in whom he then looked for symptoms of depression.[14] He found a high mean incidence of "depressive symptoms" of 61%. Furthermore, this incidence was not substantially reduced by excluding three items which seemed to be common in the scales for rating schizophrenia and depression. In a large study, Johnson found clear-cut symptoms of depression in approximately half of 37 untreated new acute schizophrenic patients and in approximately 1/3 of 168 patients with chronic schizophrenia who were experiencing relapses.[15] In this study the diagnosis of schizophrenia had been based upon the presence of Schneiderian first-rank symptoms.[16] Knights and Hirsch found that the depressive symptoms are more prevalent during the acute phase of schizophrenia and that their severity abates over time with neuroleptic treatment.[17] However, 22% of 37 schizophrenic patients were found to have developed depression de novo at a six-month follow-up interview. Roy[18] found that 39 out of 100 patients with chronic undifferentiated schizophrenia who had met the criteria of DSM-III[19] were treated for a depressive syndrome. In an outpatient study which followed 211 schizophrenic patients, Mandel et al found that approximately 25% of these patients developed symptoms of depression within five months after hospital discharge.[20] This proportion of depression was the same whether patients had been being maintained on oral fluphenazine or fluphenazine decanoate; once again, in this study it was confirmed that patients who developed depressions seemed to have had a less favorable psychiatric course in that their history was more chronic.

Siris et al[21] conducted a retrospective review of 50 hospitalized patients who had been diagnosed as having schizophrenia in accordance with the research diagnostic criteria.[13] As shown in Table 10-1, as many as 40% of these patients experienced some symptoms of depression after the resolution of their psychoses, but only 6% had the full syndromal manifestation of a major depression; 22%, however, had symptoms consistent with the diagnosis of a minor depression syndrome during the postpsychotic interval.

Taken together, the above studies, plus others of a more anecdotal nature,[22–26] present compelling evidence that a depression-like syndrome commonly complicates the postpsychotic course in schizophrenic patients.

Of course it is by no means certain that the course-related depressive syndromes in schizophrenia have a unitary basis. Most probably, they do not. Although any categories would need to be validated (and we would not yet know precisely how to distinguish such categories phenomenologically), we might speculate that there are at least four different circumstances which could lead to the development of a postpsychotic depression in schizophrenia.

First, there would be those patients for whom an affective disregulation in the direction of dysphoria is a fundamental part of their disorder. Along this line, attention, of course, has been focused on patients having "schizo-affective disorder," if such an entity truly exists,[1,2] either as a subgroup of patients with schizophrenia, as a subgroup of patients with major affective disorders, as a distinct subgroup of its own, or as a heterogeneous grouping of patients. But even beyond a group designated as schizo-affective per se, anhedonia, flattening of affect, and/or inappropriateness of affect have long been described as core symptoms of at

Table 10-1
Distribution of Depressive Symptoms in 50 Patients with a Diagnosis of Schizophrenia During Their Postpsychotic Phase of Hospitalization

Symptoms*	No. of Patients	% of Sample
1. Subjective sadness	20	40
2. Appears depressed	17	34
3. Sleep disturbance	14	28
4. Appetite/eating disturbance	2	4
5. Low energy	10	20
6. Psychomotor agitation/retardation	20†	40
7. Diminished interest/pleasure	1	2
8. Guilt/self-reproach	0	0
9. Inability to concentrate or decide (other than thought disorder)	2	4
10. Thoughts of death or suicide	2	4
11. Tearful/sad face	1	2
12. Pessimism	2	4
13. Brooding	2	4
14. Feels inadequate	0	0
15. Resentment/irritation	8	16
16. Demanding/dependent	7	14
17. Self-pity	0	0
18. Somatic concern	8	16
19. Symptoms of major depression syndrome†	3	6
20. Symptoms of minor depression syndrome§	11	22

*Symptom definitions taken from research diagnostic criteria.
†Agitation only, 12 (24%); retardation only, 6 (12%); both, 2 (4%).
‡Symptom 1 plus at least four of symptoms 3–10.
§Symptom 1 plus at least two of symptoms 3–18.

least some schizophrenic patients. If such is the case, adjunctive use of antidepressant medications may well be helpful to a number of these patients in whom dysphoric affect predominates.

Second would be those cases for whom a biologically based affective disorder might occur as a side effect of neuroleptic medication. It could be speculated that the action of neuroleptics in blockading the receptors for certain brain monoamines might lead to a biologically based affective disorder as a neuroleptic side effect in some individuals. It is worthy of note in this regard that the dopamine synapse, with which the neuroleptic drugs specifically interact, has been implicated in the switch process between mania and depression.[27]

An alternative process might involve the fact that neuroleptic medications are not entirely "clean" in their spectrum of activity and may have action at noradrenergic and serotonergic loci as well as at dopaminergic sites. In line with this speculation, some clinical observations have particularly alleged that long-acting depot neuroleptic preparations may be particularly prone to cause depression in some patients.[28,29] On the other hand, such a finding is by no means clearly established, since some double-blind controlled studies have found the placebo group to demonstrate depression just as frequently as the active drug group,[30,31] and neuroleptic drugs are known to be a usable treatment for patients with agitated depressions. More recently, this issue may have been clarified somewhat by Johnson, who found that, although depression was more common in those patients who were receiving higher maintenance doses of depot neuroleptics, patients who maintained their remissions on more moderate depot antipsychotic regimens seemed to have the lowest prevalence of depressive symptomatology.[15] Again, in the subgroup of patients who might be experiencing depression as a side effect to their neuroleptic medication, adjunctive antidepressive medication might be a rational course of treatment. Plainly, of course, decreasing the neuroleptic dosage might be of substantial value in this group as well, and the clinician should be comfortable that he or she is not giving the patient more antipsychotic medicine than is necessary before beginning treatment with an additional psychopharmacological agent.

A third group of patients who may give the appearance of a postpsychotic depression syndrome would be those who are experiencing akinesia as an extrapyramidal side effect of neuroleptic medication.[32,33] Although extrapyramidal in nature, this side effect need not necessarily be accompanied by other prominent manifestations of extrapyramidal side effects and can be extremely difficult to distinguish, clinically, from a picture of depression. Akinesia is a seemingly pleasureless and/or amotivational state in which the patient seems to be a "bump on a log." Withdrawn and nonparticipating for reasons that do not often make sense to the patient himself, the patient may complain of boredom or other dysphoric affects quite akin to depression. Such a situation, when diagnosed, often responds favorably to the addition of antiparkinsonian medication. In fact, the response to antiparkinsonian medication may be quite dramatic within a period as short as a day or two. Again, decreasing neuroleptic dosage might also favorably influence a depression-like state that is the result of akinesia. The subject of akinesia is further discussed in Chapter 11.

Finally, there are doubtless also patients who are suffering from a demoralization syndrome[34] after recovery from their acute psychotic decompensation. Faced with a serious illness such as schizophrenia, and with the anticipation that it might alter life's aspirations and attainments in multiple spheres, patients might indeed have reason to become demoralized. "Coming down with schizophrenia" is bad news for the patient, just as it would be bad news to learn that one has now developed any other serious, chronic, or potentially relapsing condition. There is no special reason to presume that a pharmacological intervention would mitigate this disappointment. On the other hand, the proper form of intensive psychosocial intervention might be most rational to employ in those patients who have a demoralization syndrome. Unfortunately, we do not as yet know how properly to make the differential diagnosis between this condition and the others mentioned above for which changes in pharmacological management might well be the best course of treatment.

THE USE OF ANTIDEPRESSANTS IN SCHIZOPHRENIA

There is little evidence to support the usefulness of antidepressant drugs, when used alone, in the treatment of schizophrenia. In fact, the clear impression from the available, mostly anecdotal literature is that use of such agents in schizophrenic patients, in the absence of concomitant neuroleptic treatment, carries a grave risk of deterioration in the patient's clinical state.[35] In a review of 14 studies, in which schizophrenic patients were treated with antidepressants, this general conclusion seemed to hold up for both tricyclic antidepressants and monoamine oxidase inhibitors.[35–53] It should be noted, however, that in only one of these studies[45] were those schizophrenics treated with antidepressants noted to have symptoms of depression. Most studies involved patients described as schizophrenic, without operationalized diagnostic criteria given, who were treated with antidepressants in an unselected way. Interestingly, the one study which did note that patients were selected on the basis of demonstrating features of depression showed that these patients improved along the dimensions of those features.[45] Otherwise, antidepressant drugs in general led to activation of patients without any definite clinical improvement. Patients who deteriorated often become more irritable, accelerated, and fragmented. They tended to have increased subjective anxiety, and they tended to complain more and argue more. Often hallucinations and delusions were noted to increase, and patients were noted to become disorganized and bizarre.

The only group of patients identified as "schizophrenic" who seemed to be improved by antidepressants were those who were identified as "pseudoneurotic schizophrenics," patients who almost certainly would not be diagnosed as schizophrenic by modern criteria.[39–41,51] These were patients who lacked Kraepelinian or Schneiderian signs of schizophrenia. They were described as anxious, anhedonic patients who were prone to obsessive-compulsive symptoms and somatic preoccupations. Often in childhood they were noted to have histories of being dependent, shy, obedient, and phobic. These patients stood out from all the others in this series by showing a favorable response to antidepressant medications used alone.

A larger number of controlled studies have been done involving the coadministration of a tricyclic or similar antidepressant and a neuroleptic in patients diagnosed as having schizophrenia.[35,46,47,54–69] Among the earlier studies in this series, most were of one of two designs: studies in which amitriptyline and perphenazine were administered beginning simultaneously, and others in which a phenothiazine, usually chlorpromazine, was given for a period of time with imipramine then being added. The frequent testing of the perphenazine-amitriptyline combination was fostered by the availability of combined preparations of these two compounds being marketed by two different pharmaceutical houses. In none of these controlled studies was amitriptyline given with any neuroleptic other than perphenazine. On the other hand, imipramine was never given with perphenazine, and in only one study was imipramine begun simultaneously with a phenothiazine. Thus, unfortunately, a clear comparison could not be made in these early studies between the usefulness of amitriptyline and imipramine under these circumstances.

The early studies, however, did not demonstrate much merit to either antidepressant being used in combination with a phenothiazine. But again it must be borne in mind that depressed-appearing patients with schizophrenia were not singled out for these trials. In the case where such depressed-appearing patients were isolated, at least statistically, there was the impression that those patients, and only those patients, did appear to do somewhat better on the combination of phenothiazine and antidepressant.[54,58,61]

More recently, there has been a retrospective study that compared the usefulness to patients of amitriptyline and imipramine, in combination with a neuroleptic, for schizophrenic and schizo-affective patients with "postpsychotic depressions" in a general clinical setting.[70] The patients in this series had been diagnosed according to the Research Diagnostic Criteria.[13] Ten of the 14 patients receiving adjunctive imipramine achieved a marked improvement or remission, whereas only 2 of the 11 patients treated with amitriptyline improved that much. This difference is statistically significant. The finding, however, must be interpreted with all of the cautions appropriate to a retrospective review. Particularly, it must be noted that patient assignment was not random. In other words, there may have been a factor involved in the patients' clinical state which influenced the clinician's free drug choice—a factor which might also have had prognostic implications. Nevertheless, the fact that 12 of the 25 patients in this entire series experienced marked improvement or remission of depressive symptoms, whereas only one patient underwent a clinical deterioration, is worthy of note.

Although other recent studies have shed substantial light on the issue of treatment of schizophrenic patients with depressive features with adjunctive antidepressant medication in combination with their neuroleptic regimen, the issue of this rationale of treatment has still not been clearly resolved. Prusoff et al studied 35 well-diagnosed ambulatory schizophrenic patients who had such "depressive symptoms" as anhedonia, sadness, and anergia, which in some cases were accompanied by sleep and/or appetite disturbances.[71] These patients were treated with perphenazine, on a flexible dosage schedule, and with amitriptyline, again in a flexible dosage, or placebo then being added for a double-blind trial over the course of three to six months. Patients receiving the perphenazine-amitriptyline combination were found to report less depression, although they had greater thought disorder at the end point and more agitation. These differences were statistically significant. The authors interpreted these results as being positive, in that they had found the beneficial changes to be affecting many patients rather than just a few.

Singh et al[72] looked at the combination of trazodone (300 mg per day) or placebo with various phenothiazines in 60 chronically hospitalized "depressed" schizophrenics diagnosed in accordance with the Feighner Criteria.[73] The phenothiazines had been adjusted to each patient's own individual best dose. After a six-week trial, the trazodone-treated group was clearly and statistically better off than the placebo-treated group with reference to items related to depression. Clinical deterioration was not observed, and there were few side effects.

On the other hand, Johnson[15] followed 50 schizophrenic patients who had been diagnosed by the Feigner Criteria and who had developed an acute episode of depression. These patients were all on a depot neuroleptic to which either nortriptyline or placebo was added double-blind for five weeks. The final nortriptyline dose in this study was 150 mg per day. Johnson found no statistically significant difference in the alleviation of depression symptoms between the nortriptyline- and placebo-treated groups, although it was noted in the data that seven patients receiving nortriptyline had a "good improvement" in their mood state versus only two for placebo. It was found, however, with statistical significance that patients treated with nortriptyline developed more side effects. A cautionary note, though, with regard to the interpretation of this study is that the nortriptyline doses employed were quite high. Ordinary maximal doses of nortriptyline are in the range of 100 mg per day, and it is considered that a therapeutic window exists for plasma nortriptyline concentrations in depression, so that if this therapeutic range is exceeded the efficacy of the drug is lost.[74-76] Furthermore, with reference to both the possible exceeding of nortriptyline's therapeutic window and the incidence of side effects observed at this dose, the observation is salient that neuroleptic compounds compete for the same hepatic cytochrome P-450 system which metabolizes tricyclic antidepressants, so that higher than expected blood levels of tricyclic antidepressants are observed when they are coadministered with neuroleptic drugs.[77–80] This last factor is a cautionary one with regard to potential adverse effects in combining any tricyclic antidepressant with a neuroleptic, so that doses should be conservative, cardiograms should be monitored appropriately, and blood levels of the drugs should be obtained where practical.

A dozen controlled, double-blind studies have failed to provide evidence that the combination of a monoamine oxidase inhibitor and a neuroleptic is of particular benefit in schizophrenia.[50,51,55,56,81–88] Again it must be noted, though, that these patients in general did not include people with clear features of depression other than possible anergia or anhedonia. One study which did look specifically at the symptom of "depression" did find that symptom improved significantly when tranylcypromine was added to trifluoperazine.[51] On the other hand, the largest study in this series made a direct comparison of the chlorpromazine-isocarboxazid combination with the chlorpromazine-imipramine combination and found the phenothiazine-monoamine oxidase inhibitor combination to be inferior to the phenothiazine-tricyclic antidepressant combination, with statistical significance, on several submeasures including "agitated depression."[55] The issue of the usefulness of the monoamine oxidase inhibitors in combination with neuroleptic medication among schizophrenic patients with specific symptoms or syndromes of depression has not been investigated with a well controlled prospective study.

A review of the literature suggests that there are two specific categories of schizophrenic patients who would be poor risks for trials of an adjunctive antidepressant.[35] The first of these includes patients with marked degrees of agitation. It has been widely noted in the literature that patients with substantial degrees of agitation are noted to worsen with the introduction of antidepressant medications. Of course, in this context, agitation needs to be differentiated from the extrapyramidal neuroleptic side effect of akathisia—a differential diagnosis which is not always easy to make, or which at times may be impossible to make prospectively with certainty. Since akathisia is an extrapyramidal side effect, the most useful treatment of this form of agitation is either lowering the dose of neuroleptic medication or providing the patient with adequate amounts of an antiparkinsonian agent. Although tricyclic antidepressants may have anticholinergic properties, they are probably not very good as antiparkinsonian agents. At least this has been clearly demonstrated in the case of imipramine in combination with fluphenazine decanoate.[89] Patients switched in a double-blind fashion from benztropine (6 mg per day total dose) to imipramine (150–200 mg per day total dose) were noted to have a clear worsening of extrapyramidal side effects.[89] This may have been due either to the relative lessening of anticholinergic effect involved in that medication switch (150–200 mg of imipramine per day would have roughly the equivalent anticholinergic potency of 2 mg of benztropine per day if in vitro work can be extrapolated to the clinical situation,[90]) to an increase in the blood concentrations of the neuroleptic after the introduction of the tricyclic antidepressant due to the fact that they both compete for the same hepatic enzyme system,[80,91] or to both.

The second group of patients with schizophrenia who are a poor risk for an antidepressant medication trial includes those schizophrenic patients with a premorbid history of childhood asociality. These are patients who never had a history of reasonable social adjustment, even in childhood, and who were always picked on, scapegoated, and excluded. Later, when psychotic, they tended to be vague, perplexed, fragmented, and fearful.[92] When such patients are treated with antidepressant medications, they often tend to have exacerbations of their psychosis.[39,40,93–97] At times this deterioration tended to follow a biphasic course, with the patient's mood at first brightening, but after a couple of weeks the patient became substantially more psychotic in a way that was difficult to manage with neuroleptics.[92]

In conclusion, several points should be emphasized in the treatment of symptoms or syndromes of depression in schizophrenia. First is the issue of differential diagnosis between depression and the extrapyramidal side effect of akinesia in patients receiving neuroleptic medication. Akinesia can look very much like depression and, at times, may be virtually indistinguishable clinically. Therefore, the first step in treating an apparent depression in the course of schizophrenia is to make sure that the patient is receiving an adequate dose of anticholinergic antiparkinsonian medication. In conjunction with this, it is important as well to be sure that the patient is not receiving a higher dosage of neuroleptic medication than is necessary to control manifestations of psychosis. Such an approach might also be helpful to any patients who are experiencing depression itself as a side effect to neuroleptic medication on a biochemical basis—if, indeed, this theoretical possibility occurs in some individuals.

After the akinesia side effect has been ruled out, if the patient still manifests a depression of a magnitude that suggests treatment, it is possible that the addition of an antidepressant medication may be helpful. Under this circumstance, there are more data to support the addition of a tricyclic antidepressant than to support the addition of a monoamine oxidase inhibitor.[35,98] By all means, the neuroleptic medication should be continued during the antidepressant trial. Patients should be closely monitored for side effects since the neuroleptic and the tricyclic antidepressant interfere with each other's metabolism, so that the patient may well have higher concentrations of each of these drugs in his system than would otherwise be anticipated. With this in mind, a gradual addition of tricyclic antidepressant is probably best. Antidepressant medication should then be maintained for at least two months (barring exacerbations or side effects) before the conclusion is reached that its addition was ineffective (S. G. Siris, unpublished data).

Due to the risk of exacerbation of extrapyramidal symptoms if the antiparkinsonian medication is discontinued during a tricyclic antidepressant trial, the antiparkinsonian medication should be maintained. Certainly, of course, under these circumstances, the patient should be closely observed for increased anticholinergic side effects. In consideration of the risks of these anticholinergic side effects, highly anticholinergic neuroleptic agents (such as thioridazine or chlorpromazine) or more highly anticholinergic tricyclic antidepressants (such as amitriptyline or doxepin) should be avoided in the combined treatment period.

During such a trial, a slight recrudescence of psychotic symptoms may occur. This need not occasion a discontinuation of the trial, since such a situation may be well managed with adjustments of neuroleptic or tricyclic antidepressant dosage under close supervision. Any gross psychotic exacerbation, of course, would occasion a termination of such a trial. The occurrence of a serious psychotic exacerbation, however, among properly selected patients who are well documented to be receiving their neuroleptic medication as prescribed is apparently rare (S. G. Siris, unpublished data). So a trial of combined antidepressant-neuroleptic medication may be quite rational for schizophrenic patients whose symptoms of psychosis are currently under adequate control and who are manifesting clinically significant symptoms of depression.

Acknowledgment

Research for this chapter was partially supported by grant number 1 RO1-MH 34309 from the National Institute of Mental Health.

REFERENCES

1. Procci WR: Schizoaffective psychosis: Fact or fiction? *Arch Gen Psychiatry* 1976;33:1167–1178.
2. Pope HG, Lipinski JF: Diagnosis in schizophrenia and manic-depressive illness. *Arch Gen Psychiatry* 1978;35:811–828.
3. Eissler KR: Remarks on the psychoanalysis of schizophrenia. *Int J Psychoanal* 1951;32:139–156.
4. Semrad EV: Long-term therapy of schizophrenia, in Usdin G (ed): *Psychoneurosis and Schizophrenia.* Philadelphia, JB Lippincott Co, 1966.
5. McGlashan TH, Carpenter WT Jr: Postpsychotic depression in schizophrenia. *Arch Gen Psychiatry* 1976;33:231–241.
6. Markowe M, Steinert J, Heyworth-Davies F: Insulin and chlorpromazine in schizophrenia: A ten-year comparative study. *Br J Psychiatry* 1967;113: 1101–1106.

7. Bowers MB, Astrachan BM: Depression in acute schizophrenic psychosis. *Am J Psychiatry* 1967;123:976–979.
8. Steinberg HR, Green R, Durell J: Depression occurring during the course of recovery from schizophrenia symptoms. *Am J Psychiatry* 1967;124:699–702.
9. Shanfield S, Tucker GJ, Harrow M, et al: The schizophrenic patient and depressive symptomatology. *J Nerv Ment Dis* 1970;151:203–210.
10. Stern MJ, Pillsbury JA, Sonnenberg SM: Post-psychotic depression in schizophrenics. *Compr Psychiatry* 1972;13:591–598.
11. McGlashan TH, Carpenter WT: An investigation of the post-psychotic depressive syndrome. *Am J Psychiatry* 1976;133:14–19.
12. Carpenter WT Jr, Strauss JS, Bartko JJ: A flexible system for the identification of schizophrenia: A report from the International Pilot Study of Schizophrenia. *Science* 1973;182:1275–1278.
13. Spitzer RL, Endicott J, Robins E: Research Diagnostic Criteria: Rationale and reliability. *Arch Gen Psychiatry* 1978;35:773–782.
14. Montgomery SM: Depressive symptoms in schizophrenia. *Prog Neuropsychopharmacol* 1979;3:429–433.
15. Johnson DAW: Studies of depressive symptoms in schizophrenia. *Br J Psychiatry* 1981;139:89–101.
16. Mellor CS: First rank symptoms of schizophrenia. *Br J Psychiatry* 1970;117: 15–23.
17. Knights A, Hirsch SR: "Revealed" depression and drug treatment for schizophrenia. *Arch Gen Psychiatry* 1981;38:806–811.
18. Roy A: Depression in the course of chronic undifferentiated schizophrenia. *Arch Gen Psychiatry* 1981;38:296–297.
19. American Psychiatric Association Task Force on Nomenclature and Statistics: *Diagnostic and Statistical Manual of Mental Disorders.* ed 3. Washington, DC, American Psychiatric Association, 1980.
20. Mandel MR, Severe JB, Schooler NR, et al: Development and prediction of post-psychotic depression in neuroleptic treated schizophrenic patients. *Arch Gen Psychiatry* 1982;39:197–203.
21. Siris SG, Harmon GK, Endicott J: Post-psychotic depressive symptoms in hospitalized schizophrenic patients. *Arch Gen Psychiatry* 1981;38:1122–1123.
22. Roth S: The seemingly ubiquitous depression following acute schizophrenic episodes, a neglected area of clinical discussion. *Am J Psychiatry* 1970;127: 91–98.
23. Winokur G: Family history studies. VIII. Depression is alive and well. *Dis Nerv Syst* 1972;33:94–99.
24. DeAlarcon R: Detection and management of affective disturbances in schizophrenia, in Lader MH (ed): *Studies of Schizophrenia. Br J Psychiatry* (special publication). 1975;10:137–141.
25. Weissman MM, Pottenger M, Kleber H, et al: Symptom patterns in primary and secondary depression. *Arch Gen Psychiatry* 1977;34:854–862.
26. MacKinnon BL: Postpsychotic depression and the need for personal significance. *Am J Psychiatry* 1977;134:427–429.
27. Post RM: Biochemical changes during the switch process (pp 325–327) in Bunney WE Jr (Moderator): The switch process in manic-depressive psychosis. *Ann Intern Med* 1977;87:319–335.
28. DeAlarcon R, Carney MWP: Severe depressive mood changes following slow-release intra-muscular fluphenazine injection. *Br Med J* 1969;3:564–567.
29. Falloon I, Watt DC, Shepherd M: A comparative controlled trial of pimozide

and fluphenazine decanoate in the continuation therapy of schizophrenia. *Psychol Med* 1978;8:59–70.
30. Hirsch SR, Gaind R, Rohde PD, et al: Outpatient maintenance of chronic schizophrenic patients with long-term fluphenazine: Double-blind placebo trial. *Br Med J* 1973;1:633–637.
31. Leff JP, Wing JK: Trial of maintenance therapy in schizophrenia. *Br Med J* 1971;3:559–604.
32. Rifkin A, Quitkin F, Klein DF: Akinesia: A poorly recognized drug-induced extrapyramidal behavioral disorder. *Arch Gen Psychiatry* 1975;32:672–674.
33. Van Putten T, May PRA: 'Akinetic depression' in schizophrenia. *Arch Gen Psychiatry* 1978;35:1101–1107.
34. Sullivan HS: Psychiatric aspects of morale. *Am J Sociol* 1941;47:277–301.
35. Siris SG, van Kammen DP, Docherty JP: Use of antidepressant drugs in schizophrenia. *Arch Gen Psychiatry* 1978;35:1368–1377.
36. Overall JE, Hollister LE, Meyer F, et al: Imipramine and thioridazine in depressed and schizophrenic patients. *JAMA* 1964;189:605–608.
37. Greenblatt M, Grosser GH, Wechsler H: A comparative study of selected antidepressant medications and EST. *Am J Psychiatry* 1962;119:144–153.
38. Greenblatt M, Grosser GH, Wechsler H: Differential response of hospitalized depressed patients to somatic therapy. *Am J Psychiatry* 1964;120:935–943.
39. Fink M, Pollack M, Klein DF, et al: Comparative studies of chlorpromazine and imipramine. I. Drug discriminating patterns. *Neuropsychopharmacology* 1964;3:370–372.
40. Pollack M, Klein DF, Willner A, et al: Imipramine-induced behavioral disorganization in schizophrenic patients: Physiological and psychological correlates. *Recent Adv Biol Psychiatry* 1965;7:53–61.
41. Klein D: Importance of psychiatric diagnosis in prediction of clinical drug effects. *Arch Gen Psychiatry* 1967;16:118–126.
42. Klein DF: Psychiatric diagnosis and a typology of clinical drug effects. *Psychopharmacologia* 1968;13:359–386.
43. Leuthold CA, Bradshaw FJ Jr, Arndt GW, et al: Behavioral evaluation of imipramine and nialamide in regressed schizophrenic patients with depressive features. *Am J Psychiatry* 1961;118:354–355.
44. Simpson GM, Amin M, Angus JWS, et al: Role of antidepressants and neuroleptics in the treatment of depression. *Arch Gen Psychiatry* 1972;27:337–345.
45. Pishkin V: Concept identification and psychophysiological parameters in depressed schizophrenics as functions of imipramine and nialamide. *J Clin Psychol* 1972;28:335–339.
46. Hanlon TE, Nussbaum K, Wittig B, et al: The comparative effectiveness of amitriptyline, perphenazine, and their combination in the treatment chronic psychotic female patients. *J New Drugs* 1964;4:52–60.
47. Chouinard G, Annable L, Serrano M, et al: Amitriptyline-perphenazine interaction in ambulatory schizophrenic patients. *Arch Gen Psychiatry* 1975;32:1295–1307.
48. Kamman GR, Freeman JG, Lucero RJ: The effect of 1-isonicotynl 2-isopropyl hydrazide (IIH) on the behavior of long-term mental patients. *J Nerv Ment Dis* 1953;118:391–407.
49. Hoshino A, Cease EA: Iproniazid phosphate in the treatment of the chronic hospitalized schizophrenic. *Am J Psychiatry* 1958;114:1111.
50. Sharpley P, Mena A, Schiele BC, et al: A comparison of pargyline and tranylcypromine with and without the addition of trifluoperazine: A double blind study. *Curr Ther Res* 1964;6:344–352.

51. Hedberg DL, Houck JH, Glueck BC Jr: Tranylcypromine-trifluoperazine combination in the treatment of schizophrenia. *Am J Psychiatry* 1971;127: 1141–1146.
52. Guertin WH, Regnier WO, Good RW, et al: Response of chronic schizophrenics to monoamine oxidase inhibitor. *Dis Nerv Syst* 1960;21: 330–332.
53. Bennett IF, Cohen D, Starer E: Isoniazid in treatment of the chronic schizophrenia patient. *Arch Neurol Psychiatry* 1954;71:54–65.
54. Michaux MH, Kurland AA, Agallianos DD: Chlorpromazine-chlordiazepoxide and chlorpromazine-imipramine treatment of newly hospitalized, acutely ill psychiatric patients. *Curr Ther Res* 1966;8:117–152.
55. Casey JF, Hollister LE, Klett CJ, et al: Combined drug therapy of chronic schizophrenics. *Am J Psychiatry* 1961;17:997–1003.
56. Bennett JL, Hamilton LD: Sequential use of antidepressant drugs with chlorpromazine in chronic schizophrenia. *Psychiatr Q* 1963;37:53–66.
57. Agallianos DD, Ota KY, Quinn MF, et al: Drug combination in the treatment of newly admitted acutely ill psychiatric patients. *Curr Ther Res* 1964; 6:626–637.
58. Kurland AA, Hanlon TE, Ota KY: Combinations of psychotherapeutic drugs in the treatment of the acutely disturbed psychiatric patient, in Vinar O, Votava Z, Bradly PB (eds): *Advances in Neuropsychopharmacology*. Amsterdam, North-Holland Publishing Co, 1971, pp 419–424.
59. Becker RE: The drug treatment of schizophrenia with depression: Is polypharmacy necessary? Scientific exhibit at the 129th Annual Meeting of the American Psychiatric Association, Miami Beach, FL, May 1976.
60. Hanlon TE, Ota KY, Agallianos DD: Combined drug treatment of newly hospitalized acutely ill psychiatric patients. *Dis Nerv Syst* 1969;30:104–116.
61. Hanlon TE, Ota KY, Kurland AA: Comparative effects of fluphenazine, fluphenazine-chlordiazepoxide and fluphenazine-imipramine. *Dis Nerv Syst* 1970;31:171–177.
62. Claghorn JL, Schoolar JC, Ryan JW, et al: Combined therapy in chronic schizophrenics stabilized on phenothiazine tranquilizers and given BL-KR140 or imipramine or placebo concurrently. *Curr Ther Res* 1967;9:576–578.
63. Chen CH, Holstein AP, Prasad PS: Etrafon in regressed schizophrenic patients. *Curr Ther Res* 1965;7:318–319.
64. Collins AD, Dundas J: A double-blind trial of amitriptyline/perphenazine, perphenazine, and placebo in chronic withdrawn inert schizophrenics. *Br J Psychiatry* 1967;113:1425–1429.
65. Lapolla A: A double-blind evaluation of chlorpromazine versus a combination of perphenazine and amitriptyline. *Int J Neuropsychiatry* 1967;3: 403–405.
66. Oltman JE, Friedman S: Perphenazine-amitriptyline in the treatment of schizophrenia. *Am J Psychiatry* 1966;123:607–609.
67. Vestre ND, Dehnel LL, Schiele BC: A sequential comparison of amitriptyline, perphenazine and the amitriptyline-perphenazine combination in recently admitted anergic schizophrenics. *Psychosomatics* 1969;10:296–303.
68. Simpson GM, Krakov BL, Kunz-Bartholini E: A controlled trial of combined medications on behavioral and extrapyramidal effects. *Acta Psychiatr Scand* 1970;212(Suppl):20–27.
69. Becker RE: Evaluation of an amitriptyline-perphenazine combination in chronic schizophrenia. *Am J Psychiatry* 1970;127:827–831.
70. Siris SG, Rifkin AE, Reardon GT: Response of post-psychotic depression to adjunctive imipramine or amitriptyline. *J Clin Psychiatry*, 1982;43:485–486.

71. Prusoff BA, Williams DH, Weissman MM, et al: Treatment of secondary depression in schizophrenia. *Arch Gen Psychiatry* 1979;36:569–575.
72. Singh AN, Saxena B, Nelson HL: A controlled clinical study of trazodone in chronic schizophrenic patients with pronounced depressive symptomatology. *Curr Ther Res* 1978;23:485–501.
73. Feighner JP, Robins E, Guze SG, et al: Diagnostic criteria for use in psychiatric research. *Arch Gen Psychiatry* 1972;26:57–63.
74. Siris SG, Glassman AH, Stetner F: The value of plasma concentrations in assessing the effects of tricyclic antidepressants, in Schoolar JC, Claghorn JL (eds): *The Kinetics of Psychiatric Drugs.* New York, Brunner/Mazel, 1979.
75. Kragh-Sorenson P, Hansen C, Baastrup P, et al: Self inhibiting action of nortriptyline's antidepressive effect at high plasma levels. *Psychopharmacologia* 1976;45:305–312.
76. Kragh-Sorenson P, Asberg M, Hansen C: Plasma nortriptyline levels in endogenous depression. *Lancet* 1973;1:113–115.
77. Vandel B, Vandel S, Allers G, et al: Interaction between amitriptyline and phenothiazine in man: Effect on plasma concentration of amitriptyline and its metabolite nortriptyline and the correlation with clinical response. *Psychopharmacology (Berlin)* 1979;65:187–190.
78. Nelson JC, Jatlow PI: Neuroleptic effect on desipramine steady-state plasma concentrations. *Am J Psychiatry* 1980;137:1232–1234.
79. Kragh-Sorenson P, Borga G, Carle L, et al: Effect of simultaneous treatment with low doses of perphenazine on plasma and urine concentrations of nortriptyline and 10-hydroxynortriptyline. *Eur J Clin Pharmacol* 1977;11: 479–483.
80. Siris SG, Cooper TB, Rifkin AE, et al: Plasma imipramine concentrations in patients receiving concomitant flupenazine decanoate. *Am J Psychiatry* 1982; 139:104–106.
81. Buffaloe EJ, Sandifer MG: A study of combined therapy with stelazine and "Parnate" (SKF 385) in chronic anergic schizophrenics. *Am J Psychiatry* 1961; 117:1030–1031.
82. Vogt AH: The use of stelazine and parnate in chronic, withdrawn patients. *Am J Psychiatry* 1961;118:256–257.
83. Schiele BC, Vestre ND, MacNaughton DV: Treatment of hospitalized schizophrenics with trifluoperazine plus tranylcypromine: A double-blind controlled study. *Compr Psychiatry* 1963;4:66–79.
84. Reinhardt RF, Schiff SB, Sinnett ER: The use of triflupromazine with iproniazid for the treatment of chronic schizophrenic patients. *Am J Psychiatry* 1959;116:68–69.
85. Mena A, Heistad G, Schiele BC, et al: A comparison of tranylcypromine alone with tranylcypromine plus trifluoperazine in the treatment of chronic outpatients: A double-blind controlled study. *J Neuropsychiatry* 1964;5: 542–550.
86. Hordern A, Somerville DM, Krupinski J: Does chronic schizophrenia respond to a combination of a neuroleptic and an antidepressant? *J Nerv Ment Dis* 1962;134:361–376.
87. Hordern A, Somerville DM: Clinical trials in chronic schizophrenia. *Med J Aust* 1963;1:40–43.
88. Janecek J, Schiele BC, Bellville T, et al: The effects of withdrawal of trifluoperazine on patients maintained on the combination of tranylcypromine and trifluoperazine: A double-blind study. *Curr Ther Res* 1963;5: 608–615.

89. Siris SG, Rifkin AE, Reardon GT, et al: Comparison of imipramine and benztropine in the prevention of extrapyramidal side effects to fluphenazine. *Psychopharmacol Bull,* 1983;19:129–131.
90. Snyder SH, Yamamura HI: Antidepressants and the muscarinic acetylcholine receptor. *Arch Gen Psychiatry* 1977;34:236–239.
91. El-Yousef MK, Mainer DH: Tricyclic antidepressants and phenothiazines. *JAMA* 1974;229:1419.
92. Klein DF: *Psychiatric Case Studies: Treatment, Drugs and Outcome.* Baltimore, The Williams & Wilkins Co, 1972, pp 89–124.
93. Pilkington TL: A report on "Tofranil" in mental deficiency. *Am J Ment Defic* 1962;66:729–732.
94. Davies TS: A monoamine oxidase inhibitor (Niamid) in the treatment of the mentally subnormal. *J Ment Sci* 1961;107:115–118.
95. Klein DF: Psychiatric diagnosis and a typology of clinical drug effects. *Psychopharmacologia* 1968;13:359–386.
96. Kramer JC, Klein DF, Fink M: Imipramine as an adjunct to phenothiazine therapy. *Compr Psychiatry* 1962;3:377–380.
97. Klein DF, Fink M: Psychiatric reaction patterns to imipramine. *Am J Psychiatry* 1962;119:432–438.
98. Brenner R, Shopsin B: The use of monoamine oxidase inhibitors in schizophrenia. *Biol Psychiatry* 1980;15:633–647.

CHAPTER 11

LONG-TERM DRUG TREATMENT OF SCHIZOPHRENIA

ARTHUR RIFKIN
SAMUEL G. SIRIS

There are few areas in psychopharmacology that are as taxing to the skill of the psychiatrist as the long-term treatment of schizophrenia. There are disorders that are more dramatic and present the need for quick action to ameliorate severe symptoms, such as mania and acute or exacerbating schizophrenia, but in several ways the clinician has an easier job of it when faced with these acute and severe disorders. First of all, the symptoms to be treated are clearly present, and the desired end point of treatment is equally clear. If the patient with mania is assaultive, has grandiose delusions, and has not slept for several nights, whether drug treatment is effective or not will be seen easily. If the treatment is ineffective, the clinician will know that a change should be made quickly, and the efficacy of the new treatment can be gauged quickly. There are clear target symptoms that are usually amenable to drug treatment. Second, the severity of the symptoms focus attention on reducing them, and if the price is mild to moderate adverse reactions, this is not considered too important in the face of such overwhelming symptoms. If, en route to calming the assaultive patient with mania or acute schizophrenia, we produce mild to moderate akinesia, dry mouth, drowsiness, stiffness, etc, we would still consider treatment successful and worth continuing if the assaultiveness stopped. With this attitude the clinician has a somewhat freer hand in medicating the patient. Third, drug treatment is for the short haul, so the impact on social and vocational functioning is not too relevant; the severe symptoms are so disruptive of social and vocational functioning that what the drugs may do to worsen it are not of concern at the moment. Finally, the patient and his or her family are preoccupied with the severe symptoms and are likely to be in a state of crisis. They turn to the doctor to relieve the crisis, and if he or she is successful, as is usually the case, there is much relief and gratitude, which helps them accept treatment and the doctor's authority, and they do not question his or her sincere desire to be helpful.

These conditions are not present when providing long-term drug treatment. The crisis has passed. The patient and his or her family now have to settle in for the long haul. Often, the hope of complete amelioration of symptoms and complete return of good functioning has been dashed; the irritants that were ignored during the crisis—from minor adverse reactions to dissatisfaction with the doctor's manner—are no longer ignored; balancing the risk/benefit ratio is much more difficult; there often are less clear-cut symptoms to aim at; and perhaps most important, the body of scientific knowledge that the doctor can lean on to guide treatment is far more skimpy than what we know about drug treatment of acute disorders, so that the clinician must worry more about whether he or she is doing the right thing.

Also, and this may seem too obvious, chronic conditions last longer than acute ones. However messy and difficult it is to treat acutely ill persons, we can count on the problem ending soon, especially if the acute treatment is given on an inpatient service where, these days, the length of stay is rarely long.

Why is it that we know so much more about acute rather than chronic treatment? The number of studies of short-term treatment of schizophrenia is enormous, even if we limit it to well-designed and well-executed double-blind, controlled studies, whereas the number of good long-term studies is a relative handful. By logic, the opposite should be true. The sheer number of important questions to answer about long-term treatment is far greater than for short-term treatment. As already mentioned, nuisance adverse reactions are not too important in short-term treatment, but may be crucial for the long haul. Constant dry mouth may seem more important to the patient than a return of psychotic symptoms, of which he may have only a dim memory. Slight sleepiness that was unnoticeable or even welcomed on the ward during the acute episode may make it very difficult for the patient to perform his work. Impotence, which is not even thought of during the acute phase, may erode a poor marriage during the chronic phase. The need for many studies to assess the risks and benefits of various treatments is more necessary for long-term treatment.

If the patient is stable and has no symptoms, or few, so that the goal of treatment is to prevent worsening, the research is more difficult. The problem of finding the right dose to test is harder. When treating acute symptoms, the dose can be adjusted within a fixed range to find what dose provides the most relief with the least adverse reactions. That dose is likely to be different among patients. If the design required a fixed dose, and if it was set too low, a true drug-placebo difference would be less demonstrable. If it was set too high, the adverse reactions would be shown to be more of a problem than they need be. It is an advantage to be able to adjust dose according to the needs of each patient. In a study of long-term treatment, in which the goal is not reduction of symptoms, but prevention of worsening, adjustment of dose is more limited. There is no way of knowing that the dose may have been too low until worsening occurs, ie, there are no target symptoms. The dose could be adjusted according to the severity of adverse reactions, but that is not easy since almost all patients have some adverse reactions, and without target symptoms, we do not know how many adverse reactions and at what severity we should urge the patient to tolerate.

Therefore, in such studies, a dose range is chosen — fairly arbitrarily as will be seen — and several studies should be done at different ranges to establish a dose-response relationship. This is even more necessary for long-term than for short-term treatment.

Many persons in long-term treatment do not worsen, more than the number of persons with acute symptoms who do not improve. By the nature of the disorder the effect of long-term treatment is less than that of treatment of the acute episode. This means that to demonstrate a drug effect, if one truly exists, requires more subjects in long-term treatment. The smaller the effect, the more subjects it takes to show mathematically that the results could not have been due to chance. It takes many more subjects to demonstrate the efficacy of a vaccine to prevent pneumococcal pneumonia than it does to test whether a new antibiotic is an effective treatment, because most people will not get pneumonia without the vaccine, and most persons with pneumococcal pneumonia would not improve rapidly spontaneously.

So, if logic determined what studies were done, we would do many more on long-term than on acute treatment because we have more questions to answer.

The reason why relatively few long-term studies are done becomes painfully clear to those of us who attempt them. By definition they are longer, which increases administrative difficulties exponentially. It is much more difficult to keep a patient in a study for 52 weeks than for 6 weeks, especially if the latter study is done on an inpatient service. Dropouts can ruin a study. Not only do they add to the expense and time that must be spent adding more patients to the study so that an adequate sample is reached, but they also make it difficult to interpret the results of the study. The logic of clinical research is that we do a study on a small group of people and generalize the results to a large group. This logic is appropriate only if we know that the small group is a good example of the large group. There are two ways of determining that a sample is a good representation of a population. If we knew what characteristics of people with schizophrenia affected drug treatment, we could measure those characteristics in the sample and generalize only to the population of persons with schizophrenia who have the same measurements on these characterizations. For example, there are some data to show that persons with schizophrenia who had very poor social adjustment before the onset of their psychotic symptoms respond less well to antipsychotic drugs than do other persons with schizophrenia.[1] If we wanted to know how well this group responded to long-term treatment (the present data refer to short-term treatment), we would select a sample with premorbid asociality. If we wanted to know whether this characteristic was important in long-term treatment, we would be sure that the sample had both types of schizophrenia so that comparisons could be made. The logic of the mathematics which we use to determine the probability that our results are not due to chance requires that subjects be assigned to the treatments to be compared randomly, ie, without bias. If we know that some variable such as premorbid asociality is likely to affect outcome, we should randomly assign the treatments within those with premorbid asociality and those without. Otherwise, there is the chance that more patients with premorbid asociality will get treatment A rather than treatment B. Then, if treatment A does less well, we do not know whether this is because treatment A is worse than treatment B, or because the patients given treatment A were less responsive to treatment.

This system of randomizing separately within relevant categories or studying one category works only if we know what characteristics are important to drug responsiveness. But we can never be sure that we know all of these characteristics. As will be shown below, we actually know very few, so how can we be sure that the sample we test is characteristic of an identifiable population?

The answer is that we depend on randomization to even things out. If there are unknown characteristics influencing drug responsiveness, they will most likely be equally distributed between treatment groups if we randomly assign them. We know that if we randomly assign subjects, treatments are unbiased, but we can never be sure that dropouts are an unbiased group; ie, those who drop out may be different in their drug responsiveness than those who remain. If the drop out is due to an unexpected move to another city, that is not likely to be related to drug treatment. However, if all dropping out is due to anger at the treatment, or an upsurge of suspiciousness due to an impending relapse, this clearly is related to the drug treatment, and losing data from that person irreparably harms the study. Therefore, a large number of dropouts is fatal to a study. Naturally, dropouts are more of a problem in long studies than in short ones.

All of these technical problems of doing research of long-term treatment have been mentioned to give a flavor of the many difficult problems in this area, to account for the poverty of studies, and to evoke the proper skeptical attitude for the next section, which is a discussion of the relevant research trials.

REVIEW OF CLINICAL RESEARCH

We shall review here the published double-blind, controlled studies of long-term drug treatment of schizophrenia that we consider most important, taking into account the difficulties in performing and evaluating such studies that were discussed above.

The first large study with clearly described methodology was by Engelhardt and associates,[2] using patients attending an outpatient clinic at Kings County Hospital in Brooklyn, NY.[2] They compared two active drugs, chlorpromazine and promazine, with placebo for a period of a year. Promazine was used as an antipsychotic drug in those years. Today it is not, because it is not as effective as many other drugs. The results of this trial were that patients receiving chlorpromazine had statistically significantly fewer relapses than did those on placebo. The promazine group was intermediate and not statistically significantly different from the other groups.

The earlier literature on long-term antipsychotic drug effects is best appreciated in its historical context. Before the introduction of antipsychotic drugs, psychodynamic approaches were the most utilized treatment modality in the treatment of schizophrenia. Although the utility of dynamic approaches had never been rigorously evaluated empirically in schizophrenic patients, clinicians were concerned that sedative or other properties of neuroleptic drugs might render psychotherapy less valuable. Drug treatment was initially seen as a method for rectifying acute symptoms rather than as a strategy, in and of itself, for long-term treatment. The Engelhardt study was the first to begin to dispel the notion that long-term medication was unnecessary or even harmful to the patients' progress, but conviction on this point required more time, more studies, and more accumulated general clinical experience on the part of practitioners.

This first study also showed us the problems of doing this sort of research. In the early 1960s in the United States, the diagnosis of schizophrenia was made very loosely. After Bleuler's contention that the basic psychopathological feature was loosening of associations, and that with this feature came a very wide variety of other clinical features, it became a mark of clinical astuteness to detect the "subtle thought disorder." As a result, schizophrenia blossomed. The rate was twice that of the United Kingdom. In later years, the diagnosis was narrowed; in DSM-III, such persons with a mild thought disorder without clear-cut psychotic symptoms are not categorized as having schizophrenia, as they are not elsewhere in the world.

However, when the study of Engelhardt et al was done, the diagnoses were based upon the clinical diagnosis in the hospital records, which by today's standards would include many persons with nonschizophrenic disorders. The fact that despite this problem a difference was found shows the strength of chlorpromazine's effect in preventing relapse, since the data from those without schizophrenia would serve to dilute the apparent drug effect.

There was a very high rate of dropouts, which makes interpretation of the results difficult. This points out a general problem in this field. Patients with schizophrenia are notorious for their fluctuating cooperativeness with treatment; in fact, if we wished to act like Bleuler (tongue in cheek) and were tempted to proclaim the one basic feature of schizophrenia, it would be that in every area it fluctuates. It is difficult to gather a sample of persons with schizophrenia and have them agree to participate in research, and it is even harder to keep them in a long-term study that requires regular visits. This means that the population to which we are entitled to generalize from our sample may not be too like the population of people with schizophrenia in general, ie, our results may be applicable to those who are particularly cooperative.

Leff and Wing, in Great Britain, compared an active drug, chlorpromazine or trifluoperazine, to placebo in 35 outpatients with schizophrenia.[3] Despite the small sample size, those given active drug for a year had a statistically significantly lower rate of relapse. There are several interesting features about this study. The 35 subjects were chosen out of a pool of 116 eligible patients because they were thought to have an intermediate prognosis. The premise was that patients with a good prognosis do not require long-term drug treatment; patients with a poor prognosis clearly do. Therefore, to put someone from either group in the study, where they would be randomized to active drug or placebo, was unethical because half would get the wrong treatment.

Their predictions about prognoses were accurate: 67% of the poor prognosis patients relapsed within the year versus 27% of those with a good prognosis. We should look carefully at this argument, because it is believed commonly and has implications for treatment. There is a basic flaw in their position: they confuse prognosis with drug responsiveness. The only accurate way of determining drug responsiveness is a study comparing the drug with a placebo or, in some instances, another active drug. Prognosis is something different: the course of the patient. Knowing that a patient has 67% or a 27% chance of relapsing during the next 12 months does not tell us whether he or she would benefit from drug treatment. The authors assume that the poor prognosis group does better on drugs, and the good prognosis group is not benefited. That is not necessarily so. Only a clinical trial can determine that. If those with the poor prognosis were entered into the study, it is possible that no difference would have been found between placebo and the active drug. In fact, some clinical trials in very chronic patients have not shown any response to a known active agent because this was a group selected to be nonresponsive to drugs. If they had been drug responsive they would not have been long-term hospitalized patients (as was the case in Leff and Wing's study).

Similarly, the good prognosis cohort, assumed to be unneedful of drugs, may have done even better on the active treatment. A relapse rate of 27% is better than 67%, but still far from acceptable.

Another interesting feature of this study is that they chose subjects who were free of psychotic symptoms at baseline. As will be seen later, there is only one other study that has done that. It may be true that the need for long-term treatment is different depending on whether or not the patient is still psychotic. Is schizophrenia like pneumococcal pneumonia or sarcoidosis; ie, once successfully treated is the illness gone, or is it a chronic illness whose underlying pathology is always present and whose symptoms fluctuate? If the former, then patients without symptoms would be free of the disorder and not require long-term treatment.

The evidence from this study, where 83% of those given placebo and 33% of those on active drug relapsed within a year, is that even if a patient is in remission from psychotic symptoms, there is a need for further drug treatment. And even with drug treatment, the chance of relapse is high.

The most impressive study of long-term treatment of schizophrenia in terms of sheer number of subjects was done by Hogarty and associates.[4] They accomplished the incredible feat of following 374 subjects for two years. The patients were recently discharged from a state hospital and came for treatment in one of three outpatient clinics run by the state. They were randomly assigned to one of two conditions of drug treatment—chlorpromazine or placebo—and one of two conditions of sociotherapy—frequent or minimal. The sociotherapy when given was individual casework and vocational counseling done by social workers. The dose of chlorpromazine was low by contemporary standards—the mean was slightly less than 300 mg per day.

After two years, it was seen that placebo was a terrible treatment—80% had relapsed—and chlorpromazine was a poor treatment—48% had relapsed. This difference is statistically significant.

The results of the psychotherapy are less clear cut. Overall, there was no statistically significant difference between the groups, although there was a trend for those receiving casework and chlorpromazine to do better than those receiving chlorpromazine alone. If the data from the first six months are ignored, then there is a statistically significant psychotherapy effect. How legitimate is it to analyze data this way? What conclusions may be drawn? This is called a post hoc analysis because an hypothesis is tested—comparing psychotherapy versus minimal contact during the 6th to 24th months—that was not considered before the study was done (an a priori hypothesis). By the usual canons of science, only an a priori hypothesis is definitively tested, to the extent that any one study can say anything definitively, because we are testing the likelihood that we can predict the future. A post hoc test only looks at the past and finds interesting associations, a far less stringent test. For example, if you noticed that today, when you wore a red tie, there were more red cars than usual on the highway while you drove to work, that might amuse you as an interesting coincidence. But, if the next day, you made a prediction that if you wore a blue tie, you would see more blue cars than usual (assuming that you had an accurate knowledge of the usual colors of cars you saw daily), and that was borne out, you would be entitled to a much stronger sense that something very strange was happening.

The importance of post hoc analysis is to uncover important hypotheses to test a priori in another study. It may well be true that psychotherapy does affect relapse rate and that its benefit is not seen during the first six months, but it would take future research to determine that.

The authors did not restrict the study to patients who had or had not remitted, nor did they analyze their results according to that factor. This study remains the most impressive evidence that antipsychotic drugs are helpful in preventing relapse for two years after inpatient treatment.

Hogarty et al also analyzed data on the adjustment of those patients who did not relapse.[5] They found that, when analyzed separately, drugs and psychotherapy conditions had no effect, but when taken together, they did. Chlorpromazine and casework were better than chlorpromazine alone, and placebo without casework was better than the combination. These data have been cited to support the opinion that the patient with schizophrenia should be treated as an outpatient with the combination of drugs and psychotherapy. We could point out that the data could technically be taken to mean that the patient should be treated with neither, but since placebo is clearly an inferior treatment, this combination is not advisable.

These data must be considered as quite nondefinitive, because they constitute an atypical sample, the patients who did not relapse. For the placebo group that represents only 20% of the patients and 52% of those given chlorpromazine; they are a subgroup of the original sample, but most importantly, they are no longer a randomly chosen group because they are survivors of a randomly selected group. That is, we have no way of knowing whether the patients in the different treatment groups are similar to begin with, and we cannot know whether they end up differently because of their treatment or other relevant factors that differentiated them.

Rifkin and colleagues[6] did a study of long-term treatment focusing not only on the question of whether drug was better than placebo in patients with schizophrenia who were in remission from their psychotic symptoms, but also on whether depot medication would be superior to oral. The supposition was that depot medication would be superior to oral medication if "active drug" was at all better than placebo, because noncompliance in regularly taking medication is thought to be a common problem.[6]

The sample was selected to include patients who were in full remission from all psychotic symptoms within a period of one year of their admission to inpatient treatment, and who were currently receiving outpatient treatment in the aftercare clinic of the hospital. This clinic offered a rich array of therapeutic services in addition to drug treatment, such as individual and group psychotherapy, rehabilitative activities and counseling, and social activities. The major question, as with Leff and Wing,[3] was to determine whether patients in remission required drug treatment. Leff and Wing's study had used a small sample, a sample not representative of the full range of patients with schizophrenia, ie, they did not include patients judged to have a particularly good or bad prognosis. The duration of observation was one year. Patients were randomized to placebo, oral fluphenazine, or depot fluphenazine decanoate.

With dummy pills and injections, the study was double blind. The ratio of fluphenazine decanoate to oral fluphenazine was fixed at 0.5 mg to 5 mg per day. The dose varied according to the psychiatrist's judgment between 0.5 mL and 2.0 mL of fluphenazine decanoate every two weeks or 5–20 mg of oral fluphenazine per day.

The total sample was 73 patients. The relapse rate in the actively treated group was quite low and equal: fluphenazine decanoate, 9%; oral fluphenazine, 11%. Those given placebo had a much higher relapse rate—64%. The difference in relapse ratio between placebo and active drug groups was statistically significant.

In Göttingen, West Germany, Müller and associates[7] did a similar study, comparing fluphenazine decanoate with placebo in remitted patients with schizophrenia for one year. In 38 patients, 6% of those given fluphenazine decanoate relapsed, versus 81% of those on placebo.

Rifkin et al[6] found that a high percentage of patients given fluphenazine decanoate had to be withdrawn from the study because of severe akinesia. Müller et al,[8] in a subsequent presentation of their data, found also that many patients on the depot drug developed what they considered to be pharmacogenic depression. They noted that such "depressions" tended to respond to an antiparkinson drug and not to a tricyclic antidepressant. It is likely that the two research groups were seeing the same problem—akinesia/depression. These results suggested that fluphenazine decanoate was particularly likely to produce akinesia or depression. This question is addressed further below.

The last study to be cited comparing an active drug with placebo was done by Hirsch and co-workers.[9] Using patients with chronic schizophrenia who were attending an outpatient clinic and receiving fluphenazine decanoate, they randomly assigned them to continue the depot active drug or placebo injections under double-blind conditions. They observed the patients for nine months. By then, 66% of those on placebo had relapsed, versus 8% on the active drug. This difference is clearly of clinical importance and is also statistically significant. This large difference was found even though most of the subjects on fluphenazine decanoate received a dose of 25 mg monthly—a lower dose than in other studies.

So far, all studies have shown that long-term treatment is far superior to placebo. Is there a group for whom drugs are not helpful? For patients whose prognosis is so excellent that little need to be done to improve it, there is too little to be gained by using drugs. In criticizing the study of Leff and Wing,[3] we discussed how drug responsiveness must be distinguished from prognosis and how the two should be examined separately. In their study, they assumed that those with a good prognosis did not need long-term medication, and those with a good prognosis did need it. Our point is that if there is an association between prognosis and drug responsiveness, this should not be assumed, but tested.

Kane and colleagues tested the hypothesis that patients with schizophrenia who had the best prognostic indicators would not require long term treatment.[10] This was part of the study of Rifkin et al[6] in which we compared two active treatments, oral fluphenazine and depot fluphenazine decanoate to placebo for one year in patients who were in full remission from their psychotic symptoms. We segregated those patients who should have the best prognosis: those with complete recovery from one episode and no premorbid mental difficulties. Our original plan was to randomize them into the three treatment groups as we did for all other subjects, but we found that such good prognosis patients were too rare. It would take far too long to enter sufficient patients to test the hypothesis. Therefore, we collapsed the two active treatments into one and used the depot drug only if we thought it likely that the subject would not take oral medication reliably. As it is, it took five years to collect the data. During that time, we were able to enter only 28 patients from an aftercare clinic attended by about 700 patients, which shows how unusual such good prognosis patients are. Of the 17 patients placed on placebo, 7 (41%) relapsed. None of the 11 subjects given active fluphenazine relapsed. This difference is statistically and clinically significant. It appears, then, as far as one study can be definitive, that even such carefully selected patients, who might be expected to do so well and not need medication, do need it and do poorly without it. Follow-up information was obtained for a mean of 3.5 years. Surprisingly, 69% had a relapse—either during the study or afterward—and half had a third episode. This suggests that if followed for a substantial period, even patients with good prognostic features tend to have repeated episodes. The follow-up data reinforce the conclusion from the drug trial that such good prognosis patients, as other patients with schizophrenia, do better on long-term medication. Although the sample is small, none of the 11 subjects given active drug relapsed. This is close to the figure of about 10% for those subjects without such good prognostic features, who in the same study were given active drug[6] after remission and similar to the 6% relapse reported by Müller et al,[7] who also used subjects in remission. The only contrary finding was by Leff and Wing,[3] who found a 33% relapse rate in patients in remission on active drug. The Leff and Wing study is not directly comparable to the others because the sample was selected more carefully to exclude patients who did not have an intermediate prognosis. Their reason for excluding those with a good prognosis was their belief that such patients clearly did not need medication. They found that after one year, 27% of them had relapsed, considerably more that the 0% relapse in the good prognosis patients of Kane et al.[10]

Such a comparison is suggested only to tantalize and should not be taken seriously, because the samples may be quite different, relapse was not defined operationally, and we are not sure what treatment (if any) the good risk patients of Leff and Wing[3] received.

The placebo-controlled studies described so far have been for periods of nine months to two years, and all indicate that drug treatment is far superior to placebo. If that question seems answered, we may ask further, for how long should drug treatment be continued? There is very little information about this. Anecdotal reports suggest that there is continued high risk for relapse even after many years, but studies are rare. Cheung[11] took 30 patients with schizophrenia who were receiving antipsychotic drugs and who had been in full remission for three to five years and, under double-blind conditions, randomized them to a benzodiazepine drug or to an antipsychotic. The benzodiazepine was used as an active placebo to mimic the sedative adverse reaction of antipsychotics and to better preserve the double-blind conditions. Eight of 13 subjects on the benzodiazepine relapsed, versus 2 of the 15 on the antipsychotic. The period of observation was 18 months. This difference in rates of relapse is statistically significant. Although the number of subjects is small, the one controlled, double-blind study looking at relapse after many years tells us that we can have no assurance that the need for medication can be thought to diminish.

A less adequately controlled study of the consequences of stopping long-term treatment was done by Johnson.[12] He compared patients who stopped depot antipsychotic drugs after one to four years with a control group, still on drugs, matched by age, sex, and duration of illness. There were more relapses among those who were withdrawn from the antipsychotics. This finding is suggestive only, because the subjects were not randomly assigned to the two groups, so we cannot be sure whether they differed in ways other than their drug treatments. However, it does add some support to the more definitive study of Cheung,[11] indicating that it is not safe to stop drugs after many years.

The studies cited so far all support the position that antipsychotic drugs prevent relapse during long-term treatment. If our only concern were to reduce the risk of relapse, the best means would be to continue drug treatment indefinitely. However, treating a person with a mental disorder is much more complex than that. We must not focus too restrictedly on one aspect. Relapse is important, but so are other considerations. The most obvious one is adverse reactions—safety for the short and long term. This topic is presented in other chapters, so we shall just summarize the major adverse reactions that are most relevant to long-term treatment.

Sedation is the most common adverse reaction and, perhaps, the most neglected. Other toxicities are more dramatic and more threatening to well being and present more complex questions of management, such as prescribing an antidote. However, chronic low-level sedation can be extremely debilitating, and when the patient and doctor no longer recognize it as an adverse reaction, but come to think of it as part of the disorder or part of the patient's personality, it can have harmful attitudinal effects. This issue merges into the question of akinesia, which is also often mistaken for psychopathology.

A chronic dry mouth is torture, but low-level torture. The patient often stops complaining about it because it does not do any good.

Akathisia is easily mistaken for agitation or anxiety. Impotence and diminished sexual drive sustained over months to years helps to corrode relationships and removes a source of pleasure in persons whose sources of pleasure are usually diminished to start with. Few persons with schizophrenia are rewarded by outstanding vocational, artistic, or social attainments. To take away the basic pleasure of sexual gratification is a considerable loss.

Tardive dyskinesia is considered the major impediment to long-term use of antipsychotic drugs. It is paradoxical that during the last 10–15 years, when clinical research demonstrated the benefits to be obtained from long-term use of antipsychotic drugs, we also have learned much more about the danger of such treatment, viz, from tardive dyskinesia. We now have more reasons to use antipsychotics for many years and more reasons not to. Assessing the risk/benefit ratio seems to grow more difficult, not less.

We suspect that tardive dyskinesia has hogged center stage excessively. The less frightening adverse reactions such as akinesia, drowsiness, restlessness, dry mouth, impotence, and so on may cumulatively be more of a problem, both in altering the patients quality of life and in inducing noncompliance with treatment. We should make every effort to relieve or reduce these "minor" toxicities. Cholinergic drugs such as neostigmine and bethanechol often are helpful for dry mouth, urine retention, and constipation. Reduction of dose and/or antiparkinson drugs are helpful for the extrapyramidal symptoms such as akinesia and akathisia (not to mention for dystonias). There is no antidote for sedation, except to keep the dose as low as possible and to use a high-potency antipsychotic. We may divide the antipsychotics into the low-potency groups of chlorpromazine and thioridazine (to cite the most commonly prescribed) and the high-potency drugs, which include the rest. For example, haloperidol and fluphenazine are about 50 times more potent than chlorpromazine or thioridazine; trifluoperazine is 20 times more potent, molindone is 10 times more potent, etc. The high-potency drugs are less sedating and more likely to cause extrapyramidal side effects. The latter may be controlled by antiparkinson drugs, whereas sedation has no antidote. In most instances, it is better to use a high-potency drug with an antiparkinsonian agent.

The review of studies of long-term drug treatment so far has shown that active drugs are better than placebo. What follows is a critique of important studies regarding the choice of drug, dosage, and route of administration.

Considered a major advance at the time was the introduction of depot antipsychotics that obviate the problem of covert noncompliance. In Europe, more than in the United States, depot drugs became very commonly used. Has this hope of improved benefit materialized? We have seen already in the study of Rifkin et al[6] that oral fluphenazine was not inferior to depot drug in preventing relapse over one year.

Del Guidice[13] reported a comparison of fluphenazine enanthate to oral fluphenazine for one year in patients recently discharged from inpatient treatment. There was a very high relapse rate on oral treatment (85%), and 40% relapsed on the depot drug. This difference is statistically and clinically significant, but puzzling because of the very high relapse rate on oral drug.

Falloon and associates,[14] compared pimozide with fluphenazine decanoate in 41 patients with schizophrenia. There was no statistically significant difference in relapse rates during the one-year study, but those on the depot drug had more depressive symptoms ($P < 0.05$), whereas those on the oral drug had fewer adverse reactions ($P < 0.02$). These data are difficult to interpret. The sample size was small. The finding of no difference between treatments must be tempered because the actual difference was substantial: 24% relapsed on pimozide, whereas 40% relapsed on depot fluphenazine. The power of the statistical test to show that such a difference was not due to chance was very low—a serious problem in clinical research with small samples comparing two active treatments. Their finding of more depressive symptoms in the group given depot fluphenazine is also difficult to evaluate because some subjects were given adjunctive antidepressants.

Hogarty and associates,[15] using a substantial sample size of 105 patients, compared two drugs—oral fluphenazine and depot fluphenazine decanoate—and two levels of psychosocial treatment—weekly casework and a social club versus routine surveillance, which meant much less psychosocial attention. The study was done in outpatients followed for two years. The modal dose of the depot drug was 25 mg every two weeks, and 10 mg of the oral drug per day. There was not statistically significant difference between the two drug treatments or the two psychosocial conditions, nor was there a significant interaction between the drug and psychosocial conditions. There was a striking finding: after the eighth month, no patient on fluphenazine decanoate with the high amount of social therapy relapsed. The trend for the depot drug and social therapy to be the best treatment was not statistically significant. To have an 80% chance of having detected a statistically significant difference at the 5% level, a sample size of 243 would have been necessary—assuming that the percentages in each group would have remained the same. This illustrates the difficulty in answering questions when attempting to study several factors.

Another intriguing finding was that those who relapsed on fluphenazine decanoate were more likely to be depressed than those relapsing on oral fluphenazine, whereas the latter were more likely to have more psychotic symptoms than the former. This raises the question of whether depot fluphenazine is depressogenic, a suggestion first made based on anecdotal data by De Alarcon and Carney.[16]

This question was assessed in a study that soon followed. Schooler et al,[17] in a large, multihospital effort, compared fluphenazine decanoate with oral fluphenazine for one year in 214 recently discharged patients with schizophrenia. The overall relapse rate was 28%. There was no statistically significant difference between drug groups, nor was there any difference in the occurrence of affective symptoms or social adjustment. Thus, they did not confirm the finding by Hogarty et al[14] of more depression in the depot group.

The clear trend in comparisons of depot versus oral antipsychotics is that there is no difference. Why should this be so? If noncompliance is the problem we thought it was, why then should we not see few relapses on depot? One possible explanation is that those patients who agree to participate in studies are the more cooperative patients who regularly take their pills. Missing doses may not predispose to relapse. Comparisons of patients who agree and do not agree to participate in trials have not shown differences in factors that might lead to the belief that one group is more cooperative than the other.

This question raises the further question of the relationship of dose to outcome. The first question to ask of a treatment is if it works. The next is to establish to optimal dose, ie, the dose that maximizes efficacy and minimizes adverse reactions.

Few studies have addressed this question directly. Kane and coworkers[18] investigated whether a 10-fold dilution of fluphenazine decanoate (2.5 mg/mL) was an effective agent compared with placebo. Patients with schizophrenia in good remission were treated openly with low-dose fluphenazine decanoate. Those who remained well after six months were randomized, under double-blind conditions, to remain on the active drug or to receive placebo injections. Of 14 patients, 6 relapsed—all on placebo, a statistically significant difference. This showed that very low-dose fluphenazine was better than placebo. The next step was to compare the low dose with standard dose. This study has been completed recently, and preliminary results are available.[19]

Outpatients with schizophrenia at three institutions who were in full or partial remission, were treated with a standard dose of fluphenazine decanoate (12.5 to 50 mg every two weeks) or one-tenth of that dose. In the low-dose group, 26 of 62 patients had 31 relapses requiring 7 rehospitalizations. In the standard-dose group, only 3 of 64 patients had 4 relapses, and none required rehospitalization. This difference is highly significant—clinically and statistically. Using a life table analysis of cumulative relapse, 56% of the low-dose cohort relapsed, versus 7% of the standard-dose cohort, ($P < 0.001$). Clearly, there is a dose effect.

The purpose of the study was not only to evaluate the effect of dose on relapse rate. It was anticipated that such a low dose would do as well as a standard dose; the relapse on the low dose might be relatively easily treated, whereas the lower dose might improve social and vocational functioning because of fewer adverse reactions. Preliminary data analysis suggests that this is true: social and vocational functioning was better on the low dose. Also, there were fewer dyskinetic symptoms on the low dose, suggesting that tardive dyskinesia would be less frequent.

It is too early to say what place, if any, very low dosage has in long-term treatment. Other studies are ongoing using a one-fifth dilution. In the ensuing years, we should know much more about the role of dose.

Baldessarini and Davis[20] performed a valuable service in reviewing all published studies comparing an antipsychotic with placebo, using random assignment, following successful treatment of an acute episode with drugs, having at least 10 patients in each treatment group, and followed for at least one month (the average was 10). Relapse rates on placebo ranged from 18 to 57% (average, 54%); relapse rates on drugs (all phenothiazines) ranged from 0 to 50% (average 11.3%). The mean difference was 39.7%, ie, overall there is a 40% improvement due to drug treatment.

Baldessarini and Davis found no statistically or clinically significant association between relapse rate on drug, or the difference in relapse rates between drug and placebo, and dose. In chlorpromazine units, the range of doses used was 100 to 2500 mg per day. Thus, aside from the studies already cited by Kane et al [18,19] which used very low dose, the equivalent of 30–40 mg of chlorpromazine per day, there is no evidence that dose within a wide range is important. This conclusion should not be understood to mean that in the individual patient dose might not be crucial. It does mean that the clinician should be humble and realize how little we know about the details of long-term treatment.

A different type of strategy is the use of intermittent drug treatment, ie, using an antipsychotic when relapse appears imminent and stopping it when remission appears firmly established.

Preliminary data from a trial of this approach were presented recently by Carpenter and associates.[21] Subjects were recently discharged patients who were removed from antipsychotic medication for 28 days and then, provided they had not relapsed, were randomized into two groups. One group received continuous medication. Patients in the other group, the targeted cohort, were treated with drugs only if, based on the clinical judgment of the treating psychiatrist, relapse appeared imminent. The drug was stopped when the patient reached stabilization. Fifty-five patients entered the first phase of discontinuing drug. Sixty-nine percent did not relapse—or, what seems to us more important, 31% did. Four of the relapsers required hospitalization. This does not strike us as a worthwhile therapeutic procedure because of the high relapse rate, although we understand that it does enable the detection of those patients who do not require medications, and, for the purposes of research design, it enables the establishment of a clinical baseline. It may also be useful as a strategy of finding tardive dyskinesia since it appears in some patients only when antipsychotic medication is withdrawn. But, these gains appear to us to be outweighed by the high risk of relapse, especially since it occurs so soon after the previous episode.

Results in the second phase, the comparison of the two treatment approaches, are available for six months of treatment for 41 patients. There are no statistically significant differences between the groups in rating scale measures of psychopathology, in the number of hospitalizations, or in the number of days in the hospital. As expected, there was a marked difference in the number of weeks on medication and in the cumulative dose; patients in the targeted group had less time on medication and lower cumulative doses.

This interesting approach deserves a full evaluation, and the results from this study and other similar studies are awaited eagerly.

Other than the difference in route of administration (oral versus depot), we have treated all antipsychotic drugs as if they were the same.

There is no evidence from the voluminous literature of comparing antipsychotics to support the idea that one is more effective than another.

One of the surprises and disappointments in psychopharmacology has been that no antipsychotic which followed the original, chlorpromazine, has been more effective, although many are equally effective. It seems that there is a ceiling beyond which we cannot go. Perhaps this is due to the way we discover new agents. Lacking an animal model of schizophrenia or an understanding of its biochemical basis, we have no rational means to develop new drugs, except by either using compounds that are similar to known antipsychotics by their pharmacological profile or by trying agents that have been developed for other disorders, eg, lithium, propranolol, or benzodiazepines.

The only important differences found to date among antipsychotics have been in their relative propensity to cause adverse reactions, which, as previously discussed, should influence the choice of agent. In keeping with this, we notice that the trend in studies of long-term treatment is to go from a low potency drug (chlorpromazine) in early studies to high-potency agents in later studies. This reflects clinical practice, and we think that it is a change for the better. The total load of adverse reactions is usually less with a high-potency drug with an antiparkinson drug than with a low potency drug with or without the antiparkinson drug.

Given this lack of differential drug responsiveness among antipsychotics in the treatment of acute psychoses, there is little reason to expect the case to be different in long-term treatment. Comparing one drug with another has been done mainly to support the application of a manufacturer for approval of a new drug. As expected, persistent differences have not been found.

A possible exception to the monotonous uniformity of new antipsychotic drugs is molindone, which unlike other drugs is associated with weight loss.[22-25] The manufacturer reports that tardive dyskinesia has not been seen with molindone. This would be hard to understand since the drug does block the postsynaptic dopamine receptor, and the finding is probably due to relative lack of use of the compound, but for the present it is an intriguing finding.

Flupentixol decanoate is a long-acting depot drug commonly used outside of the United States; several studies have compared it with fluphenazine. In a typical study, Knights and associates[26] compared the two drugs in 57 patients just before their discharge from inpatient treatment and continued treatment and double-blind observations for six months. A large proportion (30%) dropped out. Among the remaining patients, there was no significant differences between the two treatment groups. Seven percent relapsed—a low number, but difficult to evaluate because of the high number of dropouts—and about half developed some symptoms of depression. Flupentixol decanoate appears to be equally effective to fluphenazine decanoate. There are suggestions that it may be active in depression, but this study and others do not support, as yet, the differential usefulness as compared with other antipsychotics.

Not all patients receiving long-term treatment are in remission or even stabilized with mild symptoms. One treatment approach for these patients has some degree of clinical testing during long-term treatment; very high dosage, sometimes called megadosage. Lehman and coworkers[27] studied 40 patients who were unresponsive to standard treatment. At first all were treated with very high doses of fluphenazine decanoate—100 mg or more every three weeks. Then they were randomized to remain on the high dose or return to standard dose. The period of observation was six months. The mean dose of the high-dose group was 225 mg every two weeks, and that of the standard-dose group was 25 mg every two weeks. No differences on any important measures of clinical effect were found when averages were examined; however, the standard dose group had more variance, ie, to a statistically significant degree more patients on the standard dose got better and worse. Overall, this does not support the strategy of megadose.

Dencker et al, in Sweden, have had wide experience with megadose, and they recently described their results during long-term treatment in anecdotal fashion.[28] Fourteen patients were kept on megadose for four to eight years because of their unresponsiveness to standard treatment and responsiveness to megadose. Dosage was usually 250–500 mg of fluphenazine enanthate per week. Few had extrapyramidal symptoms, although four had mild tardive dyskinesia. The only possibly significant adverse reactions to such massive dosage were mild skin changes on the buttocks. This report highlights one of the "difficulties" in choosing the best dose: antipsychotic drugs are so relatively safe within an enormous dose range that the clinician has an embarrassment of choices. We can think of no other class of drugs whose range of safe application is so wide. It gives the burden of testing clinical efficacy within a wide range. But, at present there are more data supporting the safety of megadosage than its advantage over standard dosage.

The clinician does not have the luxury of waiting until definitive research has been done before making decisions. We cannot tell our patients to return in five years when more data will be at hand. It seems less beneficial to be too conservative and refrain from using treatments not yet clearly shown helpful than it is to attempt to achieve remission with treatments whose supporting evidence is anecdotal. Megadosage is a case in point. It appears to be safe, even if its efficacy is in doubt.

PREDICTORS OF RESPONSE TO LONG-TERM TREATMENT

Without burdening the reader with a literature review of plausible predictors, we can assert with confidence that no predictor has been shown with any degree of confidence to apply to efficacy of long-term treatment. Apart from the need to better drugs, our best hope for improved treatment is to be able to predict which drug fits which patient. Even given the terrible results from placebo treatment—Hogarty et al[4] found that 20% did not relapse two years after discharge from inpatient treatment—if we could accurately determine in advance who this 20% are, much drug treatment would be avoided. Similarly, substantial minorities of patients do well on very low dosage,[10] but we cannot predict who they are.

Less validated by clinical research is the common clinical experience of changing from drug to drug in a particular patient and finding one that appears to work better than others. At present, we must rely upon hit and miss to find the best drug. There is an enormous need for more studies of what to do when standard treatment does not work.

PSYCHOSOCIAL TREATMENT

This chapter is devoted to drug treatment, but something could be mentioned about psychosocial treatment. Two questions are crucial. Does psychotherapy ameliorate chronic symptoms or improve social/vocational functioning? We have reviewed already two studies by Hogarty et al[4,15] in which psychosocial treatment was experimentally tested over a long period. In neither study was psychosocial treatment shown to be effective, although there were interesting trends. Stein and Test,[29] in an ambitious attempt at demonstrating the benefit of an integrated approach of a variety of psychosocial treatments within a community, showed that their program was superior to a comparison group given more standard inpatient and aftercare treatment. Unfortunately, drug treatment was not controlled or even examined. It is difficult to interpret the results of psychosocial treatments of schizophrenia without taking drug treatment into account since drug treatment has been shown repeatedly to affect outcome, whereas the influence of psychosocial variables remains to be unequivocally proven.

In this context should be mentioned the works of Brown and coworkers,[30] who present interesting data about the interaction between aspects of the patient's family life and drug treatment on outcome. They show that families with high degrees of "expressed emotion" have patients who are at higher risk of relapse, and that drug treatment is important in protecting the patient from the high expressed emotion family, whereas drug treatment is not helpful in low expressed emotion families. These widely quoted conclusions must be considered nondefinitive because the drug treatment was not assigned randomly. The interaction of expressed emotionality and drug treatment on outcome is the result of nonexperimental data. We hope that this important hypothesis will soon receive adequate testing.

The remaining important study in this area is a comparison of family therapy in the home versus standard office-based treatment of the patient alone.[31] Family-based treatment was superior on several measures of psychopathology and social functioning. Concerning drug treatment, the authors say that all patients received adequate doses of antipsychotic drugs—although they do not document this. As mentioned before, drug treatment is such a crucial factor in outcome of long-term treatment that it is difficult to assess the impact of psychosocial treatments unless drug treatment is in some fashion accounted for. We look forward to more and better designed studies to elucidate the role of psychosocial treatment. Few, if any, experienced clinicians think that psychosocial treatments are unimportant, but solid evidence to select the more valuable treatments has been in very short supply. It makes sense to us that actively involving family members and going into homes where a more accurate picture of the family may be seen than in the clinician's office are valuable.

CONCLUSIONS

One fact stands out as definitively established from all the studies reviewed and from our clinical experience: antipsychotic drug treatment helps to prevent psychotic relapses in schizophrenia. We do not know for how long this benefit lasts; more cogently, we do not know when it is safe to stop drug treatment. We suspect that protection against relapse lasts many years or vulnerability lasts for many years.

We also have very little information about the optimal dose. Within a wide range of doses, the protection afforded by drugs seems equal. The only exception are the data from Kane et al,[19] which showed that very low dosage is less protective of relapse than standard dose; but even here, there are possible off-setting advantages to very low dose such as better social functioning and fewer dyskinetic movements.

What are the dangers of drug treatment? There are several—predominantly from sedation and neurological adverse reactions—although judicious use of drugs with sensitivity to those adverse reactions that mimic psychopathology (ie, akathesia and akinesia) enable most patients who benefit from long-term drug treatment to enjoy that benefit without excessive cost.

Further, of the multitude of antipsychotic drugs available, we have little reason to choose one rather than another. Most patients do better on the high potency drugs because of less sedation, whereas the increased risk of neurological side effects can be ameliorated or stopped altogether by antiparkinson drugs.

The topics of tardive dyskinesia and behavioral adverse reactions to these drugs are presented in other chapters and will not be repeated here except in capsule, apodictic fashion.

Tardive dyskinesia occurs in about 20% of patients treated with long-term antipsychotic drugs, but in the vast majority of instances it is mild. There is no evidence that continued treatment leads inevitably to worsening. Our reaction to tardive dyskinesia perhaps has been excessive. The risk of tardive dyskinesia is often less than the risk of stopping drug treatment.

The high frequency of extrapyramidal side effects is, on the other hand, often not recognized or adequately seen for the serious harm they may do to treatment. We recommend that clinicians be rather "quick on the trigger" to use antiparkinson drugs and stop them with caution.

What, then, do we recommend in more specific terms? It is one thing to document available evidence and present the pros and cons of various treatments; we should also be willing to stick out our necks and be more specific.

(1) Treat all patients who have had a recent episode of schizophrenia, whether in full remission or not, with antipsychotic drugs for one to two years, at least, at a dose equivalent to about 200–500 chlorpromazine units.
(2) Do not hesitate to extend this period if the patient's past episodes have been disastrous.
(3) Do not hesitate to alter the drug and dosage to find a maintenance treatment that is well tolerated. Individualize treatment based on past experience with this patient and according to current symptoms and adverse reactions.
(4) Use concomitant antiparkinson drugs if there is any suggestion of extrapyramidal side effects. We usually use them prophylactically.
(5) If antiparkinson drugs or antipsychotic drugs are stopped, observe the patient frequently.
(6) Educate the patient and his or her family about drug treatment. Considering the rapid turnover of psychiatrists in most clinics and the inadequacy of record keeping, often the best way to preserve the important knowledge of what is best for (or worst) for this person is for the patient and/or the family to know it and educate the psychiatrist. For the same reason, nonmedical clinicians should be knowledgeable about their patients' drug histories.
(7) Use depot preparations if there is any doubt about compliance.
(8) Do not accept chronic psychotic symptoms as untreatable unless a wide range of standard and nonstandard treatment has been tried (see Chapter 9).
(9) Do not automatically discontinue drug treatment if tardive dyskinesia appears. Assess carefully which is the greater

risk: dyskinesia (usually mild) or likelihood of relapse and its consequences.

We have led you through a bewildering thicket of facts and opinions, and we hope we have left, along with bewilderment, some light. Treating chronic disorders is not easy, but in this case it should be gratifying to know that we can usually significantly ameliorate a very nasty illness.

REFERENCES

1. Klein DF, Rosen B: Premorbid asocial response to phenothiazine treatment among schizophrenic inpatients. *Arch Gen Psychiatry* 1973;29:480–485.
2. Engelhardt DM, Freedman N, Rosen B, et al: Phenothiazines in prevention of psychiatric hospitalization. III. Delay of prevention of hospitalization. *Arch Gen Psychiatry* 1964;11:162–169.
3. Leff JP, Wing JK: Trial of maintenance therapy in schizophrenia. *Br Med J* 1971;3:599–604.
4. Hogarty GE, Goldberg SC, Schooler NR, et al: Drug and sociotherapy in the aftercare of schizophrenic patients. II. Two year relapse rates. *Arch Gen Psychiatry* 1974;31:603–608.
5. Hogarty GE, Goldberg SC, Schooler NR, et al: Drug and sociotherapy in the aftercare of schizophrenic patients. III. Adjustment of nonrelapsed patients. *Arch Gen Psychiatry* 1974;31:609–618.
6. Rifkin A, Quitkin F, Rabiner CJ, et al: Fluphenazine decanoate, oral fluphenazine and placebo in remitted schizophrenics. I. Relapse rates after one year. *Arch Gen Psychiatry* 1977;34:43–47.
7. Müller P, Kind J, Lohrengel H, et al: Prophylactic treatment of schizophrenic psychosis: Preliminary report. *Nervenarzt* 1977;48:560–561.
8. Müller P, Kind J, Steuber H: Pharmacogenic depressive syndromes in the course of schizophrenic psychoses. Presented at the Annual Meeting of the American College of Neuropsychopharmacology, New Orleans, LA, Dec 1977.
9. Hirsch SR, Gaind R, Rhode PD, et al: Outpatient maintenance of chronic schizophrenic patients with long-acting fluphenazine: Double blind placebo trial. *Br Med J* 1973;1:633–637.
10. Kane J, Rifkin A, Quitkin F, et al: Fluphenazine v. placebo in patients with remitted, acute, first episode schizophrenia. *Arch Gen Psychiatry* 1982;39: 70–73.
11. Cheung HK: Schizophrenics fully remitted on neuroleptics for 3–5 years-to stop or continue drugs? *Br J Psychiatry* 1981;138:490–494.
12. Johnson DAW: Further observations on the duration of depot neuroleptic maintenance therapy in schizophrenia. *Br J Psychiatry* 1979;135:524–530.
13. Del Giudice J, Clark WG, Gocha EF: Prevention of recidivism of schizophrenia treated with fluphenazine enanthate. *Psychosomatics* 1975; 16:32–36.
14. Falloon I, Watt DC, Shephard M: A comparative controlled trial of pimozide and fluphenazine decanoate in continuation treatment of schizophrenia. *Psychol Med* 1978;8:59–70.
15. Hogarty GE, Schooler NR, Ulrich R, et al: Fluphenazine and social therapy

in the aftercare of schizophrenic patients. *Arch Gen Psychiatry* 1979;36: 1283–1294.
16. De Alarcon R, Carney MWP: Severe depressive mood changes following slow-release intramuscular fluphenazine injection. *Br Med J* 1969;3:564–567.
17. Schooler NR, Levine J, Severa JB, et al: Prevention of relapse in schizophrenia: An evaluation of fluphenazine decanoate. *Arch Gen Psychiatry* 1980;37:16–24.
18. Kane J, Rifkin A, Quitkin R, et al: Low dose fluphenazine decanoate in the maintenance treatment of schizophrenia. *Psychiatry Res* 1979;1:341.
19. Kane JM, Rifkin A, Woerner M, et al: Low-dose neuroleptics in out-patient schizophrenics. *Psychopharm Bull* 1982;18:20–21.
20. Baldessarini RJ, Davis JM: What is the best maintenance dose of neuroleptics in schizophrenia. *Psychiatry Res* 1980;3:115–122.
21. Carpenter WT Jr, Stephens JH, Rey AC, et al: Early intervention versus continuous pharmacotherapy of schizophrenia. *Psychopharm Bull* 1982;18: 21–23.
22. Clark ML, Huber WK, Sabata K, et al: Molindone in chronic schizophrenia. *Clin Pharmacol Ther* 1970;11:668–688.
23. Gallant DM, Bishop MP: Molindone: A controlled evaluation in chronic schizophrenic patients. *Curr Ther Res* 1968;10:441–447.
24. Gallant DM, Bishop MP, Steele CA, et al: Molindone: A cross-over evaluation of capsule and tablet formulations in severely ill schizophrenic patients. *Curr Ther Res* 1973;15:915–918.
25. Gardos G, Cole JO: Weight reduction in schizophrenics by molindone. *Am J Psychiatry* 1977;134:302–304.
26. Knights A, Okasha MS, Solch MA, et al: Depressive and extrapyramidal symptoms, and clinical effects: A trial of fluphenazine versus flupenthixol in maintenance of schizophrenic outpatients. *Br J Psychiatry* 1979;135:515–523.
27. Lehman E, Quadheck G, Tegeler J, et al: Wirkeingskifferenzen bei Hoch-und Standarddosierung von Patienten-Merkmalon. *Pharmakopsychiat-Neuropsychopharmakol* 1980;13:117–129.
28. Dencker SJ, Enoksson P, Johansson R, et al: Late (4–8 years) outcome of treatment with megadoses of fluphenazine enanthate in drug-refractory schizophrenics. *Acta Psychiatr Scand* 1981;63:1–12.
29. Stein LI, Test MA: Alternative to mental hospital treatment. *Arch Gen Psychiatry* 1980;37:392–397.
30. Brown GW, Birley JLT, Wing JK: Influence of family life on the course of schizophrenic disorders: A replication. *Br J Psychiatry* 1972;121:241–248.
31. Falloon LRH, Boyd JL, McGill CW, et al: Family management in the prevention of exacerbations of schizophrenia: A controlled study. *N Engl J Med* 1982;306:1437–1440.

CHAPTER 12

ADVERSE PSYCHOLOGICAL (OR BEHAVIORAL) RESPONSES TO ANTIPSYCHOTIC DRUG TREATMENT OF SCHIZOPHRENIA

THEODORE VAN PUTTEN

All useful medicines have adverse effects. Therefore the antipsychotic drugs must have adverse psychological (or behavioral) effects. The questions are as follows. How often does this occur? What is the nature of these adverse effects? What is their mechanism? How should they be managed?

This is a controversial and ill-studied area in which there are many assertions, dramatic case reports, and little evidence. This chapter will attempt a balanced review.

Do Antipsychotic Drugs Promote Depression?

Depression occurs frequently in the course of schizophrenic illness: at the very beginning, during the acute episode, in the wake of more florid symptoms ("postpsychotic depression"), and during maintenance treatment – whether patients receive antipsychotic medications or not.[1-3] The question is whether antipsychotic drugs promote depression in some patients. The question is an important one since some schizophrenics do just as well (or badly) without antipsychotic drugs, and some schizophrenics could be managed with intermittent treatment.

During the neuroleptic era, reports of "postpsychotic depression" have multiplied, the reported incidence varying from 0 to 50% with an average of about 25%.[3] Depression becomes a serious problem in 25% to

50% of drug-maintained outpatients and is a frequent cause of readmission.[2-4] Falloon et al[5] and Knight et al[6] monitored depression in drug-maintained outpatients for 12 and 6 months, respectively, and both noted depression in approximately half the patient sample. In the study by Falloon,[5] more patients required inpatient treatment for depression than for schizophrenic relapse.

Anecdotal and uncontrolled reports have attributed depression, and even suicide,[7] to antipsychotic drugs—particularly long-acting fluphenazine enanthate or decanoate.[7-14] The high prevalence of depression in drug-free patients, both first illness patients and relapsed chronic schizophrenics, indicates, however, that a significant proportion of depressive symptoms are not drug related.[1,2] In fact, Hirsch et al[1] found that schizophrenic patients given fluphenazine decanoate maintenance treatment were prescribed antidepressant medication and/or were readmitted to the hospital for depression less often than patients given placebo maintenance.

The real questions are: Are some medications, such as fluphenazine decanoate, more likely to promote depression, and are higher doses of antipsychotic drugs more likely to promote depression than lower doses?

Dose Comparison Studies

Controlled dosage comparison studies in chronically hospitalized, treatment-refractory schizophrenics[15-27] indicate, on balance, that higher doses do not result in increased depression. These results, however, may not generalize to the usual newly admitted or readmitted schizophrenic. For one thing, the patient's drug absorption, metabolism, and tissue levels—and so his or her response—may be different. For another, depression is difficult to diagnose in the chronically ill with their blunted affect. Further, side effects associated with high dose might seem more depressing to a person who is expected to live and make it on his own outside of the hospital than for an institutionalized patient.

Indeed, the findings for the controlled dose comparison studies in patients whose conditions are more acute are somewhat different. Both Goldstein et al[25] and Quitkin et al[26] report increased depression in groups of the high-dosage patients; Goldstein et al report increased depression primarily in "good premorbid" men, and Quitkin et al report increased depression in patients who developed akinesia despite prophylactic procyclidine (66% of Quitkin's sample happened to be good premorbid patients as well). Wijsenbeck et al,[27] however, found no difference in depression ratings between those on 60 mg and those on 600 mg of trifluoperazine.

In outpatients there are no controlled dosage comparison studies which comment on depression. Johnson,[2] in a naturalistic study of outpatients maintained on depot fluphenazine or flupenthixol, noted that among those patients who relapsed, depression was more common ($P < 0.05$) in those on higher doses of neuroleptic (fluphenazine, >12.5 mg in weekly equivalents of decanoate). There was no difference in the frequency or severity of depression between patient groups on the two depot drugs.

On balance, it seems reasonable to infer that higher doses of antipsychotic drugs are more likely to promote depression, particularly in cases with a relatively good prognosis.

Are Long-Acting Injectable Phenothiazines More Depressogenic Than Tablets?

Two controlled studies[28,29] compared fluphenazine decanoate with oral fluphenazine in discharged schizophrenic patients who were in the average prognostic range; in each study half of the patients received placebo injections and active tablets, and vice versa. In the Hogarty et al[28] study, among patients who relapsed, those treated with depot fluphenazine decanoate had a higher incidence of affective symptoms than did those treated with fluphenazine tablets. Those who relapsed on the fluphenazine tablets were more psychotic, suggesting that they had stopped their tablets (probably as a result rather than a cause of relapse). In addition, family histories in the decanoate relapse group tended to be positive for affective disorder, thus suggesting a "relapse vulnerability." Schooler et al,[29] however, in a different sample with a near identical study design, did not find more depression in the depot fluphenazine group. (Interestingly, the oral fluphenazine dosage in the Schooler et al[29] study was higher: 24 mg per day versus 10 mg per day in the Hogarty et al[28] study. The decanoate dosage was roughly the same.)

Falloon et al[5] also compared (double blind) orally given pimozide with fluphenazine decanoate in schizophrenic outpatients. He found a significantly ($P < 0.05$) greater proportion of depressed patients in the fluphenazine decanoate group at one year.

Overall, patients on depot fluphenazine are probably at greater risk of developing depression than are those on tablets. This is almost certainly not because of some intrinsic pharmacologic property of fluphenazine decanoate. Rather, patients on tablets can stop them if the drug effect is disagreeable, whereas with the decanoate there is no turning back. Also, at least in the United States, those with a history of noncompliance tend to be treated with fluphenazine decanoate; these may be the very patients who stopped their medication because of a dysphoric response.[30]

Akinesia and Depression

Since there is indication that higher doses of antipsychotic drugs place patients at greater risk of depression, it is reasonable to postulate that some side effect (such as akinesia) is central to some drug-induced depressions.

Schizophrenic patients with postpsychotic depression have been described as "wooden" in appearance,[31] motorically "inactive or retarded," lacking in initiative to perform routine tasks,[32] experiencing overwhelming fatigue and neuroasthenic symptoms, [33,34] "hypersomnic," and "emotionally withdrawn."[35] Nearly all reports comment on the patient's disinclination to speak.[3] All of these symptoms, however, *can* be manifestations of antipsychotic drug-induced akinesia.[36] Indeed, persons with Parkinson's disease regularly experience "a blunting of interest and drive, amounting to apathy, a limitation in intellectual activity, and an apparent slowing of thought process and memory."[37] There is a high incidence of depression associated even with the early stages of parkinsonism,[38] and the depression of Parkinson's disease seems out of proportion to the physical handicap.[39]

In our own work,[40] out of a total of 94 schizophrenic inpatients, 28 developed a mild akinesia and 32 never developed extrapyramidal symptoms. Those who developed akinesia became less psychotic, but they also experienced a significant, although modest, increase in depression ratings. Vigorous treatment of the akinesia with trihexyphenidyl resulted in significant improvements in depression, somatic concern, anxiety, emotional withdrawal, blunted affect, and motor retardation on both physicians' and nurses' ratings. A high association between akinesia and both objectively rated and subjectively experienced sedative effect indicates that an "akinetic depression" is not likely if the patient does not look or feel drowsy. The 32 nonakinetic patients also became less psychotic, but not more depressed.

Some of the akinetic patients who did *not* become more depressed did experience dysphoria, stating that they felt "blah," "listless," "tired" or that they had no "interest," "life," or "ambition," but they did not complain much and specifically denied sadness or depression. Some of them seemed quite accepting of these feelings, and it appears that both the patient and the doctor can get used to a mild akinesia.

Rifkin and associates[40a] compared fluphenazine decanoate and oral fluphenazine with a placebo in remitted schizophrenics who were in an aftercare clinic. Remission was defined as the absence of signs of psychosis—delusions, hallucinations, bizarre behavior, or disorganized speech. In addition to medication, these patients received a rich spectrum of clinical services: supportive psychotherapy, vocational rehabilitation, social groups, supervised apartments, etc.

All patients received daily tablets and biweekly injections, some active, some placebo, in double-blind fashion. Thirty-five percent of the patients assigned to fluphenazine decanoate (but none of the patients on oral fluphenazine) developed disabling akinesia even though they received prophylactic procyclidine. (The dose of fluphenazine decanoate ranged between 0.5 and 2.0 mL (12.5 to 50 mg), and all akinetic patients were managed with 0.5 mL before it was decided to withdraw the patient because of disabling akinesia.) The akinetic patients became significantly (although modestly) more depressed and withdrawn when compared to their own baseline and to the survivors who did not develop akinesia.[40a,b]

Patients with "akinetic depression" do not tell us that they are depressed because of the akinesia. What is beguiling is that they speak of loss, of personal failure and humiliations, of personal inadequacy and lack of meaning—in short, the psychodynamics of "postpsychotic depression."[3] We are not saying that patients are not right about their situation; we can say that they no longer speak that way when the akinesia is corrected.

If an extrapyramidal symptom, particularly akinesia, is associated with depression (or if patients experience it as depression), then populations of schizophrenics stabilized on antiparkinson drugs should experience depression upon antiparkinson withdrawal. This is so. In two different samples (one in Boston,[41] the other in Greece[42,43]) of chronic schizophrenic patients stabilized on antiparkinson drugs, sudden or gradual double-blind withdrawal of antiparkinson drugs did result in increased anxiety, depression, and general dysphoria and suffering.[41–43]

Johnson,[2] in a naturalistic study of schizophrenic outpatients, also found the presence of extrapyramidal symptoms (type not specified) to be significantly ($P < 0.001$) related to depression. There was also a trend, not reaching significance, for more severe extrapyramidal symptoms to correlate with more severe depression. It is important to note, however, that those patients successfully maintained in remission by depot injections had the lowest prevalence of depression.

In a substudy, Johnson[2] administered orphenadrine, 50 mg twice daily (an antiparkinson drug), or placebo to 40 depressed schizophrenic patients maintained in remission with depot injections and free from *overt* extrapyramidal symptoms. More patients (8 versus 3) in the orphenadrine group experienced "good improvement," but the difference was not significant. Orphenadrine improvers experienced significantly more subjective "muscular weakness and stiffness," suggesting that their depression may have been akinesia-based.

In sum, the risk of depression appears increased by higher doses of neuroleptic. Further extrapyramidal symptoms, particularly akinesia, appear associated with increased depression ratings in schizophrenic patients during all stages of their illness. If antipsychotic drugs do promote depression in some patients, this is likely part of, or a reaction to, akinesia. It is unclear if antipsychotic drugs can promote depression without akinesia, akinesia being much underdiagnosed.

At a practical level, if a schizophrenic patient becomes depressed during the course of antipsychotic drug therapy, the clinician should first consider the possibility that this is a "toxic" drug effect. The fact that the depression may be "understandable" or that the schizophrenic himself attributes it to his circumstances should not be accepted at face value. The response to a brief course of vigorous treatment with an antiparkinson drug should distinguish between akinetic depression and depression due to some other cause.

Akinesia

Akinesia, just by itself and without depression, may be the most toxic behavioral side effect.

Akinesia is defined by Rifkin et al as a "behavioral state of diminished spontaneity characterized by few gestures, unspontaneous speech and, particularly, apathy and difficulty with initiating usual activities."[36] So defined, this side effect of antipsychotic drugs often goes unrecognized.

Rifkin and associates,[40a,b] in an aforementioned study, had to withdraw 35% of patients on fluphenazine decanoate maintenance because of disabling akinesia even though they received a low dose (0.5 mL or 12.5 mg) and prophylactic procyclidine. Rifkin and associates,[44] in another study, withdrew antiparkinson drugs from long-term aftercare patients stabilized on antipsychotic drugs. After three weeks, 27% of patients on procyclidine placebo developed akinesia. The magnitude of these figures derived from raters sensitive to akinesia indicates that akinesia often goes undiagnosed.

Even mild akinesia is socially disabling. Akinetic apathy and lack of spontaneity are mistaken for the negative symptoms of schizophrenia and add to the notorious social and emotional disability of schizophrenic patients on maintenance therapy. Most important, the onus of detection is on the physician, for the patient seldom complains. Indeed, even when asked if he feels "slowed up" or "sluggish," the patient often denies any difficulty whatever and is seemingly locked in some peaceful apathetic remoteness.

These are bold assertions, born more from clinical experience than controlled investigation. But there is some controlled evidence that akinesia has far-reaching consequences.

Falloon et al[5] compared the social outcome of schizophrenic patients maintained either on pimozide or fluphenazine decanoate. At one year those on pimozide were rated significantly more favorable on aspects of sociability, use of leisure, warmth of personal relationships, household tasks, and child rearing. This could not be related to superior antipsychotic effect (both pimozide and fluphenazine decanoate scored the same on schizophrenic symptomatology), but did seem related to the patients on pimozide experiencing *less* extrapyramidal rigidity. The authors speculated that akinetic "flatness of expression" and "psychomotor retardation" were responsible for the poorer social adjustment on depot fluphenazine. Barro et al,[45] in an open trial, also showed that, for matched long-stay schizophrenics, pimozide was superior to haloperidol and penfluridol in terms of nurses' ratings of social function. A particular feature of this study was the finding that gestures and movements were more appropriate on pimozide. An akinetic poverty of spontaneous movement could be very influential in social adjustment. Argyle[46] has shown that nonverbal signals may have a far greater impact than verbal ones for assertiveness and friendship.

It is, of course, notoriously difficult to differentiate schizophrenic apathy and blunting from extrapyramidal side effects. Nevertheless, we fear that some, perhaps even many, schizophrenics are entrapped in akinesia. In a recent survey of community board and care facilities, the residents with schizophrenia were being maintained on an average of 760 mg (standard deviation 540 mg) of chlorpromazine equivalent per day, and 59% appeared to be at least mildly akinetic.[47] (There is the dark thought that akinetic apathy and lack of initiative may even be welcomed because they promote organizational efficiency.)

Detection of akinesia It would help to have a measure that distinguishes between akinesia and the negative symptoms of schizophrenia or the psychomotor retardation of depression. Constriction of handwriting (micrographia) turns out *not* to be a reliable correlate[48]; neither is antipsychotic drug or prolactin plasma level.[49]

One useful correlate of akinesia is a subjective sense of sedation. When rated at 9:00 AM (12 hours after H.S. dose), 88% of the akinetic patients rated themselves as slightly drowsy, as opposed to 18% of the nonakinetic patients.[30]

Leg crossing may be another useful correlate. Most persons (except the very obese and tense) will cross their legs when seated in a comfortable chair; persons with Parkinson's disease do not.[50]

Figure 12-1 shows the relationship between severity of akinesia and the percentage of schizophrenic patients crossing their legs (as rated during a brief interview ranging between 5 and 20 minutes). About 80% of nonakinetic schizophrenic patients cross their legs when seated in a comfortable chair, but only 10% of patients with mild akinesia cross theirs.

The point is that if a schizophrenic patient does not cross his legs during a brief interview, there is a good chance that he experiences a drug-induced akinesia.

Subjective Responses to Antipsychotic Medication

Subjective response is not be be equated with patient satisfaction or with a patient's attitudes toward drug treatment. A patient who finds the medication helpful (a syntonic response) may still regard the tablet as a daily reminder of mental or moral weakness and may be thoroughly

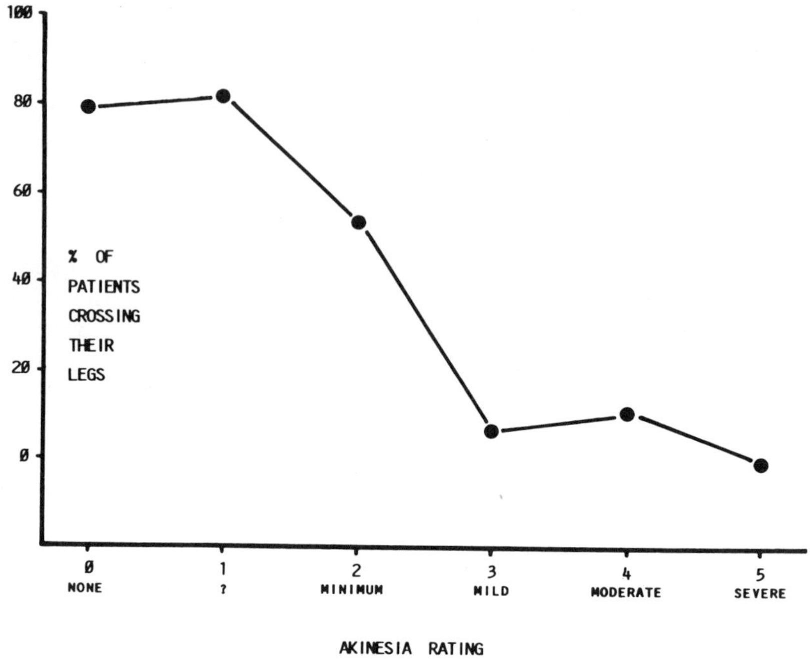

Figure 12-1 Percentage of patients crossing their legs versus severity of drug-induced akinesia (N = 130).

unhappy with his treatment. Similarly, a patient with a dysphoric response to medication may, particularly if he has a concerned physician, be satisfied with his care.

Dysphoric responses to antipsychotic drugs have received little systematic inquiry. Yet they are important; no matter how much a patient improves behaviorally, in the end we have to pay attention to how he feels.

Dysphoric responses to medication erode the quality of life. Lack of vigor, ever-present fatigue, lack of interest or motivation, muscular cramps and achiness, inner restlessness or impatience, and vague complaints of "just not feeling right" are feeling states that schizophrenics often (correctly) attribute to their medications. Hogarty (personal communication) even speaks of a "neuroleptic-induced anguish" which, in his opinion, is poorly captured with the conventional rating scales.

At times, dysphoric responses interfere with work. For a night watchman, a mild dysphoric drug-induced lethargy might be more disabling than his voices, with which he usually manages to cope. Minimizing dysphoric response without unduly compromising the desired antipsychotic effect is the art of pharmacotherapy.

Studying the schizophrenic's subjective response to antipsychotic medication is, ironically, a rather new idea. Heretofore, the profession has not been very sensitive to subjective responses to antipsychotic medication. Certainly in public mental hospitals the emphasis, understandably, has been on control of psychotic symptoms. Complaints of drug-induced dysphoria are often given short shrift, if acknowledged as drug related at all.

In general, drug-induced dysphoria, when it has been recognized, has been regarded as a small price to pay for improvement in florid psychotic symptoms. Many schizophrenic patients, however, have little grasp of their circumstances and deny that anything is wrong in the first place; for such patients side effects easily become the central drug experience, rather than a discomfort to be tolerated on the road to recovery.

Value judgments are involved. A few angry ex-patients have gone to the courts complaining, in effect, that doctors are not sensitive to drug-induced dysphoric states. They equate their past treatment with "psychiatric assault," "chemical straightjacketing," and "chemical lobotomy." American courts are listening—and intervening in physicians' decisions to medicate the mentally ill. Some of the testimony makes compelling reading. From a young woman:

> My tongue was so fuzzy, so thick, I could barely speak. Always I needed water and even with it my loose tongue often could not shape the words. It was so hard to think, the effort was so great; more often than not I would fall into a stupor of not caring or I would go to sleep . . . I could not focus my blurred eyes to read and I always fell asleep at a film. People's voices came through filtered, strange. They could not penetrate my Thorazine fog; and I could not escape my drug prison.
>
> Yet to detail the physical suffering caused by these drugs is to touch only on one aspect of the pain they cause. Psychologically and emotionally they are devastating. They cause sensations—drowsiness, disorientation, shakiness, dry mouth, blurred vision, inability to concentrate—that would be enough to unnerve the strongest among us . . . It is common practice among psychiatrists *not* to inform their patients that the disturbing things they are experiencing are drug induced . . . My hands would shake as I held a coffee cup, my legs would beat a wild tattoo on the floor, and sometimes I would fall asleep in the middle of a conversation. I knew I was deteriorating, going slowly, surely insane. No one thought it necessary to advise me otherwise. "But why do you *think* people are looking at you strangely?", Dr. Sternfeld would ask. Why indeed?

From a young man:

> After 10 days or so, the effects of the Prolixin began building up in my system and my body started going through pure hell. It's very hard to

> describe the effects of this drug and others like it, that's why we use strange words like "zombie." But in my case the experience became sheer torture. Different muscles began twitching. My mouth was like very dry cotton no matter how much water I drank. My tongue became all swollen up. My entire body felt like it was being twisted up in contortions inside by some unseen wringer . . . But most disturbing of all was that I feared that all these excruciating experiences were in my mind, or caused by my mind—a sign of my supposed sickness . . . (Testimony before the Senate subcommittee, 1977[51].)

Even allowing for a certain amount of histrionic exaggeration, few would doubt that these patients were improperly medicated, however well-intentioned their physician may have been. Clearly a good clinical outcome is unlikely with such obvious drug-related dysphoria and gross side effects.

Dysphoric Response and Outcome

Even with moderate dosages and no gross side effects, a substantial minority of schizophrenic patients have a dysphoric response. These patients complain that the medication "keeps me closed in" . . . "makes me feel spacey" . . . "takes me away from my normal frame of mind" . . . "slows my thinking" . . . "makes my whole body feel like it is in a physical prison" . . . "makes me confused." The majority of these dysphoric responders do not regard the medication as helpful.

To what degree are the patient's perceptions of drug effect in agreement with the professional's? The correlations between subjective response in two inpatient samples (one treated with haloperidol, 10 mg daily, the other with thiothixene, 0.44 mg/kg) and the doctors' and nurses' ratings of improvement are shown in Table 12-1.

These correlations indicate a respectable agreement, both at the beginning and end of treatment, between subjective response and staff's ratings of improvement—with two different drugs in two different samples. Put another way, if the patient finds the medication helpful (a syntonic response), the staff's ratings bear him out; conversely, patients with a dysphoric response are seen by the staff as doing less well.

Since many dysphoric responders (about 65% in both samples) stopped medication very early in their treatment course, we do not know whether they could profit from antipsychotic medication. Those dysphoric responders who did complete four weeks of inpatient treatment tended to have a poorer outcome—by both doctors' and nurses' criteria.[52]

May and Van Putten's unreplicated work[56] should not be taken to imply that patients with a dysphoric response should not be given antipsychotic drugs. Some patients with a dysphoric response do eventually make their peace with antipsychotic medication and experience good symptomatic improvement—often, in our experience, with very low

Table 12-1
Correlations (*r*) Between Total Subjective Response and Outcome, Both Measured at the Same Time.

	Haloperidol Sample				
	Doctor			*Nurse*	
Subjective Response	*BPRS Total*	*CGI*	*Total MACC*	*Total NOSIE*	*CGI*
7 days	0.441	0.444	0.294	0.153	0.400
P	0.025	0.05	n.s.*	n.s.	0.05
28 days	0.534	0.609	0.377	0.377	0.469
P	0.005	0.001	0.01	0.01	0.01

	Thiothixene Sample				
	Doctor			*Nurse*	
Subjective Response	*BPRS Total*	*CGI*	*Total MACC*	*Total NOSIE*	*CGI*
48 hours	0.562	–	0.200	–	–
P	0.005		n.s.		
28 days	0.381	0.387†	0.361	0.283	0.403
P	0.05	0.025	0.05	n.s.	0.01

*n.s., Not significant.
†One extreme outlier deleted (including outlier $r = 0.290$, $P < 0.05$)
Abbreviations: BPRS = Brief Psychiatric Rating Scale, CGI = Clinical Global Impression, MACC = Mack Behavior Adjustment Scale, NOSIE = Nurses Observation Scale for Inpatient Evaluation.

doses, eg, thioridazine, 50 mg daily, or fluphenazine decanoate, 5 mg intramuscularly every two weeks. Others experience fair symptomatic improvement but at the expense of ongoing dysphoria. If such persons were floridly psychotic and dangerous to others in their unmedicated state, then their dysphoria is clearly "worth it."

It is important that dysphoric responses to antipsychotic medication need to be acknowledged; that dysphoric responders, at least when compared with syntonic responders, tend to have a poorer outcome; either noncompliance[52a] or less symptomatic improvement.

Mechanisms of dysphoric response In our experience, dysphoric responses to antipsychotic medication tend to be associated with extrapyramidal symptoms—notably akathisia.[30,52] Even with an antiparkinson drug, a persisting akathisia is, in our experience, not uncommon.

This observation—intractable akathisia despite the maximal allowable doses of antiparkinson drug—may raise the question of whether it was the doctor or the patient who was so sensitive to akathisia. The reported incidence of side effects depends on how side effect data are elicited. Side effects are elicited with increasing frequency depending on whether one relies on spontaneous complaints, general questions ("How do you feel?"), or specific questions. For akathisia, the staff asked, "Do you feel restless or jittery inside; is it difficult to sit still?" In addition, the physician was probably more sensitive to side effects. For example, if a patient mentioned feeling "strange," "frightened," or "weird," the physician would first rule out akathisia by asking specific questions; in doubtful cases amelioration by antiparkinson drug would then support a diagnosis of akathisia.

The point is that if the possibility of akathisia is elicited by specific questions, it will be found to occur much earlier than commonly supposed and, at least in our experience, is an important contribution to dysphoric response.

Double-blind withdrawal of antiparkinson drugs If extrapyramidal symptoms are easily elaborated into dysphoric feeling states, withdrawal of antiparkinson drugs should result in dysphoria. This is so. When Jellinek et al[41] substituted placebo for antiparkinson drug, 62% of patients on long-term antipsychotic drug therapy experienced pronounced adverse effects. Many of the symptoms were psychopathologic—eg, anxiety, depression and hallucinations. Some patients developed strange complaints; they complained of feeling "keyed up," "edgy and nervous," "strange," and "drained," and one felt "drunk with pain in my chest and head." Manos and associates[42,43] confirmed these findings: in their study, 22.6% of patients even developed psychotic symptoms that the investigators related to extrapyramidal reactions. For example, one patient stated that "pliers are squeezing my body"—a probable psychotic elaboration of an extrapyramidal side effect.

Drug-Induced Exacerbations of Psychotic Illness Secondary to Side Effects

Dramatic exacerbations of psychosis have been observed particularly with the high-potency drugs. Since such exacerbations were reversed by antiparkinson drug and not by placebo, it seems reasonable to assume that they were an expression of extrapyramidal involvement—most likely akathisia.[53,54]

For a case example, a 48-year-old woman was admitted with a well-organized delusional system to the effect that a NASA computer controlled her mind and actions. She was somewhat excited, but conversed quite rationally as long as the delusional system was avoided. On the fifth day after an injection of fluphenazine enanthate, 25 mg, she burst into my office panic-stricken. She was extremely agitated and talking in pressured fashion. "I was hit by ultrasonic sound. A war machine has been used against me. You can get polio with these lasers. Please, can't you see I'm wasting away. Touch me . . . " No rational contact could be established. She had a mild parkinsonian tremor of her fingers and would not sit down. One hour after biperiden, 5 mg given intramuscularly, she was a changed person. She felt "relaxed" and spoke very coherently. Six hours after the biperiden, moderate anxiety recurred. A placebo injection had no effect.

Injection of antiparkinson drug (biperiden) in many of those who experienced an exacerbation of psychosis improved psychotic symptoms, anxiety, depression and eliminated such peculiar complaints as "feeling swollen up inside," "tightness inside," and feelings of extreme "fear" and "confusion." Such feeling states as "it's a horrible feeling; I can't describe it," or "if this feeling continues, I'd rather be dead," or "it feels like I will explode into a thousand pieces" were not unusual and were abolished (or at least diminished) by biperiden.

The point is that thought-disordered expressions of extrapyramidal effect can take strange forms, that such effects can be terrifying, and that a worsening of psychosis should always raise the question of a trial of treatment with antiparkinson drug.

Failure to Improve (or Worsening) Secondary to High Plasma Levels

All that appears to be firmly established in the literature is that plasma levels of antipsychotic drugs vary enormously among patients. This raised the hope that plasma levels, rather than dosage, could guide the clinician. (It has also been assumed that patient noncompliance is not a factor in plasma level variability: probably a large assumption.)

Much of the past research on the relation between plasma levels of antipsychotic drug and clinical change has been difficult to interpret because of shortcomings with the assays or design deficiencies (lack of fixed-dose design, contamination with other treatments, etc).[55,56]

Recent fixed (or constant)-dose studies with fluphenazine,[57] haloperidol,[58,59] and chlorpromazine[60] do suggest a "therapeutic window" beyond which patients either do not respond or become worse.

In a fixed-dose study with chlorpromazine patients with high plasma levels (>300 pmol of chlorpromazine) became distinctly worse. (Two became assaultive, one became agitated and menacing, one cut his clothes into little pieces, and one ceased to have any spontaneous behavior.) Patients who became worse on higher plasma levels shared certain characteristics: They were clinically inaccessible and severely thought disordered; they asked for more medication; and their illness, in retrospect, was only minimally sensitive to treatment with antipsychotic drug.[60]

In a haloperidol study by Bjorndal et al,[59] three of 12 patients on high dose (120–240 mg) and high plasma levels (>100 ng/mL) "exhibited attacks of violent aggression during which they struck fellow patients and staff and damaged furniture." These attacks disappeared after a 50% reduction in dose. Further, depression items (somatic concern, anxiety, guilt feelings, and depressive mood) increased significantly during high dosage and high plasma level treatment in the nonresponders. Side effects were also more prominent in the high-dose group: sedation (5 of 12 patients), muscular weakness and a tendency to fall (2 patients), and epileptic attacks (1 patient). Patients in the standard dose group (12–36 mg per day; mean, 15 mg per day) had lower plasma haloperidol levels, improved more, and had fewer side effects. These patients also were at least moderately ill and "relatively treatment resistant" to neuroleptic medication.

The mechanism behind the presumed behavioral toxicity at high plasma levels is unknown. It may well be that these patients, whose illness is only partially sensitive to medication, become worse because of the stress of side effects that they, because of their thought disorder, cannot communicate. It should also be kept in mind that behavioral toxicity at high plasma levels is supported by only about a dozen cases (in those studies with either a fixed or constant dose).

The notion of behavioral toxicity at high plasma levels would appear to be contradicted by the literature on megadoses in chronic patients. This literature, on balance, indicates that some chronic treatment-resistant patients do improve more at very high doses (eg, fluphenazine 800-1200 mg/day).[60a] However, this improvement is relative; these patients do not improve to the point where they can be discharged. In the author's experience with megadoses in treatment-refractory cases who have been chronically hospitalized, megadoses can result in some further improvement, but at the expense of considerable akinesia. After treatment with megadoses, these patients are rated improved in the sense that there is "less of them": they spend more time sitting, are less excited and speak less, but they remain very psychotic. Thus, in the treatment-resistant patient with florid symptoms, the "toxicity" at higher plasma levels might serve some "therapeutic" purpose.

So far, it seems that a plasma level might be useful in ruling out surreptitious noncompliance or the remote possibility that the drug is not being absorbed; if the plasma level is unexpectedly high and the patient is doing poorly, a trial reduction in dosage seems prudent.

"Supersensitivity Psychosis"

Tardive dyskinesia is considered to be a supersensitivity of dopaminergic neurons in the basal ganglia. Similarly, if supersensitivity of dopaminergic neurons within the mesolimbic system were to occur, then there might be a "tardive psychosis." Such an iatrogenic psychosis, like tardive dyskinesia, might require increasing amounts of neuroleptic for suppression, and a decrease or discontinuation of neuroleptic drug would result in immediate and new florid symptomatology. This frightening hypothesis was first raised by Ungerstedt and Ljungberg in 1977.[61]

Chouinard and Jones[62] reported on 10 patients who required continual increases of antipsychotic drug to control florid symptoms. After three or more years these patients seemed to require 234 (standard deviation, 217) mg of fluphenazine enanthate to control florid symptoms of schizophrenia. Small decreases in drug resulted in the rapid emergence of florid symptoms, and eight patients had tardive dyskinesia.

Fortunately, such increasing dosage requirements in schizophrenic outpatients are not common experience. Also, high doses often reflect the physician's desperation in those whose illness is only partially sensitive to antipsychotic drug. Lastly, we have seen patients who develop delusional ideas about the dosage of medication they believe they require.

At this time, it seems wise to have an open mind about the possibility of "supersensitivity psychosis" and to investigate those rare cases that seem to require continual increases of neuroleptic.

Conclusion

The above review indicates that behavioral toxicity to antipsychotic drugs is a murky and poorly explored area. Scattered anecdotal case reports give no idea about prevalence, and not all are compelling.

Some anecdotally reported adverse mental reactions to antipsychotic drugs have all the earmarks of a toxic psychosis with clouded sensorium, vivid visual and auditory hallucinations, confusion, memory impairment, slurred speech, etc.[53] El-Yousef and co-workers[63] have reported an anticholinergically based exacerbation of psychosis in patients maintained on moderate dosages of antipsychotic drugs and antiparkinson agents. These exacerbations were reversed by physostigmine, a cholinergic agent.

Others[64-66] have attributed neuroleptic-induced exacerbations of schizophrenia to a subtle interaction between antipsychotic drug effect and premorbid personality. In this psychodynamic view, exacerbations of the disease process occur because the pharmacologic action of the drug has particular emotional meaning and significance to the subject.

Judging from our clinical work and a review of the literature, the following practical guidelines emerge with regard to behavioral toxicity:

- Neuroleptic-induced depression can occur and the risk of depression and extrapyramidal symptoms particularly (akinesia) seems increased by high doses.
- Neuroleptics can also improve mood. Populations of schizophrenics treated with antipsychotics experience less

depression than populations treated with placebo.

- If a schizophrenic patient becomes depressed during the course of antipsychotic drug treatment, an "akinetic depression" should be considered. If such a patient appears at all akinetic, a vigorous trial of treatment with an antiparkinson drug should distinguish between akinetic depression and depression due to some other cause.
- Akinesia, as a "behavioral state of diminished spontaneity characterized by few gestures, unspontaneous speech, and, particularly, apathy and difficulty with initiating usual activities,[36] is often unrecognized and is socially disabling.
- Dysphoric responses to antipsychotic drugs are not uncommon and augur a poor outcome: either noncompliance or, if the dysphoric response persists, less symptomatic improvement than is seen with syntonic responders.
- Dysphoric responses are often extrapyramidally based and should be given a vigorous trial of treatment with antiparkinson drugs. Some dysphoric responders seem to do well on very low doses of antipsychotic drug.
- Many chronic patients stabilized on antiparkinson drugs derive ongoing therapeutic benefit from the combination. Withdrawal of antiparkinson drugs results in increased anxiety, dysphoria, depression, somatic preoccupation, and psychotic symptoms.
- Behavioral deterioration at unexpectedly high plasma levels of haloperidol, chlorpromazine, and fluphenazine may occur. The mechanism is unknown.

REFERENCES

1. Hirsch SR, Gaind R, Rhode PD, et al: Outpatient maintenance of chronic schizophrenic patients with long-acting fluphenazine: Double-blind placebo trial. *Br Med J* 1973;1:633–637.
2. Johnson DAW: Studies of depressive symptoms in schizophrenia. I. The prevalence of depression and its possible causes. II. A two-year longitudinal study of symptoms. III. A double blind trial of orphenadrine against placebo. *Br J Psychiatry* 1981;139:89–101.
3. McGlashan TH, Carpenter WT Jr: Postpsychotic depression in schizophrenia. *Arch Gen Psychiatry* 1976;33:231–239.
4. Mandel MR, Severe JB, Schooler NR, et al: Development and prediction of postpsychotic depression in neuroleptic-treated schizophrenics. *Arch Gen Psychiatry* 1982;39:197–203.
5. Falloon I, Watt DC, Shepherd M: A comparative controlled trial of pimozide and fluphenazine decanoate in the continuation therapy of schizophrenia. *Psychol Med* 1978;8:59–70.
6. Knight A, Okasha MS, Salih MA, et al: Depressive and extrapyramidal

symptoms and clinical effects: A trial of fluphenazine vs. flupenthixol in maintenance of schizophrenic outpatients. *Br J Psychiatry* 1979;135:515–523.

7. DeAlarcon R, Carney WMP: Severe depressive mood changes following slow-release intra-muscular fluphenazine injection. *Br Med J* 1969;3:564–567.
8. Ray I: Amotivational syndrome. *Can Med Assoc J* 1972;107:279.
9. Keskiner A: A long-term follow up of fluphenazine enanthate treatment. *Curr Ther Res* 1973;15:305–313.
10. Johnson J: Depressive changes after fluphenazine treatment. *Br Med J* 1969;3: 718.
11. Marjot DH: Depression following fluphenazine treatment. *Br Med J* 1969;3: 780.
12. Segal M, Ropschitz DH: Depressive changes after fluphenazine treatment. *Br Med J* 1969;4:159.
13. West D: Dangers of fluphenazine. *Br J Psychiatry* 1970;117:718–719.
14. Lambert PA, Marcon G: Fluphenazine enanthate given to inpatients and outpatients. *Dis Nerv Syst* 1970;31(Suppl A):63–65.
15. Prien RF, Cole JO: High dose chlorpromazine therapy in chronic schizophrenia. *Arch Gen Psychiatry* 1968;18:481–495.
16. Prien RF, Levine J, Cole JO: High dose trifluoperazine therapy in chronic schizophrenia. *Am J Psychiatry* 1969;126:305–313.
17. Clark ML, Ramsey HR, Ragland RE, et al: Chlorpromazine in chronic schizophrenia: Behavioral dose-response relationships. *Psychopharmacology (Berlin)* 1970;18:260–270.
18. Clark ML, Ramsey HR, Rahhal DK, et al: Chlorpromazine in chronic schizophrenia. *Arch Gen Psychiatry* 1972;27:479–483.
19. Brotman RK, Muzekari LH, Shanken PM: Butaperizine in chronic schizophrenic patients: A double-blind study. *Curr Ther Res* 1969;11:5–8.
20. Carscallen HB, Rochman H, Lovegrove TD: High dosage trifluoperazine in schizophrenia. *Can Psych Assoc J* 1968;13:459–461.
21. Itil TM, Saletu B, Hu W, et al: Clinical and quantitative EEG changes at different dosage levels of fluphenazine treatment. *Acta Psychiatr Scand* 1971;47:440–451.
22. Itil TM, Keskiner A, Heinemann L, et al: Treatment of resistant schizophrenics with extreme high dosage fluphenazine hydrochloride. *Psychosomatics* 1970;11:456–463.
23. Simpson GM, Amin M, Kurz-bartholini E, et al: Problems in the evaluation of the optimal dose of a phenothiazine (butaperazine). *Dis Nerv Syst* 1968; 29:478–484.
24. McClelland HA, Farquharson RG, Leyburn P, et al: Very high dose fluphenazine decanoate. A controlled trial in chronic schizophrenia. *Arch Gen Psychiatry* 1976;33:1435–1439.
25. Goldstein MJ, Rodnick EH, Evans JR, et al: Drug and family therapy in the aftercare treatment of acute schizophrenia. *Arch Gen Psychiatry* 1978;35: 1169–1177.
26. Quitkin F, Rifkin A, Klein DF: Very high dosage vs standard dosage fluphenazine in schizophrenia. *Arch Gen Psychiatry* 1975;32:1276–1281.
27. Wijsenbeck H, Steiner M, Goldberg SC: Trifluoperazine: A comparison between regular and high doses. *Psychopharmacology (Berlin)* 1974;36:147–150.
28. Hogarty GE, Schooler NR, Ulrich R, et al: Fluphenazine and social therapy in the aftercare of schizophrenic patients: Relapse analyses of a two-year controlled study of fluphenazine decanoate and fluphenazine hydrochloride.

Arch Gen Psychiatry 1979;36:1283–1294.
29. Schooler NR, Levine J, Severe JR, et al: Prevention of relapse in schizophrenia: An evaluation of fluphenazine decanoate. *Arch Gen Psychiatry* 1980;31:16–24.
30. Van Putten T, May PRA, Marder SR, et al: Subjective response to antipsychotic drugs. *Arch Gen Psychiatry* 1981;38:187–190.
31. Steinberg HR, Green R, Durell J: Depression occurring during the course of recovery from schizophrenic symptoms. *Am J Psychiatry* 1967;124:699–792.
32. Wildroe HJ: Depression following acute schizophrenic psychosis. *J Hillside Hosp* 1966;15:114–122.
33. Kayton L: Good outcome in young adult schizophrenia. *Arch Gen Psychiatry* 1973;29:103–110.
34. Sachar EJ, Mason JW, Kolmer HS, et al: Psychoendocrine aspects of acute schizophrenic reactions. *Psychosom Med* 1963;25:510–537.
35. Stern MJ, Pillsbury JA, Sonnenberg SM: Postpsychotic depression in schizophrenics. *Compr Psychiatry* 1972;13:519.
36. Rifkin A, Quitkin F, Klein DF: Akinesia. *Arch Gen Psychiatry* 1975;32: 672–674.
37. Marsden CD, Parkes JD: Success and problems of long-term levodopa therapy in Parkinson's disease. *Lancet* 1977;1:345–349.
38. Celesia GG, Wanamaker WM: Psychiatric disturbances in Parkinson's disease. *Dis Nerv Syst* 1972;33:577–583.
39. Robins AH: Depression in patients with parkinsonism. *Br J Psychiatry* 1976; 128:141–145.
40. Van Putten T, May PRA: "Akinetic depression" in schizophrenia. *Arch Gen Psychiatry* 1978;35:1101–1107.
40a. Rifkin A, Quitkin F, Rabiner CJ, et al: Fluphenazine decanoate, fluphenazine hydrochloride given orally, and placebo in remitted schizophrenics. I. Relapse rates after one year. *Arch Gen Psychiatry* 1977;34:43–47.
40b. Rifkin A, Quitkin F, Klein DF: Fluphenazine decanoate, oral fluphenazine, and placebo in treatment of remitted schizophrenics. II. Rating scale data. *Arch Gen Psychiatry* 1977;34:1215–1219.
41. Jellinek T, Gardos G, Cole JO: Adverse effects of antiparkinson drug withdrawal. *Am J Psychiatry* 1981;138:1567–1571.
42. Manos N, Gkiouzepas J, Logothetis J: The need for continuous use of antiparkinsonian medication with chronic schizophrenic patients receiving long-term neuroleptic therapy. *Am J Psychiatry* 1981;138:184–188.
43. Manos N, Gkiouzepas J, Tzotros T, et al: Gradual withdrawal of antiparkinson medication in chronic schizophrenics: Any better than the abrupt? *J Nerv Ment Dis* 1981;169:659–661.
44. Rifkin A, Quitkin F, Kane J, et al: Are prophylactic antiparkinson drugs necessary? *Arch Gen Psychiatry* 1978;35:483–489.
45. Baro F, Van Lommel R, Dorn R, et al: Pimozide treatment of chronic schizophrenics as compared with haloperidol and penfluridol maintenance treatment. *Acta Psychiatr Belg* 1972;72:199–214.
46. Argyle M: Non-verbal communication and verbal disorder. *Psychol Med* 1978;8:551–554.
47. Van Putten T, Spar JE: The board and care home. *Hosp Comm Psychiatry* 1979;30:461–464.
48. Shackman DR, Van Putten T, May PRA: Micrographia and akinesia. *Am J Psychiatry* 1979;135:839–840.
49. Van Putten T, May PRA, Wilkins JN: Importance of akinesia: Relationship to plasma CPZ and prolactin levels. *Am J Psychiatry* 1980;137:1446–1448.

50. DeJong RN: *The Neurologic Examination,* 3rd Ed. New York, Harper and Row, 1967, pp 398–400.
51. Testimony of Janet Gotkin and Wade Hudson Before the Senate Subcommittee to Investigate Juvenile Delinquency, August 18, 1975, in Drugs in Institutions: Hearings Before the Subcommittee to Investigate Juvenile Delinquency. Washington, DC, Government Printing Office, 1977, pp 14–15, 33.
52. Van Putten T, May PRA, Marder SR: Response to antipsychotic medication: The doctor's and the consumer's view. *Am J Psychiatry* in press.
52a. Van Putten T, May PRA, Marder SR, et al: Subjective response to antipsychotic drugs. *Arch Gen Psychiatry* 1981;38:187–190.
53. Van Putten T, Mutalipassi LR, Malkin MD: Phenothiazine induced decompensation. *Arch Gen Psychiatry* 1974;30:102–105.
54. Van Putten T, Mutalipassi LR: Fluphenazine enanthate induced decompensation. *Psychosomatics* 1975;16:37–40.
55. Davis JM, Erikson S, Dekirmenjian H: Plasma levels of antipsychotic drugs and clinical response, in Lipton MA, DiMascio A, Killam KF (eds): *Psychopharmacology: A Generation of Progress.* New York, Raven Press, 1978, pp 905–915.
56. May PRA, Van Putten T: Plasma and saliva levels of chlorpromazine in schizophrenia: A critical review of the literature. *Arch Gen Psychiatry* 1978; 35:477–480.
57. Dysken MW, Javaid JI, Change SS, et al: Fluphenzaine pharmacokinetics and therapeutic response. *Psychopharmacology (Berlin)* 1981;73:205–210.
58. Magliozzi JR, Hollister LE, Arnold KV, et al: Relationship of serum haloperidol levels to clinical response in schizophrenic patients. *Am J Psychiatry* 1981;138:365–367.
59. Bjorndal N, Bjerre M, Gerlach J, et al: High dosage haloperidol therapy in chronic schizophrenic patients: A double-blind study of clinical response, side effects, serum haloperidol, and serum prolactin. *Psychopharmacology (Berlin)* 1980;67:17–23.
60. Van Putten T, May PRA, Jenden DJ: Does a plasma level of chlorpromazine help? *Psychol Med* 1981;11:729–734.
60a. Klein DF, Gittelman R, Quitkin F, et al: *Diagnosis and Drug Treatment of Psychiatric Disorders: Adults and Children,* ed 2. Baltimore, Williams and Wilkins, 1981, pp 88–91.
61. Ungerstedt V, Ljungberg T: Behavioral patterns related to dopamine neurotransmission: Effect of acute and chronic antipsychotic drugs. *Adv Biochem Psychopharmacol* 1977;16:193–199.
62. Chouinard G, Jones BD: Neuroleptic-induced supersensitivity psychosis: Clinical and pharmacologic characteristics. *Am J Psychiatry* 1980;137:16–21.
63. El-Yousef MK, et al: Reversal of antiparkinsonian drug toxicity by physostigmine: A controlled study. *Am J Psychiatry* 1973;130:141–145.
64. Nevins DB: Adverse response to neuroleptics in schizophrenia. *Int J Psychoanal Psychother* 1977;6:227–241.
65. Sarwer-Foner GJ: Some comments on the psychodynamic aspects of the extrapyramidal reactions. *Rev Can Biol Extrapyramidal Sys Neuroleptics* 1961; 20:527–533.
66. Sarwer-Foner GJ: On the mechanisms of action of neuroleptic drugs: A theoretical psychodynamic explanation. *Recent Adv Biol Psychiatry* 1963:6: 217–232.

CHAPTER 13

TARDIVE DYSKINESIA: A REVIEW OF CURRENT KNOWLEDGE

JOHN M. KANE
BRUCE J. KINON

Tardive dyskinesia has been a topic of increasing concern over the past decade.[1] The literature on diagnosis, epidemiology, and treatment as well as papers relating to putative pathophysiological mechanisms have mushroomed in recent years. The reasons for this include the fact that tardive dyskinesia is generally felt to be an iatrogenic condition resulting from the administration of a class of medications referred to as neuroleptic or antipsychotic. In addition, this toxic effect occurs in a group of patients who by and large benefit considerably from the administration of these agents, which are otherwise generally well tolerated. A good deal of confusion has also existed in the literature because the scope and severity of the problem has not been clearly established. The fact that no effective and safe treatments for tardive dyskinesia have been established has added to the concern regarding its occurrence. It might also be suggested that American psychiatry, heavily influenced by the psychoanalytic tradition, has remained somewhat more uncomfortable than other medical specialities in dealing with difficult benefit-to-risk issues in pharmacologic treatment. A good deal of interest in tardive dyskinesia can also be traced to assumptions regarding its etiology and the relevance of changes in neurochemical receptors to both this toxic effect and the therapeutic effect of neuroleptic drugs.

To put tardive dyskinesia in the proper perspective, it is important to provide as background a summary of the data supporting the efficacy of neuroleptics in the treatment of schizophrenia. Numerous well-controlled, double-blind investigations have demonstrated the efficacy of neuroleptics in the treatment of schizophrenia.[1] These studies have been widely reviewed, and pharmacotherapy remains the mainstay of treatment for this disorder.[2] Fewer investigations have been carried out regarding the long-term efficacy of these agents; however, there appears to be little question regarding the benefits of maintenance antipsychotic drugs in reducing the risk of psychotic relapse.[2,3]

Although relapse rates vary among drug-treated patients between studies, this phenomenon may very well be related to such issues as chronicity, level of remission, age, sex, and diagnostic criteria. The route of administration and compliance in taking medication may also play some role. (Differences have also been apparent between studies in relapse rates among patients taking placebo, and similar factors may account for this variation.) Given the relatively small sample size in many of these studies, the differences in proportion relapsing in either drug or placebo-treated groups from study to study is also not surprising from a statistical standpoint. The fact that in many of these studies a substantial subgroup of patients receiving long-term neuroleptic treatment relapse despite this and the fact that among placebo-treated patients there is also a small subgroup of patients who do not experience relapse has led some critics to question the true "value" of antipsychotic drug maintenance treatment. It is clear, however, that in the overwhelming majority of controlled trials a statistically significant drug-placebo difference has been demonstrated.[3] In addition, attempts at identifying factors that may be helpful in predicting outcome among drug or placebo-treated schizophrenics have by and large been unsuccessful. A recent investigation suggests that even among first episode acute-onset schizophrenics (generally felt to have the best prognosis) a statistically significant drug-placebo difference was apparent during the one year following recovery.[4] Given the data available, there is little to argue against the use of neuroleptic maintenance treatment in well-diagnosed schizophrenic patients who have demonstrated clinical benefit from such agents.

In recent years, "second-generation" maintenance studies have been undertaken to assess in a methodologically sophisticated way other potential factors that may play a role in outcome, eg, family and social interactions, putative neurobiological factors, drug metabolic factors, and the application of more sophisticated diagnostic assessment and criteria. In addition, largely due to the risk of tardive dyskinesia, increasing attention has been given to strategies that might ultimately reduce cumulative neuroleptic exposure. Attention is being given to identifying minimum effective dosage requirements for maintenance treatment,[5] to establishing alternative strategies other than continuous drug administration,[6] and to identifying schizophrenic subtypes that may benefit from other somatic treatment besides neuroleptics.[7] Although much of the impetus for these efforts has arisen out of the concern regarding tardive dyskinesia, it remains unclear to what extent cumulative neuroleptic exposure accounts for the variance in tardive dyskinesia prevalence rates. This topic will be discussed in more detail below.

Differential Diagnosis

The difficulties inherent in the differential diagnosis of tardive dyskinesia have complicated research on incidence, prevalence, severity, and treatment outcome.

The term tardive dyskinesia should be reserved for describing abnormal involuntary movements that appear after several months or years of treatment with antipsychotic medications and are felt to be attributable to treatment with these agents. Tardive dyskinesia may be permanent or reversible (the proportion of cases which are reversible appears to be substantial; however, accurate estimates are difficult to obtain since longitudinal data are largely lacking). Tardive dyskinesia is characterized by a variable mixture of orofacial dyskinesia, chorea, athetosis, dystonia, tics, and facial grimacing. The most typical or characteristic features of tardive dyskinesia are the orofacial and lingual movements, frequently referred to as the buccolingual masticatory triad. Tardive dyskinesia is frequently insidious in onset, and initially the movements may be subtle or difficult to detect without a systematic examination. One of the most characteristic signs is a curling or twisting movement of the tongue, sometimes with protrusion from the oral cavity or resulting in extending the cheek outward. Pouting, puckering, sucking or smacking lip movements are frequently seen. Chewing or lateral movements of the jaw may occur. Blepharospasm, arching of the eyebrows, and a variety of movements that could be described as grimaces can also occur. Movements of the extremities can also be seen in tardive dyskinesia, and truncal movement has been observed as well. Movements of the fingers or toes may be observed, and postural disturbances of the neck and trunk, including torticollis, retrocollis, rocking and swaying, or pelvic movements can also be seen. Disturbances of respiratory rhythm have also been attributed to this condition. Abnormal involuntary movements that have been attributed to neuroleptic administration have also been reported in children, usually after the withdrawal of these agents, and are generally characterized by chorea of the extremities, athetosis, and myoclonus. Although orolingual movements are felt to be unusual in children, they do occur, and facial tics may be quite common in children. It is sometimes confusing to clinicians that movements of tardive dyskinesia can worsen with emotional stress, decrease with relaxation, drowsiness, or sedation, and uniformly disappear during sleep. This has led some clinicians to conclude at times that these movements were "psychogenic" in origin. In this regard, however, tardive dyskinesia resembles other choreoathetotic syndromes that are clearly disorders of the central nervous system. Movements may be enhanced or evoked, at times, by repetitive motor activity in other body parts or concentration on a specific task. It has been widely observed that patients with tardive dyskinesia are frequently unaware of their movements until they are pointed out to them. Patients with severe forms of this disorder can be severely disabled as a result of their condition.

As we shall discuss in more detail below, it is likely that many cases diagnosed as tardive dyskinesia represent movement disorders unrelated to the administration of neuroleptic medications. Patients exhibiting abnormal involuntary movements who have received neuroleptic medication must be evaluated in a systematic fashion to rule out the presence of other neuromedical conditions which might produce abnormal involuntary movements. The development in recent years of several rating scales for the assessment of tardive dyskinesia has led to the utilization of these scales in some cases as a "diagnostic tool." [8] Rating scales should not be used in this fashion, but may be useful as a screening device to identify those patients who manifest signs and symptoms that might be associated with a specific illness. The diagnosis, however, requires further investigation and preferably a longitudinal perspective. A frequent problem in establishing whether movements are due to the administration of neuroleptic medication is the lack of a documented, careful neurological evaluation before the initiation of such drug treatment. If this were systematically done in psychiatric patients, the presence of preexisting movement disorders could be better appreciated.

It is likely that the majority of cases of abnormal involuntary movements appearing in patients taking neuroleptics are, in fact, related in some way to the administration of these drugs, but this does not minimize the importance of identifying to the extent possible that subgroup which does not have true tardive dyskinesia. This term should be reserved for only those cases in which a clear-cut association between the movements and the administration of neuroleptic medication is apparent.

There remains considerable debate over to what extent schizophrenic patients unexposed to antipsychotic drugs may represent a group with a significant prevalence of abnormal involuntary movements. Descriptions of some movement disorders date back to Kraepelin[9] and Bleuler,[10] and this concern continues to be apparent in the literature.[11] At the present time it is extremely difficult to find suitable subjects for such an investigation since most persons with schizophrenia who have been ill for any length of time have been exposed to neuroleptic medications. In addition, as we shall review below, the evidence, although epidemiological, from numerous prevalence surveys is extremely compelling in supporting the role of neuroleptic medication as a major factor in the production of these movements disorders.

Parkinsonian side effects are a frequent occurrence in patients receiving neuroleptic treatment.[1] These effects may be more apparent during the early stages of treatment; however, it has become clear in recent years that even patients undergoing long-term maintenance treatment with neuroleptics can continue to manifest clinically significant extrapyramidal side effects.[12] Since parkinsonism and tardive dyskinesia can coexist in some patients,[13] a degree of diagnostic confusion often results. In addition, some patients are exquisitely sensitive to switching from one state to the other (ie, a patient with obvious abnormal involuntary movements who then receives a sufficient dose of neuroleptics to mask the abnormal involuntary movements may become severely parkinsonized). Bradykinesia, rigidity (including so-called cogwheeling), and tremor (particularly of the hands, although also of the tongue and other body areas) can be seen. A manifestation of extrapyramidal side effects in patients receiving neuroleptics which is not seen in adult idiopathic parkinsonism is akathisia, a syndrome of motor restlessness usually manifested by a patient's subjective need to move or objective evidence of restlessness with crossing and uncrossing of the legs, pacing, and inability to sit still. This can also be seen in some patients with tardive dyskinesia and may add to diagnostic difficulties. (Akathesia has been seen in post-encephalitic parkinsonism.) Acute dystonias—slow, sustained movements frequently seen in the neck or trunk or eye muscles (occulogyric crises)—can be dramatic and subjectively very distressing. Recently, descriptions have appeared in the literature of "persistent" or "tardive" dystonias,[14] which may be analagous to tardive dyskinesia in being brought about by chronic use of neuroleptic medication and persisting after the discontinuation of neuroleptic treatment (which would not be expected in acute dystonias). The differential diagnosis of dystonias includes: hereditary torsion dystonia (dystonia musculorum deformans); nonhereditary idiopathic torsion dystonia; oromandibular dystonia; blepharospasm; and dystonias produced by infections, vascular phenomena, neoplasms, toxins, or degenerative disorders.

It has generally been felt that the parkinsonian side effects of neuroleptics can be differentiated from tardive dyskinesia on the basis of a response to anticholinergic agents or dopamine agonists. Unfortunately, this differential response is not uniform. Some patients with severe akathesia, for example, will not respond to anticholinergic agents, and this may give the clinician the impression that this is in fact tardive dyskinesia. In addition, the old notion that all cases of tardive dyskinesia will worsen upon exposure to antiparkinsonian drugs does not appear to be the case in light of recent investigations.[15]

Abnormal involuntary movements clinically indistinguishable from the movements of tardive dyskinesia are also seen in patients with idiopathic parkinsonism who receive levodopa, bromocriptine, or other agents that functionally increase dopaminergic transmission.

Choreiform movements and choreoathetic movements may also be seen in tardive dyskinesia. Other causes of such movements should be considered in evaluating an individual patient. Hereditary choreas have been described.[16,17] Drug-induced choreas have occurred with the use of oral contraceptives,[18] although this appears to be a rare condition. Choreas may result from streptococcal infections. Ten percent of patients with rheumatic fever have chorea as a sole physical sign of illness.[19] Other infectious agents (diptheria, rubella, and pertussis) are rare causes of chorea.

Chorea gravidarum is the chorea that appears during pregnancy. This is an unusual condition occurring in perhaps 1 in 2000–3000 pregnancies. There is often a history of rheumatic fever or chorea before pregnancy in such individuals. Movements of this type should disappear after delivery.

Chorea has been described in patients experiencing hypernatremia secondary to dehydration.[20] This is a situation which might occur in acutely psychotic patients with organic brain syndrome who are also severely dehydrated. Memory disturbance and laboratory features of dehydration should be apparent. In addition, myoclonus is a frequent phenomenon as well. Treatment of hypernatremia should result in improvement in the clinical picture. Systemic lupus erythematosus may produce a variety of central nervous system signs and symptoms including psychosis. Chorea has been described in patients with systemic lupus erythematosus as well. Sedimentation rate, lupus erythematosus preparation, and antinuclear antibody studies should aid in the diagnosis.

Hyperthyroidism may in rare cases cause chorea in addition to tremor.[21] A thyroid test battery should aid in the differential diagnosis.

Huntington's disease is the most widely known cause of chorea, and since these patients develop emotional disturbances that may lead to the institution of neuroleptic medication, the potential for diagnostic confusion is considerable. Chorea of the extremities is the typical movement seen in this disease. Oral facial dyskinesias are much less frequent than in tardive dyskinesia. Family history is extremely important because this condition is usually expressed in an autosomal dominant genetic fashion, although sporadic cases of Huntington's chorea with no evidence of family history have been reported. The usual age of onset is in the fourth decade; however, onset in childhood may occur in a small percentage of cases. Duration of the condition from onset until death usually averages eight years in the childhood onset form and 15 to 20 years in the adult onset form. A computer-assisted tomography scan may aid in the differential diagnosis of Huntington's chorea and tardive dyskinesia; in the former, a loss of the caudate nucleus may be apparent.

A number of movement disorders occurring in schizophrenia which may resemble extrapyramidal disturbances have been described in the literature. These are frequently categorized as "stereotypic" movements. It is our impression that although these stereotyped movements can in some cases resemble orofacial dyskinesias, they usually lack the rhythmic character frequently seen in tardive dyskinesia.

Bleuler claimed not to have observed chorea in schizophrenics and suggested that others who had noted this phenomenon were employing a different definition of the condition.[10] It is also quite likely that many movement disorders described in the old literature on schizophrenia included patients with undiagnosed neurological conditions not readily appreciated at that time.

Confusion has also arisen as to what extent the phenomena observed in tardive dyskinesia are similar to the orofacial dyskinesias sometimes observed in elderly persons not exposed to neuroleptic drugs. Dyskinesias, particularly orofacial dyskinesias, have been described in elderly persons; however, the prevalence among healthy elderly persons with no evidence of neurological or psychiatric disease is quite low.[22,23] As will be discussed below, there does appear to be an increase in prevalence in tardive dyskinesia associated with age among patients receiving antipsychotic drug treatment. However, age per se does not appear to be a significant factor in producing this increase in movement disorders, but rather appears to increase an individual's vulnerability to the toxic effect of neuroleptics. A condition referred to as Meige syndrome or oromandibular dystonia has also been described.[24] This condition appears to have a peak age of onset in the sixth decade and at times is slowly progressive with further involvement of other areas of the body. This disorder may be clinically indistinguishable from tardive dyskinesia; therefore, differential diagnosis requires knowledge of exposure to neuroleptics either before or after its development. Since many clinicians will treat spontaneous dyskinesias with neuroleptics to suppress them, the differential diagnosis may become extremely difficult if an accurate medical history is not obtained or not available.

Tics or habit spasms may be difficult to differentiate from tardive dyskinesia. Shapiro et al[25] have suggested a classifactory system for tics. Gilles de La Tourette's syndrome is an important consideration in any discussion of tardive dyskinesia since many patients with this condition are treated with neuroleptic medication and could conceivably go on to develop a superimposed tardive dyskinesia. The age of onset of Tourette's syndrome, however, is generally between 2 and 15 years. Although coprolalia and other vocal utterances are not always seen in these patients, when they do occur this is an important distinction from tardive dyskinesia. Chronic simple tic may be difficult to distinguish from tardive dyskinesia in a patient receiving neuroleptic treatment; however, this condition frequently begins during the early part of the second decade, and an accurate history should help in making the differential diagnosis.

Other disorders which should be considered in the differential diagnosis are: Wilson's disease, chronic manganese poisoning and other heavy metal toxicity, acquired hepatocerebral degeneration, postanoxic and postencephalitic extrapyramidal syndromes, and extrapyramidal syndromes associated with calcification of the basal ganglia. A variety of vascular, endocrinologic, and metabolic disorders (hypoparathyroidism, hypoglycemia, hyperthyroidism) may produce choreoathetotic movements, but these movements are more likely to be transient. Brain tumors may in rare cases cause hyperkinetic dyskinesias, and neoplasms of the thalamus or basal ganglia may be associated with involuntary movements.

The American Psychiatric Association Task Force on Late Neurological Effects of Antipsychotic Drugs[1] suggested the following as a reasonable list of studies that should be done in investigating a presumed case of tardive dyskinesia: evaluation by a neurological consultant, electrolytes, glucose, thyroid function studies, liver function tests, sedimentation rate, serum ceruloplasmin, urinary copper, electroencephalograph, and in selected cases, a computer-assisted tomography scan.

Prevalence and Risk Factors

Kane and Smith[26] reviewed 56 prevalence surveys of tardive dyskinesia carried out over a 20-year period. The mean prevalence among the patient populations exposed to neuroleptics (involving a total of 34,555 persons) was 20% (uncorrected for presumptive rates of spontaneous dyskinesias). Among 19 samples of untreated persons (psychiatric and nonpsychiatric patients not exposed to neuroleptics), the mean prevalence of "spontaneous" dyskinesias was 5%. The prevalence estimates among treated populations varied from 0.5% to 56%. These wide variations in prevalence estimates have led to considerable confusion in arriving at a concensus regarding the scope of the problem. Since there are no established or universally accepted criteria for the diagnosis of tardive dyskinesia, it is likely that diagnostic criteria have varied from one study to the next. A particularly difficult problem is the diagnosis of the mild or questionable case. Prevalence varies markedly with the symptom severity required to identify a "case." Two prevalence surveys by Smith et al[27,28] highlight the importance of this consideration. Prevalence in these two studies varied from more than 60% to less than 5% depending upon the criterion selected.

Recent studies have tended to be based on a detailed and standardized examination of each patient and generally report higher prevalence rates. It is apparent that those studies employing a nominal ("yes/no") categorization report a lower prevalence rate than those studies employing an ordinal (severity) categorization.

It also appears that the reported prevalence of tardive dyskinesia has increased during the past decade. The average prevalence for the 23 studies reported between 1960 and 1969 was 14.6% whereas that for the

33 studies reported between 1970 and 1979 was 23.9% (t=2.50, $P<0.02$).

Several factors might have led to a "true" increase in prevalence of tardive dyskinesia since the early 1960s. If the disorder is persistent in some cases, prevalence would increase even if incidence remained stable. In addition, increasing numbers of patients have been exposed for longer durations since the introduction of neuroleptics over 25 years ago. Higher doses of medication may have been employed in recent years, and new classes of drugs have been introduced, particularly the so-called high-potency neuroleptics. These agents appear to have different binding characteristics in dopamine systems, and this may have played some role in the increased prevalence reported in the literature; however, this remains to be clearly demonstrated.

Other factors accounting for variations in prevalence rates include differences in demographic characteristics from one population to the next, differences in diagnostic composition, length of treatment, degree of response to treatment, current and prior neuroleptic dose, etc. Those reports with the highest prevalence figures tend to come from chronically ill, public hospital populations.

The prevalence of abnormal involuntary movements in untreated patient populations has been reported in several studies. The mean prevalence reported in these studies which include a total sample of 11,000 patients is 5% (standard deviation, 9%). This would suggest that approximately one in four individuals who appear to have tardive dyskinesia due to neuroleptic exposure may in fact be experiencing abnormal involuntary movements for other reasons. One might suggest then that a best estimate of a "true" corrected rate of drug-related tardive dyskinesia is about 15% (20% minus 5%). At the present time our ability to separate this group remains limited, although one obvious measure would be to exclude other neuromedical disorders before and during neuroleptic drug treatment.

It is not ideal to contrast prevalence rates in populations exposed to neuroleptics with patients who have been drug free. These populations may differ in a variety of variables other than exposure to neuroleptics. Even contrasts between treated and untreated samples within the same study suffer from similar problems. Ideally, patients would have to be randomly assigned to drug or no drug treatment in large numbers for long periods of time to assess the role of neuroleptic treatment in the development of tardive dyskinesia. Despite this, it is our impression that the epidemiological data implicating neuroleptic treatment as the single most significant etiological factor in the development of abnormal involuntary movements are compelling.

Those few surveys among untreated populations which have reported a very high prevalence have generally included patients with "organic" disorders, or senile dementia. Although one might argue that schizophrenia is a form of dementia, there are important differences between the "dementia" of schizophrenia and that involved in senile dementia of the Alzheimer's type, or multiinfarct dementia. Unfortunately, most of the surveys in populations not exposed to neuroleptic treatment have included institutionalized subjects, either in hospitals or in nursing homes. It would be valuable to have additional data on the prevalence of abnormal involuntary movements among individuals who have not been institutionalized. Varga et al[29] recently reported a prevalence of at least 10% of oral dyskinesias of the type described as characteristic of tardive dyskinesia in elderly patients (over age 65) not exposed to any medications. These patients were examined in nursing homes or in senior citizen centers. Kane et al[30] recently reported on a sample of 127 healthy elderly volunteers examined in senior citizen groups (average age, 72.5 years; standard deviation, 7.3 years). Four percent of these persons had abnormal involuntary movements which would be considered mild in severity. If questionable cases were included, the prevalence was increased to 8%.

It is our impression from this literature that the aging process itself can produce involuntary movements clinically indistinguishable from tardive dyskinesia; however, these movements are relatively uncommon. On the other hand, if one examines elderly patients institutionalized for dementia or other neurological conditions, the prevalence of abnormal involuntary movements appears to be much higher.

Risk Factors in the Development of Tardive Dyskinesia

Kane and Smith[26] have reviewed risk factors discussed in the literature, focusing on studies that reported the frequency of a putative risk factor in both a dyskinetic group and a comparable nondyskinetic control group. Several risk factors suggested by early, uncontrolled studies have gained wide acceptance, despite the lack of supporting evidence from such comparisons.

It is widely assumed, given the epidemiologic evidence implicating neuroleptic drugs in the development of tardive dyskinesia, that the risk of this disorder increases with increasing drug exposure. This relationship clearly has some intuitive appeal; however, dose-response curves usually plateau so that increasing doses beyond a certain point no longer increase the likelihood of a given effect. In the case of tardive dyskinesia increasing doses may even mask an existing dyskinesia, further complicating interpretation of existing data.

Since the development of tardive dyskinesia is relatively infrequent, (ie, 15% corrected prevalence), attempts at identifying dose-response curves are made difficult. In addition, most of the available data are retrospective in nature, and there are serious methodological problems in attempting to assess pharmacological variables retrospectively.

It is interesting, however, that very few controlled investigations have suggested a statistically significant relationship between cumulative dose of neuroleptics or length of neuroleptic exposure and the development of tardive dyskinesia. Studies that have reported such a relationship have generally focused on patients with relatively brief (or low total dose) exposure. This observation may be meaningful in terms of identifying a dose-response relationship for tardive dyskinesia. Of the 18 studies reviewed by Kane and Smith[26] which explored the relationship between cumulative drug dose and tardive dyskinesia prevalence, 4 reported a significant positive relationship and 14 did not.

The possibility that maximum dose received may bear a relationship to tardive dyskinesia has also been explored in a handful of studies. It is difficult, however, to assess this relationship given the interindividual differences in drug absorption and metabolism after the same oral dose. This factor has been suggested to some extent by the increase in prevalence over the past decade, which may have also coincided with greater utilization of "high-dose" or "megadose" treatment strategies (although there is little evidence demonstrating their value).

Smith et al [31] reported a significant positive correlation between maximum daily amount of neuroleptic (minimum duration for this dose was not defined) and severity of facial dyskinesia scores. Crane[32] reported that maximum daily dose (defined as highest dose prescribed for at least six months) was correlated ($r=0.19$; $P<0.01$) with the presence of tardive dyskinesia, controlling for age, and with tarkive dyskinesia ($r=0.17$; $P<0.01$), controlling for current dose. Two other studies that examined this issue found no significant relationship.[33,34]

Studies exploring the length of drug treatment as a risk variable can be criticized for the same methodological problems as those involving cumulative dose. Kane and Smith[26] found six studies that reported increasing length of exposure to be a significant risk factor (two of these involved patient samples with relatively brief exposure). Fifteen studies found no statistically significant relationship.

Several studies[35–38] suggest that a substantial percentage of patients in whom tardive dyskinesia develops manifest it within three years of drug exposure. Since duration of drug treatment before tardive dyskinesia is overestimated in most studies (dating emergence of tardive dyskinesia retrospectively is difficult), it is likely that these estimates are conservative. If there were a period of maximum risk for the development of tardive dyskinesia (for example, from three to five years of drug exposure), it would be difficult to identify this period from data available in the literature.

There is some suggestion that, once developed, tardive dyskinesia might become more severe or more persistent with continued drug exposure; however, these possibilities remain to be fully explored. It is important to emphasize that some reports indicate that tardive dyskinesia can remit even with a stable dose of neuroleptic medication being continued.

Increasing age has been one of the most consistently reported risk factors in the development of tardive dyskinesia. Dating the onset of tardive dyskinesia is often problematic (in retrospective surveys), making overestimation of age at onset likely. To explore age effects, adequate sampling is essential. Kane and Smith[26] defined an adequate age distribution as one including a sufficient sample of a least three decades, one of which is the 30s or 40s. A total of 30 studies presented controlled data on current age and tardive dyskinesia. Of 20 studies with adequate age distributions, 13 reported a statistically significant association between increasing age and prevalence rates of tardive dyskinesia, whereas none of 10 reports that involved inadequate age distributions found a significant age relationship.

The rise in prevalence with age, however, may not reflect a parallel increase in incidence. A recent review by Smith and Baldessarini[39] suggested a strong correlation between age and severity of tardive dyskinesia and a strong inverse relationship between rates of spontaneous remission of tardive dyskinesia and advancing age. Greater likelihood of persistence might contribute to higher prevalence rates in older age groups, even if incidence were not affected by age.

A variety of neurochemical changes have been reported to occur with age. It seems reasonable to assume that some degree of neuronal plasticity or adaptability is lost with age. Other possible factors are age-related changes in drug metabolism (which may lead to higher drug blood levels), slower clearance, and altered rates of production of some metabolites. The increase in prevalence of tardive dyskinesia in older age groups remains a striking finding and may provide some clues to etiology or pathophysiology.

A recent comprehensive review (J.M. Smith and D.D. Dunn, unpublished data) summarize data on female sex as a risk factor from 31 published reports. In aggregate, these data comprised 33 samples including more than 15,000 patients. In 29 (87.9%) of these 33 samples, the prevalence of tardive dyskinesia was higher in women than in men ($P<0.001$, sign test). The average unweighted ratio of female to male prevalence for the 31 samples in which this value could be computed was 1.68, and in only 9 samples was the ratio 2 to 1 or higher.

The results of a recent series of studies[26] have suggested that the magnitude of sex differences in tardive dyskinesia is dependent both on the age range of the sample and the severity of the criterion used to define the disorder.

It appears that women do have a somewhat higher overall prevalence of tardive dyskinesia than men; however, sex samples were not always matched by age and dose. Since it appears that the ratio of female to male cases increases as the criterion used to define tardive dyskinesia becomes more conservative; the more severe forms of the disorder are apparently more likely to develop in women (in a ratio of 3 or 4 to 1). Whether the sex differences in relation to tardive dyskinesia are epiphenomena of differing drug histories or reflect underlying neurobiological differences between the sexes remains to be determined.

With regard to drug type as a risk factor in the development of tardive dyskinesia, there is at present little systematic evidence implicating any one neuroleptic as carrying more risk than any other. Of the fifteen studies reviewed by Kane and Smith,[26] which included some controlled data on drug type and tardive dyskinesia prevalence, five reported significant findings. Four of these studies, however, suggested depot fluphenazine as carrying the increased risk. It is difficult to interpret these findings, since injectable preparations of fluphenazine may reduce noncompliance in pill taking among both inpatient and outpatient schizophrenics (which has been estimated to involve 30 to 50% of patients). It is therefore possible that any suggested association of tardive dyskinesia with a depot preparation of fluphenazine may be at least partially related to compliance. In addition, given large individual differences in drug metabolism, it is particularly important to consider the role of parenteral routes of administration in increasing actual "neuroleptic exposure" in the brain. Although there have been some suggestions from preclinical work that neuroleptics may differ in their propensity to produce dopamine receptor hypersensitivity in animal models of tardive dyskinesia (eg, sulpiride, molindone, clozapine) there are as yet no clinical data to further test the implications of these findings.

At the present time, we must conclude that there is no convincing evidence that any specific neuroleptic or class of neuroleptics carries a lesser risk of tardive dyskinesia. Clearly, to establish such a difference, a large-scale, methodologically sound, epidemiological study would be necessary. It is likely that patients are given specific neuroleptics for clinical reasons, and one would have to assume some degree of random assignment as well as control over compliance and blood levels to make meaningful comparisons among drugs.

At present, there are also no controlled data suggesting an association between neuroleptic polypharmacy and an increased risk for the development of tardive dyskinesia; however, the use of polypharmacy should be avoided if at all possible, since it makes understanding of specific drug response more difficult.

Several early investigations on risk factors in tardive dyskinesia had suggested organic brain dysfunction as a risk factor in the development of tardive dyskinesia. Unfortunately, various presumed measures of brain disease or dysfunction have been used, and in many of the studies interpretation is complicated by the fact that the dependent variables were assessed after the development of tardive dyskinesia. A variety of criteria have been used to define groups of patients with presumptive central nervous system dysfunction (eg, diagnosed organic brain syndrome, clinical signs of organicity, abnormal electroencephalogram, computed tomography scan, neuropsychological tests, etc). Clearly, it would be difficult to draw conclusions from the studies employing these types of criteria even if significant relationships were found. However, the majority of studies in the literature do not report a significant association between these factors and the risk of tardive dyskinesia.[26] The elimination of false-positive tardive dyskinesia diagnoses is particularly difficult when considering underlying neurologic disease as a risk factor, particularly in prevalence surveys where detailed medical histories and longitudinal follow-up are not available. It is possible that studies with more sophisticated methodology will in fact identify central nervous system factors that predispose patients to the development of tardive dyskinesia; however, this remains an unproven hypothesis. It is clear from the literature that not all patients develop tardive dyskinesia, and it is likely that individual vulnerability plays a major role.

The hypothesis that patients who show a greater sensitivity to early extrapyramidal side effects of neuroleptics would also have a greater risk of developing tardive dyskinesia with further exposure to neuroleptics has some appeal. This notion is consistent with the hypothesis that both effects are the result of dopamine receptor blockade. It is clear, however, that tardive dyskinesia develops in only a minority of patients who first manifest extrapyramidal side effects. There are few data in the literature which explore this question. In a sample of over 300 patients, Jus et al[40] reported that prevalence of a previous history of neuroleptic-induced extrapyramidal side effects was the same in patients with and without tardive dyskinesia. Kane et al,[41] reporting preliminary results from an ongoing prospective study, suggested that those patients who developed tardive dyskinesia with less than two years of drug exposure were particularly likely to have had a history of significant extrapyramidal side effects. This might suggest the strategy of identifying patients at high risk by looking at those individuals who appear to have developed tardive dyskinesia with relatively little neuroleptic exposure. Further work is necessary to clarify this association. This does not suggest, however, that those drugs with less propensity to produce extrapyramidal side effects are necessarily less likely to produce tardive dyskinesia. At present (as indicated above) there are no systematic data to suggest that this is the case.

The consideration of anticholinergic, antiparkinsonian drugs as a risk factor in the development of tardive dyskinesia is complicated by the possible role of extrapyramidal side effects in indicating vulnerability. One might assume that those patients manifesting extrapyramidal side effects are those patients most likely to receive antiparkinsonian agents. This is not always the case, since many clinicians use these agents prophylactically; however, it is possible that an association which might be evident between antiparkinsonian drug use and tardive dyskinesia development could be really an epiphenomenon of vulnerability to extrapyramidal side effects.

Those studies in the literature which do explore the relationship between antiparkinsonian drugs and tardive dyskinesia do not allow any clear conclusions.[26] Investigators differed on the variable that was employed in these studies (eg, current antiparkinsonian drug use, total amount received, duration of administration, mean daily dose of antiparkinsonian agents, etc). The majority of studies that have explored this issue did not find a significant relationship between antiparkinsonian drug administration and presence or severity of tardive dyskinesia.

The observation that anticholinergic agents frequently (although not consistently) exacerbate already manifest tardive dyskinesia has led many to assume that these agents were indeed a risk factor. The fact that these agents exacerbate tardive dyskinesia once it is apparent does not necessarily mean they play a role in producing it. In animal models of tardive dyskinesia, the concurrent administration of anticholinergic agents and neuroleptics does not consistently increase sensitivity to dopamine agonists (eg, apomorphine hydrochloride, amphetamine, or methylphenidate hydrochloride).[42–45]

The issue of drug holidays or drug-free intervals has also been discussed in the context of tardive dyskinesia. The assumption is that this strategy might reduce the likelihood of tardive dyskinesia developing. The data supporting this idea are minimal at best. In addition, repeated "on-off" manipulations of some neurochemical systems may, in fact, have a negative impact. The "kindling" of seizures by repeated dosing with a stimulant drug may be one example.[46] It is also apparent in animal models of tardive dyskinesia that supersensitivity to dopamine agonists can be demonstrated after a single dose of a neuroleptic. This is a serious theoretical problem for the clinical relevance of such models; however, it also suggests that some processes possibly relevant to the development of tardive dyskinesia may occur early in the administration of neuroleptics. The fact, however, that this supersensitivity does occur early in treatment does not necessarily mean that it is analogous to a "persistent" receptor alteration, which might be expected to be found in those patients demonstrating an irreversible movement disorder.

At the present time, there are insufficient data in the literature to draw any conclusions about drug-free intervals. A brief period of drug withdrawal may be helpful in identifying those patients with "masked" or "covert" dyskinesias, but the role of drug-free intervals in increasing or decreasing the risk of tardive dyskinesia development remains to be established. In an animal model, Bannet et al[47] found that intermittent haloperidol treatment increased tritiated spiperone binding to the same degree as that seen after continuous haloperidol therapy.

The question of psychiatric diagnosis as a risk factor has also arisen. Some anecdotal reports[48-50] have suggested that patients with affective illness may be more vulnerable than schizophrenics, but appropriate control comparisons have not been carried out. It is important to emphasize, however, that it is not unreasonable to suggest caution in the use of neuroleptic agents in the treatment of affective illnesses. Other possibly more specific agents are available, and the benefit/risk ratio in the utilization of neuroleptics may not be comparable to that in schizophrenia.

In summarizing the epidemiological data on tardive dyskinesia, it is difficult to avoid the conclusion that neuroleptics play a highly significant role in producing abnormal involuntary movements in some patients who receive them.

Although tardive dyskinesia has become a major concern in psychopharmacology, it appears that the condition does not develop in the majority of patients treated with neuroleptic medications. In addition, some neuroleptic-treated psychiatric patients who do have abnormal involuntary movements probably have them for reasons independent of the drug treatment. Our ability to tease apart this subgroup is limited at present; however, this argues very strongly for careful neurological history and examination before the institution of any neuroleptic drug treatment. It should also be stressed that the majority of cases reported in prevalence surveys are mild and that the prevalence of severe drug-induced movement disorders is probably well under 5%.

In terms of risk factors, it does appear that increasing age and female sex appear to have a relatively consistent effect in increasing the reported prevalence of tardive dyskinesia. Whether these risk factors have the same effect on incidence remains uncertain.

The issue of cumulative dose effect remains an important one. Although the literature is not convincing in suggesting the importance of cumulative dose, a good deal of further work is necessary to determine whether there is a dosage threshold for the development of tardive dyskinesia.

Pathophysiology and Etiology of Tardive Dyskinesia

Although the epidemiologic evidence implicating neuroleptic agents as a major factor in the development of tardive dyskinesia is convincing, the actual mechanism through which this effect occurs remains unknown.

Hypotheses have evolved, however, which have stimulated a considerable amount of research in this area. The fact that tardive dyskinesia can persist for many months and, in some cases, years after the withdrawal of neuroleptic medications has suggested that some relatively permanent structural alterations in the central nervous system may have occurred. Neuropathologic studies of antipsychotic drug-treated laboratory animals have not consistently demonstrated specific or localized changes in the brain.

The suggestion that the syndrome of tardive dyskinesia is associated with relative dopaminergic overactivity has been a major formulation in discussions regarding etiology. The fact that tardive dyskinesia can appear for the first time or worsen upon withdrawal of neuroleptic drugs (which are believed to be dopamine receptor blockers) lends support to this notion. In addition, as mentioned above, abnormal involuntary movements clinically indistinguishable from tardive dyskinesia can be produced by levodopa in patients treated for Parkinson's disease. In addition, agents that are felt to act as dopamine agonists or to indirectly increase dopaminergic transmission frequently will exacerbate tardive dyskinesia. The consistent observation that administration of neuroleptics can mask or suppress dyskinetic movements also supports the role of excess dopaminergic function in this disorder.

Chronic interruption of dopaminergic neurotransmission in the nigrostriatal system of rodents by either direct lesioning[51,52] or neuroleptic administration[53-55] leads to heightened sensitivity to the behavioral effects of dopamine agonists such as apomorphine. In rats, a spectrum of motor stereotypies consisting of various degrees of repetitive sniffing, gnawing, licking, and rearing in response to apomorphine appears at lower dosages and in greater intensity in the behavioral hypersensitive animal compared with controls, and attenuated forms of these behaviors may even be seen spontaneously. Behavioral hypersensitivity is presumably mediated by dopamine receptor supersensitivity, which is an increase in number of striatal postsynaptic dopamine receptors in response to the direct lesioning of presynaptic afferents[56] or chronic "chemical denervation" due to neuroleptics.[57] Such behavioral and receptor changes occur after at least seven days of chronic neuroleptic administration to rats. Increased behavior response to apomorphine, which has been reported to occur after a single dose of neuroleptic, probably is not mediated by dopamine receptor supersensitivity.[58] Behavioral hypersensitivity to dopamine agonists in rodents serves as a model for the development of tardive dyskinesia in humans.

Investigation of a threshold daily neuroleptic dose for developing behavioral hypersensitivity has not been extensively studied in animals, although available results indicate that a threshold can be demonstrated within a range of clinically relevant daily neuroleptic doses[59,60] (B. Kinon, D. Merson, and J.M. Kane, unpublished results), and that the intensity of the behavioral response increases proportionally to increasing daily dose. Behavioral hypersensitivity may also increase with duration of chronic neuroleptic treatment, as demonstrated indirectly by tolerance to the stereotypy blocking ability of teflutixol developing over continuous exposure[61] and as reported actually to intensify over a nine-week exposure to chlorpromazine.[62]

A major criticism of behavioral hypersensitivity being an animal model for tardive dyskinesia is the need to utilize a dopamine agonist to demonstrate the heightened behaviors. Some studies[63-66] suggest that certain isolated behaviors (increased locomotor activity, repetitive chewing, buccal twitching, grooming, tongue protrusion, limb movements) as well as subtle increases in total stereotypy scores (Kinon et al, unpublished results) are apparent spontaneously either during prolonged neuroleptic treatment or only after withdrawal. Although these animals show more dramatic responses to dopamine agonist challenge, these spontaneous movements may represent behavioral hypersensitivity in a less obvious form, suggesting that a valid parallel be drawn to overt tardive dyskinesia.

Treatment Approaches to Tardive Dyskinesia

Numerous treatment trials have been carried out in tardive dyskinesia. Many of these trials, however, suffer from serious methodological problems. Frequently, dyskinetic symptomatology is not well characterized, and attempts are not made to exclude false-positive cases from treatment trials. In addition, insufficient knowledge is available regarding the natural course of tardive dyskinesia, making uncontrolled trials difficult to interpret. For example, if a patient manifests tardive dyskinesia after withdrawal from a neuroleptic and one month later enters a treatment trial, any improvement that does occur would not necessarily be attributable to the experimental drug. It would seem that those patients who should be studied in attempting to identify new treatments for tardive dyskinesia would include persons with relatively persistent (duration of at least three months) dyskinesias.

The recent proposal of research diagnoses for tardive dyskinesia[67] could help in better characterizing the patient populations included in therapeutic trials. The literature is replete with instances where new treatments were reported to be efficacious on the basis of open, uncontrolled trials, but were subsequently found to have no advantage over placebo under double-blind conditions. It is also likely that patient characteristics may play some role in the potential therapeutic response to a new agent. For example, as indicated above, elderly persons may have more severe or more persistent forms of dyskinesia. One might speculate that these patients would be less likely to respond to a therapeutic agent than would younger patients.

It has also been suggested that subtypes of tardive dyskinesia exist. Some investigators have proposed a distinction between orofacial dyskinesias and dyskinesias occurring in the extremities.[68] Further study is needed to validate this distinction. Others have attempted to use pharmacological probes to subtype tardive dyskinesia.[69] For example, those movement disorders that respond to physostigmine may be distinct from those disorders that do not change after administration of this agent. The same reasoning can be applied to cholinomimetic agents, dopamine antagonists, or dopamine agonists. Much of the thinking with regard to therapeutic strategies relies heavily on the pathophysiological hypotheses described above. Many treatment strategies have attempted to stimulate cholinergic systems or to inhibit dopaminergic systems. it is clear that the single most effective strategy for reducing severity of tardive dyskinesia, at least acutely, is the administration of neuroleptic medications.[69] The majority of patients will show substantial improvement after the administration of neuroleptics. The potential problem with this treatment strategy, however, is the possibility of further exacerbation of tardive dyskinesia either by increase in severity or increase in persistence. Unfortunately, there are relatively few studies that longitudinally follow patients manifesting tardive dyskinesia who continue to receive neuroleptic treatment. From the data available, it is not at all clear that this strategy consistently leads to a worsening of the underlying condition. At the present time, since effective alternative treatments for multiepisode schizophrenic patients who benefit from neuroleptics are not available, the possibility of continuing to use neuroleptics is extremely important. Other agents that may suppress evidence of tardive dyskinesia include drugs that interfere with the synthesis or release of dopamine (ie, reserpine, tetrabenazine, alpha-methyl-para-tyrosine).

Jeste and Wyatt,[69] in reviewing therapeutic strategies against tardive dyskinesia, reported that the mean daily dosage of neuroleptics in those studies reviewed was equivalent to 304 (± 132) mg of chlorpromazine. These findings are similar to those regarding maintenance requirements of neuroleptics in the long-term treatment of schizophrenics. Baldessarini and Davis,[70] after reviewing 30 controlled long-term trials, suggested that above 300 mg of chlorpromazine per day there was no apparent relationship between neuroleptic dosage and relapse rate. Whether the dosage required to adequately suppress tardive dyskinesia is similar to the dosage necessary for the prevention of relapse in schizophrenic patients requires further study; however, this is an important question.

Neuroleptic withdrawal has been a logical strategy when possible in schizophrenic patients. Jeste and Wyatt[69] reviewed 23 treatment studies in which neuroleptics were withdrawn for periods varying from several weeks to three years. Of the patients withdrawn from neuroleptics, 36.5% had a remission of dyskinetic symptoms. Within three months of neuroleptic withdrawal approximately one-third of all patients had improvement, whereas only 3% had remission more than three months after discontinuation of neuroleptics. Unfortunately, many studies have not followed patients off of neuroleptics for a sufficient interval to accurately determine the rate of remission after extended periods of time. The question, however, is academic, for many schizophrenic patients cannot maintain remission for long periods of time without continued neuroleptic drug treatment. Putative cholinergic drugs have been widely studied in the treatment of tardive dyskinesia.

Deanol has been the subject of numerous studies since the early 1970s. Jeste and Wyatt[69] point out that in the 13 double-blind studies employing deanol only 24% of the 123 patients treated had improvement.

Physostigmine (a centrally active reversible cholinesterase inhibitor), which has been available in parenteral preparations, has been employed as an acute treatment for tardive dyskinesia with mixed results. Generally, it appears that 50% of patients will show some improvement during the 24 hours after administration of this agent. It has been suggested, however, that this effect may be due to the sedative action of physostigmine. After the cholinergic treatment strategy, choline (a naturally occurring precursor of acetylcholine) underwent several trials in the treatment of tardive dyskinesia. Approximately 50% of patients participating in such trials exhibited improvement; however, there is little evidence to suggest a correlation between plasma choline levels and clinical improvement. Choline is unfortunately an unpleasant substance to work with in that it produces a body odor in the patients who take it. This is presumed to be caused by a metabolite of choline formed in the gut (trimethylamine). Consistent with the cholinergic hypothesis of depression, it is not surprising that some investigators have reported depressed mood among patients taking choline (or lecithin). Lecithin is a naturally occurring source of dietary choline which is metabolized to choline in the intestine and liver. Lecithin does not have the undesirable effects of inducing a severe body odor and is therefore easier to work with. The overall improvement rate in the lecithin trials summarized by Jeste and Wyatt[69] was 48%. These findings may also argue for subtypes of tardive dyskinesia.

Another class of compounds which have been studied in the treatment of tardive dyskinesia are the so-called gamma-amino butyric acid (GABA)-ergic drugs. The assumption is that the stimulation of GABA-ergic systems would inhibit dopamine neurotransmission in the nigrostriatal tracts. Several agents have been suggested to exert effects in this system, although as yet drugs that are truly specific in this regard have not been well tested. Benzodiazepines and sodium valproate have been presumed to exert GABA-ergic effects, and these agents have been studied in numerous patients with tardive dyskinesia. The results with benzodiazepines as a class are better than with other nonneuroleptic compounds; however, it is difficult to interpret these results since the methodology has frequently been poor and the antidyskinetic effect that may occur with benzodiazepines could result from nonspecific sedative and muscle relaxant effects. Studies conducted to date have not made attempts to separate out these possibilities.

The stimulation of dopamine autoreceptors with very low doses of dopamine agonists (apomorphine, bromocriptine, etc) has been attempted[71](B. Kinon and J.M. Kane, unpublished data). The assumption underlying this strategy is that autoreceptor stimulation would reduce dopaminergic activity since the autoreceptors inhibit synthesis and release of dopamine. To date, studies employing this strategy have not been very encouraging (Kinon and Kane, unpublished data; G. Asnis, personal communication).

The use of high doses of dopamine agonists has also been employed in an attempt to temporarily increase dopamine levels and thereby reduce dopamine receptor supersensitivity. The assumption underlying this approach is that if chronic dopamine receptor blockade results in increased sensitivity, then chronic dopamine receptor stimulation should lead to reduced sensitivity. Alpert and Friedhoff[72,73] have reported preliminary results on this strategy which are encouraging; however, this treatment has the potential of exacerbating the psychotic disorder and has not been widely studied.

Numerous other drugs have been tried in the treatment of tardive dyskinesia. A partial list would include propranolol, lithium carbonate, pyridoxine hydrochloride, baclofen, and fusaric acid. By and large these treatments have not been widely studied, or the results have been less than encouraging.

At the present time it is reasonable to conclude that there is no proven safe and effective treatment for tardive dyskinesia; however, there remains the possibility that with better diagnoses, research design, and methodology that further advances in this area could be forthcoming.

In conclusion, research in tardive dyskinesia must proceed along three different lines concurrently. Attempts at identifying risk factors and preventing development of the disorder are clearly needed; however, data relevant to this question are difficult to obtain, and few prospective studies have been attempted. Treatment strategies should also be pursued; however, the research design and methodology in such trials need to be improved. A third focus must be a continuation of efforts to identify new antipsychotic compounds which do not produce tardive dyskinesia. Clearly a major effort on the part of clinicians must be made to reduce the nonessential use of neuroleptic and confine their use to patients who clearly need and benefit from their administration.

REFERENCES

1. *Tardive Dyskinesia,* American Psychiatric Association Task Force Report no. 18. Washington, DC, American Psychiatric Association, 1979.
2. Klein DF, Gittelman-Klein R, Rifkin A, et al: *Diagnosis and Drug Treatment of Psychiatric Disorders.* ed 2. Baltimore, The Williams & Wilkins Co, 1982.

3. Davis JM, Schaffer CB, Killian GA, et al: Important issues in the drug treatment of schizophrenia. *Schizophrenia Bull* 1980;6:70–87.
4. Kane J, Rifkin A, Quitkin F, et al: Fluphenazine vs. placebo in patients with remitted, acute first-episode schizophrenia. *Arch Gen Psychiatry* 1982;39: 70–73.
5. Kane J, Rifkin A, Quitkin F, et al: Low dose fluphenazine decanoate in maintenance treatment of schizophrenia. *Psychiatry Res* 1979;1:341–348.
6. Herz MI, Szymanski HB, Simon JC: Intermittent medication for stable schizophrenic outpatients: An alternative to maintenance medication. *Am J Psychiatry* 1982;139:918–922.
7. Hirschowitz H, Zemlan FP, Garver DL: Growth hormone levels and lithium ratios as predictors of success of lithium therapy in schizophrenia. *Am J Psychiatry* 1982;139:646–649.
8. Gardos G, Cole JO, LaBrie R: The assessment of tardive dyskinesia. *Arch Gen Psychiatry* 1977;34:1206–1212.
9. Kraepelin E: *Demential Praecox and Parafrenia.* Edinburgh, E. & S. Livingstone, 1919, pp 43–83.
10. Bleuler EP: *Demential Praecox or the Group of Schizophrenias.* New York, International University Press, 1950, pp 180–205,445–449.
11. Cunningham-Owens DG, Johnstone EC, Frith CD: Spontaneous involuntary disorders of movement. *Arch Gen Psychiatry* 1982;39:452–461.
12. Rifkin A, Quitkin F, Kane J, et al: Are prophylactic antiparkinsonian drugs necessary? A controlled study of procyclidine withdrawal. *Arch Gen Psychiatry* 1978;35:483–489.
13. Fann WE, Lake CR: On the coexistence of parkinsonism and tardive dyskinesia. *Dis Nerv Sys* 1974;35:324–326.
14. Crane GE: A classification of the neurologic effects of neuroleptic drugs, in Fann WE, Smith RC, Davis JM, et al (eds): *Tardive Dyskinesia.* New York, Spectrum Books, 1980, pp 187–191.
15. Moore D, Bowers M: Identification of a subgroup of tardive dyskinesia patients by pharmacologic probes. *Am J Psychiatry* 1980;137:1202–1205.
16. Mount LA, Reback S: Familial paroxysmal choreoathetosis, preliminary report on a hitherto undescribed syndrome. *Arch Neurol Psychiatry* 1940; 44:841–847.
17. Haerer AF, Currier RD, Jackson JF: Hereditary non-progressive chorea of early onset. *N Engl J Med* 1967;276:1220–1224.
18. Nausieda PA, Koller WC, Weiner J, et al: Chorea induced by oral contraceptives. *Neurology* 1979;29:1605–1609.
19. Paradise JL: Sydenham's chorea without evidence of rheumatic fever. *N Engl J Med* 1960;263:625–629.
20. Sparacio RB, Anziska B, Schoutta HS: Hypernatremia and chorea. *Neurology* 1976;26:46–50.
21. Klawans HL, Shenker DM: Observations on the dopaminergic nature of hyperthyroid chorea. *J Neural Transm* 1972;33:73–81.
22. Marsden C, Tarsy B, Baldessarini RJ; Spontaneous and drug induced movement disorders in psychotic patients, in Benson DF, Bloomer D (eds): *Psychiatric Aspects of Neurologic Disease.* New York, Grune & Stratton, 1975.
23. Altrocchi PH: Spontaneous orofacial dyskinesia. *Arch Neurol* 1972;26: 506–512.
24. Meige M: Les convulsions de la face une forme clinique de convulsion faciale, bilaterale et mediane. *Rev Neurol* 1910;10:437–443.
25. Shapiro AK, Shapiro ES, Bruun RD, et al: Gilles de La Tourette's Syndrome: Summary of clinical experience with 250 patients and suggested nomencla-

ture for tic syndromes, in Eldridge R, Fann S (eds): *Dystonia.* New York, Raven Press, 1976.
26. Kane JM, Smith JM: Tardive dyskinesia: Prevalence and risk factors 1959–1979. *Arch Gen Psychiatry* 1982;39:473–481.
27. Smith JM, Oswald WT, Kucharski LT, et al: Tardive dyskinesia: Age and sex difference in hospitalized schizophrenics. *Psychopharmacology* 1978;58: 207–211.
28. Smith JM, Kucharski LT, Eblen C, et al: An assessment of tardive dyskinesia in schizophrenic outpatients. *Psychopharmacology (Berlin)* 1979;64:99–104.
29. Varga E, Sugerman A, Varga V, et al: Prevalence of spontaneous oral dyskinesia in the elderly. *Am J Psychiatry* 1982;139:329–331.
30. Kane J, Weinhold P, Kinon B, et al: Prevalence of abnormal involuntary movements (spontaneous dyskinesias) in the normal elderly. *Psychopharmacology (Berlin),* 1982;77:105–108.
31. Smith RC, Strizich M, Klass D: Drug history and tardive dyskinesia. *Am J Psychiatry* 1978;135:1402–1403.
32. Crane GE: Factors predisposing to drug-induced neurologic effects, in Forest IS, Carr CJ, Usdin E (eds): *The Phenothiazines and Structurally Related Drugs.* New York, Raven Press, 1974, pp 269–279.
33. Gardos G, Cole JO, LaBrie R: Drug variables in etiology of tardive dyskinesia: Application of discriminant function analysis. *Progr Neuropsychopharmacol* 1977;1:147–155.
34. Jus A, Pineau R, LaChance R, et al: Epidemiology of tardive dyskinesia: Part II. *Dis Nerve Sys* 1976;37:257–261.
35. Faurbye A, Rasch PJ, Peterson PB, et al: Neurological symptoms in pharmacotherapy of psychoses. *Acta Psychiatr Scand* 1964;40:10–27.
36. Degkwitz R, Binsack KF, Herkert H, et al: Zum Problem der persistieren den extrapyramidalen Hyperkinesen nach langfristiger Anwendung von Neuroleptika. *Nervenarzt* 1967;38:170–174.
37. Asnis GM, Leopold MA, Duvoisin RC, et al: A survey of tardive dyskinesia in psychiatric outpatients. *Am J Psychiatry* 1977;134:1367–1370.
38. Crane GE, Smeets RA: Tardive dyskinesia and drug therapy in geriatric patients. *Arch Gen Psychiatry* 1974;30:341–343.
39. Smith JM, Baldessarini RJ: Changes in prevalence, severity and recovery in tardive dyskinesia with age. *Arch Gen Psychiatry* 1980;37:1368–1373.
40. Jus A, Pineau R, LaChance R, et al: Epidemiology of tardive dyskinesia: Part I. *Dis Nerv Sys* 1976;37:210–214.
41. Kane JM, Woerner M, Weinhold P: A prospective study of tardive dyskinesia development: Preliminary results. *J Clin Psychopharm,* 1982;2:345–349.
42. Sawyers AC, Burk HR, Ruch W, et al: Anticholinergic properties of antipsychotic drugs and their relation to extrapyramidal side effects. *Psychopharmacology (Berlin)* 1976;51:15–22.
43. Tarsy D, Baldessarini RJ: Behavioral supersensitivity to apomorphine following chronic treatment with drugs which interfere with the synaptic function of catecholamines. *Neuropharmacology* 1974;13:927–940.
44. Christensen AV, Nielsen IM: Dopaminergic supersensitivity: Influence of dopamine agonists, cholinergics, anticholinergics, and drugs used for the treatment of tardive dyskinesia. *Psychopharmacology (Berlin)* 1979;62: 111–116.
45. Smith RC, Davis JM: Behavioral evidence of supersensitivity after chronic administration of haloperidol, clozapine and thioridazine. *Life Sci* 1976;19: 725–732.
46. Post RM: Intermittent vs. continuous stimulation: Effect of time interval on

the development of sensitization or tolerance. *Lif Sci* 1980;26:1275–1282.
47. Bannet J, Belmaker RN, Ebstein RP: The effect of drug holidays in an animal model of tardive dyskinesia. *Psychopharmacology (Berlin)* 1980;69:223–224.
48. Davis KL, Berger PA, Hollister LE: Tardive dyskinesia and depressive illness. *Psychopharmacol Commun* 1976;2:125–130.
49. Rosenbaum KM, Niven RG, Hanson MP, et al: Tardive dyskinesia: Relationship with primary affective disorder. *Dis Nerv Sys* 1977;38:423–427.
50. Kane JM, Struve FA, Weinhold P, et al: Strategy for the study of patients at high risk for tardive dyskinesia. *Am J Psychiatry* 1980;137:1265–1267.
51. Ungerstedt U: Postsynaptic supersensitivity after 6-hydroxydopamine-induced degeneration of the nigrostriatal system. *Acta Physiol Scand* 1971; 82(Suppl 367):69–93.
52. Thornburg JE, Moore KE: Supersensitivity to dopamine agonists following unilateral 6-hydroxydopamine-induced striatal lesions in mice. *J Pharmacol Exp Ther* 1975;192:42–49.
53. Tarsy D, Baldessarini RJ: Behavioral supersensitivity to apomorphine following chronic treatment with drugs which interfere with the synaptic function of catecholamines. *Neuropharmacology* 1974;13:927–940.
54. Smith RC, Davis JM: Behavioral evidence for supersensitivity after chronic administration of haloperidol, clozapine and thioridazine. *Life Sci* 1976;19: 725–732.
55. Gianutsos G, Moore KE: Dopaminergic supersensitivity in striatum and olfactory tubercle following chronic administration of haloperidol or clozapine. *Life Sci* 1977;20:1585–1592.
56. Creese I, Burt DR, Snyder SH: Dopamine receptor binding enhancement accompanies lesion-induced behavioral supersensitivity. *Science* 1977;197: 596–598.
57. Burt DR, Creese I, Snyder SH: Antischizophrenic drugs: Chronic treatment elevates dopamine receptor binding in brain. *Science* 1977;196:326–328.
58. Müller P, Svensson TH, Carlsson A: Pre- and postsynaptic mechanisms in haloperidol-induced sensitization to dopaminergic agonists. *Adv Biochem Psychopharmacol* 1980;24:69–74.
59. Lautin A, Wazer D, Stanley M, et al: Chronic treatment with metoclopramide induces behavioral supersensitivity to apomorphine and enhances specific binding of ^{3}H-spiroperidol to rat striata. *Life Sci* 1980;27: 305–316.
60. Klawans HL, Carvey P, Hitri A, et al: Correlation between daily dosage of chlorpromazine and subsequent supersensitivity. *Adv Biochem Psychopharmacol* 1980;24:569–572.
61. Christensen AV, Nielsen IM: Dopaminergic supersensitivity: Influence of dopamine agonists and drugs used for the treatment of tardive dyskinesia. *Adv Biochem Psychopharmacol* 1980;24:341–349.
62. Klawans HL, Carvey P, Goetz, CG: Effect of dose, duration and type of neuroleptic in an animal model of tardive dyskinesia. *Abstr Third World Cong Biol Psychiatry* 1981;S194.
63. Clow A, Jenner P, Marsden CD: Changes in dopamine-mediated behavior during one year's neuroleptic administration. *Eur J Pharmacol* 1979;57: 365–375.
64. Waddington JL, Gamble SJ: Neuroleptic treatment for a substantial proportion of adult life: Behavioral sequelae of 9 months haloperidol administration. *Eur J Pharmacol* 1980;67:363–369.
65. Iversen SD, Howells RB, Hughes RP: The behavioral consequences of long-

term treatment with neuroleptic drugs. *Adv Biochem Psychopharmacol* 1980;24:305–313.
66. Smith RC, Leelavathi DE: Behavioral and biochemical effects of chronic neuroleptic drugs: Interaction with age, in Fann WE, Smith RC, Davis JM, et al (eds): *Tardive Dyskinesia.* New York, Spectrum Books, 1980, pp 65–88.
67. Schooler NR, Kane JM: Research diagnoses for tardive dyskinesia. *Arch Gen Psychiatry* 1982;39:486–487.
68. Barnes TRE, Kidger T: The concept of tardive dyskinesia. *Trends Neurosci* 1979;2:135–136.
69. Jeste DV, Wyatt RJ: Therapeutic strategies against tardive dyskinesia. *Arch Gen Psychiatry* 1982;39:803–816.
70. Baldessarini RJ, Davis JM: What *is* the best maintenance dose of neuroleptics in schizophrenia? *Psychiatry Res* 1980;3:115–122.
71. Tamminga CA, Chase TN: Bromocriptine and CF 25-397 in the treatment of tardive dyskinesia. *Arch Neurol* 1980;37:204–205.
72. Friedhoff AJ, Alpert M: Receptor sensitivity modification as a potential treatment, in Lipton MA, DiMascio A, Killam KF (eds): *Psychopharmacology: A Generation of Progress.* New York, Raven Press, 1978, pp 797– 802.
73. Alpert M, Friedhoff A: Clinical application of receptor modification treatment, in Fann WE, Smith RC, Davis JM, et al (eds): *Tardive Dyskinesia.* New York, Spectrum Books, 1980, pp 471–473.

INDEX